Be in Health
Bible-Based Health Restoration

May you always Be in Health!

Carol Rendlee

Be in Health
Bible-Based Health Restoration

Living in Harmony with God's Ways Regarding Health

Carol A. Rundle
3Jn2 Wellness LLC

Spirit's Sword Publishing

Be in Health: Bible-Based Health Restoration
 Living in Harmony with God's Ways Regarding Health

Copyright © 2018 3Jn2 Wellness LLC and Rev. Carol A. Rundle
ISBN: 978-1717250322
Library of Congress Number: 2018907823

All rights reserved. No part of this book may be used, stored, or reproduced in any manner: electronic, mechanical, photocopying, recording, or otherwise, without written permission from the author. A short quotation of a few sentences used for private non-commercial individual or group study, or in printed reviews is fully encouraged, and no written permission is needed in such cases.

NOTICE: The information contained in this book is intended for educational purposes only and is not meant to substitute for medical care or to prescribe treatment for any specific health condition. Please see a qualified health care provider for medical treatment. We assume no responsibility to, or liability for, any person or group for any loss, damage, or injury resulting from the use or misuse of any information in this book. No express or implied guarantee is given regarding the effects of using any of the products, methods, or recipes described herein.

The statements herein have not been evaluated by the FDA. Products and techniques mentioned are not intended to diagnose, treat, cure, or prevent any disease. Information provided here is in no way intended to replace proper medical help. Consult with the health authorities of your choice.

3Jn2 Wellness LLC is a distributor for Young Living Essential Oils, member number 2421931. That means they earn a commission on any product you purchase from YLEO through their link. This commission is paid by YLEO and does not affect the price you pay.

Published by Spirit's Sword Publishing
Tucson, AZ 85715
http://3Jn2Wellness.com
Printed in the United States of America

This book is dedicated to those yearning to live in harmony with God's ways regarding health. May your path be lighted with hope and your heart filled with God's joy unspeakable.

ACKNOWLEDGMENTS

I've been writing and teaching about God and about health for many years, but I never considered writing a book until recently. I want to thank the following for their help and inspiration.

Bob Rundle, my husband and my biggest cheerleader. Thank you for your unending love and support. I love you always.

Veda Rallins, my dear friend, for inspiring me to put in writing how I learned to Be in Health and turn it into this book. You were the impetus I needed, and I'm thankful for you.

Felicia Hermann, my friend and editor, thank you for your keen eye and quick wit, both of which keep me on my toes.

My clients, who have taught me more than words can say. I'm especially grateful for your input.

Most importantly, my heavenly Father God and my Lord Jesus Christ, without whom I can do nothing. You are the reason.

TABLE OF CONTENTS

AUTHOR'S NOTE 1

INTRODUCTION 3
    Finding My Why 4

PART 1: GOD HAS ALWAYS PROVIDED FOR THE
HEALTH AND WELLNESS OF HIS PEOPLE 7
    CHAPTER 1: What Does It Mean to Be in Health? 9
        Be in Health 10
        Avoid Evil 12
        Guarding the Heart 12
        What You See 13
        What You Hear 14
        What You Think 15
        What to Think About 16
    CHAPTER 2: God's Ways vs. Man's Ways 25
    CHAPTER 3: God's Original Eating Plan for Mankind 29
        After the Fall: Vegetables 30
        After the Flood: Meat 30
    CHAPTER 4: The Dietary Laws of the Old Testament 33
        Can Eat (Clean) 34
        Do Not Eat (Unclean) 34
    CHAPTER 5: Freedom in Christ or License to Sin? 37

PART 2: A SPIRITUAL ATTACK IS UNDERWAY 41

TABLE OF CONTENTS

CHAPTER 6: Health Care or Sick Care? 43
God's Plan for Health 43
The Health Benefits of Plants 44
Health Care in the Early Church 45
The Origin of Doctors 46
Paracelsus 48
A Dual System of Medicine Emerges 49
The Battle Against Germs 50
20th Century Health Care 51
The Creation of Cancer 52
Health Care? 53
German Influence 54
Eugenics 55
A Crackdown on Natural Healing Arts 56
Operation Paperclip 56
Use of Industrial Waste 57
Our Current System 58
What are Drugs Doing to Us? 59
Poison 'Control' 59
Drugs Contribute to Nutritional Deficiencies 60
Take Control of Your Health 61

CHAPTER 7: The Church Under Assault 63
The Spiritual Battle 63

TABLE OF CONTENTS

What is Happening to Our Food? 65

What is Organic Food? 69

Mycotoxins 70

Food Additives 70

What Can We Do About This? 71

CHAPTER 8: Healing Is in Christ 73

PART 3: WHAT I WAS EATING MADE ME SICK 77

CHAPTER 9: Why I Avoid Processed Food 79

What is Processed Food? 79

Processed Meats 79

Are Some Processed Foods Healthy? 80

Reading Labels 81

Give Up Processed Food? 81

Eat Real, Whole Food 82

CHAPTER 10: Wheat: The Staff of Life 83

How Man Changed Wheat 83

Reactions to Gluten 84

Alternatives to Gluten 84

Why I Don't Eat Grains 85

Whole Grain vs. Refined Grain 86

Is the Problem Gluten or Glyphosate? 86

Grains, Leaky Gut, and Autoimmune Disorders 87

TABLE OF CONTENTS

CHAPTER 11: Dairy Products: Yea or Nay? 89
- Cow's Milk, Goat's Milk, and Sheep's Milk 90
- The Land of Milk and Honey 91
- Why Do We Think Cow's Milk is Healthy? 92
- The History of Human Milk Consumption 92
- Why We Keep Drinking Cow's Milk 93
- Does Milk Really "Do a Body Good?" 93
- The Autoimmune Connection 95
- The Problem with Modern Dairy Products 95

CHAPTER 12: Soy: Friend or Foe? 97
- History of Soy 97
- Reasons to Consume Soy Products 98
- Impact of Soy on Hormones 99
- Other Problems with Soy 99
- Fermented vs. Unfermented Soy 100

CHAPTER 13: The Advantages of Coconut Milk 101
- What is Coconut Milk? 101
- Dairy Free 102
- Vegan Friendly 102
- Nutrient-Rich 102
- Heart Health 102
- Digestive Health 102
- Choosing Coconut Milk 103

TABLE OF CONTENTS

CHAPTER 14: Avoiding Nightshades 105
   Meet the Solanaceae Family 105
   Alkaloids 106
   Nightshade Allergy and Sensitivity 107
   Studies 108
   Avoiding Nightshades 108

CHAPTER 15: Just Say No to Bacon 109
   What Does the Bible Say? 109
   Modern Science 109
   Bottom Line 110

CHAPTER 16: The Dangers of Fast Food 113
   Lack of Nutrition 113
   Health Problems 114
   High Cost 114

PART 4: UNDERSTANDING LEAKY GUT 117

CHAPTER 17: "All Disease Begins in the Gut" 119
   Causes of Leaky Gut Syndrome 120
   8 Symptoms of Leaky Gut Syndrome 120

CHAPTER 18: Your Gut: Your Second Brain 123
   The Enteric Brain 123
   The Head Brain – Gut Brain Connection 123
   You Are What You Eat 125

TABLE OF CONTENTS

PART 5: DEALING WITH AUTOIMMUNE DISORDERS 127

CHAPTER 19: Why Does the Body Attack Itself? 129

- "All Disease Begins in the Gut" 129
- Autoimmune Disorder Begins 130
- What Causes Leaky Gut Syndrome? 130
- How to Restore the Gut 131
- What I Avoid 132
- Why I Changed What I Eat 132

CHAPTER 20: Spiritual Reasons the Body Attacks Itself 135

- Having an Autoimmune Disorder Sucks 135
- Why Isn't What I'm Doing Working? 135
- What Am I Telling My Body? 136
- Spiritual Causes of Autoimmune Disorders 136
- Who Are You in Christ? 137

CHAPTER 21: I Hurt All Over. Do I Have Fibromyalgia? 139

- What is Fibromyalgia? 139
- What Causes Fibromyalgia? 141
- How to Deal with Fibromyalgia 141

CHAPTER 22: Thyroid, Hormones, and Autoimmune 143

- Hyperthyroidism 143
- Hypothyroidism 144
- The Autoimmune Connection 145
- Getting the Right Dose 146

TABLE OF CONTENTS

    Bioidentical Hormones 146

    History of HRT 147

CHAPTER 23: What Can Be Done About IBS 149

    The Underlying Cause 149

    Symptoms.. 149

    Spiritual Causes... 151

PART 6: BE IN HEALTH 153

CHAPTER 24: Overview of the Be in Health Lifestyle 155

    Implementing the Lifestyle 155

PART 7: HOW I RESTORED MY BODY TO HEALTH 157

CHAPTER 25: How I Changed What I Eat 159

    The Be in Health Lifestyle 159

    How I Feel Living the Be in Health Lifestyle.............................. 159

    Potential Detox Symptoms 160

    What I Eat 160

    Substitutions 161

    Growing My Own Food... 163

    Tips for Healthier Cooking 164

CHAPTER 26: Food Allergy or Food Intolerance? 167

    Symptoms of Food Intolerance 167

CHAPTER 27: The Food Reintroduction Challenge.................... 171

    How I Felt on the Food Reintroduction Challenge 171

    Potential Detox Symptoms 171

TABLE OF CONTENTS

Food Reintroduction Challenge Stages 172

Step 1: Observe 173

Step 2: Eliminate 174

Step 3: Challenge 174

Mental Preparation 175

What I Ate on the Food Reintroduction Challenge 176

Completing the Food Reintroduction Challenge 176

CHAPTER 28: Cleansing and Maintaining the Colon 177

Probiotics 177

Digestive Enzymes 178

Parasite Cleanse 178

For Gallbladder Issues 178

For SIBO 179

Nutritional Supplements 179

Cleansing the Colon 180

CHAPTER 29: Benefits of Essential Oils for Body, Soul, and Spirit 183

What are Essential Oils? 183

How Essential Oils Work 183

Biblical References to Essential Oils 185

Plague Doctors 190

AROMAtherapy vs. AromaTHERAPY 193

Support Your Body 194

TABLE OF CONTENTS

    Anointing with Oil **195**

    Got Emotions? **200**

    Aroma Freedom Technique **201**

    Forgiveness **201**

    Zyto Balance Biomarker Report **203**

    Important Considerations When Purchasing Essential Oils **204**

    Can Essential Oils Be Used on Children? **204**

    Can Essential Oils Be Used During Pregnancy or While Nursing? **204**

    Conclusion **205**

CHAPTER 30: The Be in Health Meal Plan **207**

    Foods I Eat **207**

    Foods I Avoid **207**

    Water **207**

    Cooking Double **207**

    Meals **207**

    Salad Dressing **208**

    For Vegans/Vegetarians **209**

    Snack/Dessert Ideas **209**

    Be in Health Sample 7-Day Menu **210**

CHAPTER 31: My Shopping List **211**

    Food Shopping Guidelines **211**

    Be in Health Shopping List **212**

TABLE OF CONTENTS

PART 8: LIVING THE LIFESTYLE 215

CHAPTER 32: The Amazing Health Benefits of Bone Broth 217

Restore the Gut to Health with Bone Broth 217

Bone Broth Supports Immune Health 218

Taking Glucosamine & Chondroitin? 218

Look Younger, Sleep Better, Feel Better 218

Get a Jump on Detoxing with Bone Broth 219

CHAPTER 33: How to Overcome a Sugar Addiction 221

Positive Mental Attitude 221

Exercise 222

Eat Sour Foods 222

Eat Fat/Starchy Foods 222

Make Sure You're Getting Enough Minerals 222

Don't Overdo It on Fruit 223

Don't Replace Sugar with Artificial Sweeteners 223

Soothe the Detox 223

CHAPTER 34: How to Quit Coffee 225

Why Should I Quit Drinking Coffee? 225

Cold Turkey Method 226

Weaning Method 227

Benefits of Quitting Coffee 228

CHAPTER 35: Why (the Right Kind of) Fat is Healthy 229

Saturated Fats 229

TABLE OF CONTENTS

The American Heart Association Strikes Again 230

Eggs and Cholesterol 231

The Best Healthy Fats 232

Improved Health Markers 235

CHAPTER 36: Surprising Benefits of Intermittent Fasting 237

What is Intermittent Fasting? 237

Weight Loss... 228

Health Restoration 238

Spiritual/Mental Clarity 239

Making the Change... 240

CHAPTER 37: The 10 Best Anti-Inflammation Foods 241

CHAPTER 38: Food Preparation Tips 243

CHAPTER 39: Cooking with Essential Oils 245

Are Essential Oils Ingestible? 245

Tips for Cooking with Essential Oils 246

Substituting with Essential Oils... 246

CHAPTER 40: Hacks That Help Me Sleep 249

CHAPTER 41: Reducing Toxin Exposure 251

Reducing Toxins in My Environment...................................... 251

Replacing Toxic Thoughts 252

Removing Toxic People from Your Life 253

The Facts About Chemicals 254

Bayer Buys Monsanto 255

xi

TABLE OF CONTENTS

    Glyphosate/Roundup® 255

    Problems with Standard Household Cleaners 256

    Thieves® Line 257

    14 Easy, Fun, and Inexpensive Solutions 257

    Soap 259

    Oral Care 260

    Making Your Own Products 261

    Top Toxins to Avoid 261

    Toxins in Personal Care/Beauty Products 262

    Tattoos/Permanent Makeup 263

    Making the Change 264

CHAPTER 42: The Body Was Made to Move 265

CHAPTER 43: How to Eat Healthy When Eating Out 267

    Mindset 267

    I Ask for What I Want 268

    Snacks When I'm Away from Home 268

PART 9: PRACTICAL APPLICATION 271

CHAPTER 44: What is a Herxheimer Reaction? 273

    What is Happening to Me? 273

    How Do I Deal with This? 274

    Ongoing Detoxification 275

CHAPTER 45: Is Healthy Food Really Too Expensive? 277

    Types of Food 277

TABLE OF CONTENTS

Why is Most Processed Food Unhealthy? 277

Organic Food vs. Non-Organic Food 278

Are You Willing? 279

What Are You Comparing? 282

CHAPTER 46: Kitchen Makeover 281

Instead of That, Eat This 281

Kitchen Gadgets 282

Where to Shop 283

CHAPTER 47: 6 Spices to Improve and Maintain Health 285

Turmeric Root 285

Garlic 286

Astragalus Root 287

Ginger Root 287

Ashwagandha Root 288

Cinnamon Bark 288

CHAPTER 48: Apps to Help Us Get and Stay Healthy 291

EWG's Healthy Living 291

Think Dirty. 291

Non-GMO Project Shopping Guide 292

EWG's Food Scores 292

Healthyout 292

Real Plans 293

CHAPTER 49: Food - Mood - Poop Journal 295

xiii

TABLE OF CONTENTS

CHAPTER 50: Gut-Restoring Recipes 297

Applesauce 297

Avocado-Stuffed Meatballs 297

Baked Apple Smoothie 298

Carol's Homemade Holy Guacamole 299

Cauliflower Soup 299

Chia Seed Coconut Milk Pudding 300

Chicken Bone Broth 301

Cilantro Salmon Burgers 302

Coconut Milk Kefir 303

Egg Scramble with Asparagus, Avocado, and Sauerkraut 304

Farmer's Wife with Lamb Sausage 304

Fat Bombs 305

Garlicky Spaghetti Squash with Chicken, Mushrooms, Kale ... 306

Green Tea Chicken Soup 307

Kale Chips 308

Lemon Basil Chicken 308

Mayonnaise 309

Pumpkin-Ginger Soup 310

Super Restoring Smoothie 311

Sweet Potato/Beet Hash 315

Taco Salad 315

Waldorf Chicken Salad 317

TABLE OF CONTENTS

PART 10: THE BE IN HEALTH MINDSET 319

CHAPTER 51: Stop Trying to Be Perfect 321
- Where Does Perfectionism Come From? 321
- What Perfectionism Does to Us 324
- Self-Righteousness 322
- Doomed to Fail 325
- The Righteousness of God 326
- Our Response to God's Righteousness 329
- Changing Your Thoughts Changes Your Ways 329
- You Are Righteous Now 331

CHAPTER 52: Eating in Faith 333
- God Gave Us Good Food to Eat 333
- God's Health Solution #1 334
- God's Health Solution #2 335
- Rebellion Revisited 335
- Common Sense Eating 336
- Making the Change 337

CHAPTER 53: How the Soul Prospers 339
- Defining Terms 340
- How the Soul Prospers 343
- The Prosperity of the Soul 346
- Rejoice 348
- Your Identity Is In Christ 348

TABLE OF CONTENTS

Putting It All Together 350

Verses About the Soul 351

Wisdom 355

CHAPTER 54: How to Overcome Self-Sabotage 359

What is Self-Sabotage? 359

Types of Self-Sabotage 359

How to Stop Self-Sabotage 361

CHAPTER 55: Words of Life 363

CONCLUSION 367

APPENDICES 369

APPENDIX 1: Common GMO Ingredients 371

APPENDIX 2: Common Names for Sugar 373

APPENDIX 3: Common Chemicals to Avoid 375

INDEX 381

ABOUT THE AUTHOR 401

ENDNOTES 403

AUTHOR'S NOTE

Beloved, I wish above all things that thou mayest prosper and be in health, even as thy soul prospereth.
3 John 2 KJV

In the scripture verse above, God makes it clear that He wants His beloved children to prosper and be healthy. God is a God of love and He hasn't forgotten about you.

Are you a saint who's sick and tired of being sick and tired?

I was chronically fatigued, in pain, unable to hold down a job, and too tired to do the things that brought me joy. All this, plus I felt guilty and ashamed because of it.

Is this you, too? You may be blessed to learn about my journey and how I returned to being in health.

This book is based on my many years of searching and researching to restore my health. It will show you what I learned about God's original plan for health and wellness, how eating the wrong foods is the root cause of most (if not all) sickness, how and why the health care and food industries are harming us, and how to live in harmony with God's ways rather than against them regarding health. I also include some of my favorite health-restoring recipes.

Some questions this book will answer:

AUTHOR'S NOTE

- What does the Bible say about health and wellness?
- Why do so many of God's people currently find themselves in the grip of the Evil One regarding health?
- How does food affect health?
- How does toxin exposure affect health?
- What's the best way to recover from chronic illness?
- Does taking supplements and using essential oils mean I'm not trusting God?
- How can I stop doing the things that caused sickness in the first place?
- How can I succeed in changing my health for the better?

I hope you enjoy the information and I'm praying for you on your journey to wellness. May you be in health!

Carol A. Rundle
Tucson, AZ

INTRODUCTION

This book is divided into ten parts:

Part 1: God Has Always Provided for the Health and Wellness of His People. This part explains God's original plans for mankind and why many of God's people currently find themselves in the grip of the Evil One regarding health.

Part 2: A Spiritual Attack is Underway. There's something going that most of us aren't paying attention to. The current medical/health care system isn't designed to make people well. We also discuss the spiritual attack on the church via our food supply.

Part 3: What I Was Eating Made Me Sick. In this part, we get down to the nitty-gritty of what is wrong with the Standard American Diet (SAD) and how it affects health.

Part 4: Understanding Leaky Gut. Many of our modern diseases have their root in leaky gut syndrome. Eating a Standard American Diet can lead to leaky gut syndrome.

Part 5: Dealing with Autoimmune Disorders. Hints and tips to reduce discomfort.

Part 6: Be in Health. We have been promised health and healing through the finished work of Jesus Christ. The Be in Health lifestyle is a way of being. Here I show you the steps I followed to Be in Health.

Part 7: How I Restored My Body to Health. The best way to restore health to our bodies is to cooperate with God's ways of health, rather than living cross purpose to them. Something I was eating was making me sick. But what? How I figured out which foods were causing problems. Here I expand on the steps I laid out in Part 6 to restore my health, including a sample menu and a shopping list.

Part 8: Living the Lifestyle. Living in harmony with God's ways to restore health from leaky gut syndrome is, above all, a lifestyle change. It encompasses the whole man: body, soul (mind and emotions), and

INTRODUCTION

spirit (1 Thessalonians 5:23). Includes tips for succeeding with the Be in Health lifestyle. Also, learn how I reduced my toxin exposure.

Part 9: Practical Application. The best-kept secret of medicine is that the body heals itself IF we provide the right conditions and stop doing the things that caused the sickness in the first place. Includes tips to work the Be in Health lifestyle into everyday life.

Part 10: The Be in Health Mindset. Spiritual and mental insight.

There are also several appendices with lists of GMO ingredients, different names for sugar, and chemicals to avoid.

As with any new venture in life, I encourage you to be kind to yourself. No one needs a harsh taskmaster. Take the hand of your loving heavenly Father as you embark on this life-long journey into health and wellness.

There's usually a spiritual reason behind everything we see with the five senses. We can't afford to ignore either one.

Finding My Why

In the fall of 2015, I was approaching a major milestone birthday. I knew that God had been nudging me for some time to make changes in my diet (which I define as 'a way of eating'). So, as this birthday approached, I began to think about the final years of my earthly journey. I have no idea how long I will live. I only know that for as long I live, I want to be strong in spirit, mind, and body so I can walk into the good works that God has prepared for me (Ephesians 2:10).

I also knew that if I continued on the path I was on (my main food groups at the time were corn chips, ice cream, and chocolate cake; I'm not kidding), I would end up as my parents did. They both developed cancer (from which my father died) late in life; my mother died of congestive heart failure. They were both miserable in their final years. And I have their genes. But, I also knew that I could turn off those destructive genes[1] with different choices.

I already had the biggest factor for health: my spiritual relationship with my Father God. The other factors within my control were my food

INTRODUCTION

choices and toxin exposure. So, I restarted searching and researching. I became a certified health coach. I developed a way of eating and living that worked for me. That is what I'm sharing with you in this book.

As I said, my journey started because I wanted to feel better and be better for God. You <u>must</u> have a compelling reason to start your journey or you will fail. It's as simple as that. I've started and failed so many times in the past. It wasn't until I discovered my reason, my why, that I was able to succeed.

So, I encourage you to find your 'why.' Ask God to show you. He will lead you with His light. If He leads you to the Be in Health lifestyle, know that I'm here to support you. I pray for everyone who decides to live this lifestyle. If you have specific questions or want to schedule a phone conversation, please email me at Carol@3Jn2Wellness.com. Enjoy your journey!

INTRODUCTION

PART 1

GOD HAS ALWAYS PROVIDED FOR THE HEALTH AND WELLNESS OF HIS PEOPLE

"What would it mean to you to know that God had a plan from the beginning of time to heal our physical, emotional, and spiritual needs?"
Dr. David Stewart

Jesus Christ heals you!
Acts 9:34 NLT

CHAPTER 1

WHAT DOES IT MEAN TO BE IN HEALTH?

Beloved, I wish above all things that thou mayest prosper and be in health, even as thy soul prospereth.
3 John 2 KJV

Being in health means different things to different people. Let's look at it from God's perspective.

The English word 'prosper' in 3 John 2 is the Greek word *euodoō*, which means "to have a prosperous, successful journey." The English Standard Version translates this verse, "Beloved, I pray that all may go well with you and that you may be in good health, as it goes well with your soul."

Being in health and prospering are results of the soul prospering. Does your soul hate parts of your body? Is it ignoring the spirit? When your soul prospers, health and prosperity (all things going well with you, which is the definition of wellness) will follow.

Note the distinction between spirit and soul. See 1 Thessalonians 5:23 and Hebrews 4:12. Your soul is the part of you that gives life and movement to your body, and thoughts and emotions to your mind. The heart is the innermost part of the soul. The spirit is the gift from God when one becomes born again (see Acts 2:4). All humans and animals have soul life. Only those born again (Romans 10:9) have spirit life.

In order to be in health, the soul must be prospering, doing well. So, let's find out what the Bible means by "be in health."

CHAPTER 1 – WHAT DOES IT MEAN TO BE IN HEALTH?

Be in Health

The first use of "be in health" is in Genesis 43:28 where it's translated "in good health." The Hebrew word is *shalom*. You may be familiar with this word. It means not only peace (quiet, tranquility, contentment), but also completeness, soundness (in body), welfare (health and prosperity), and friendship. It means to be whole (also called saved). I've heard it described as 'nothing missing, nothing broken.'

Psalm 42:11 shows us where health comes from.

> *Psalm 42:11 KJV*
> *Why art thou cast down, O my soul? and why art thou disquieted within me? hope thou in God: for I shall yet praise him, who is the health of my countenance, and my God.*

Bullinger's Companion Bible translates the last part as, "Who is the salvation of me, and my God."

The New International Version (NIV) of this verse is,

> *Psalm 42:11 NIV*
> *Why am I discouraged? Why is my heart so sad? I will put my hope in God! I will praise him again—my Savior and my God!*

The psalmist is talking to himself when he addresses his soul. He asks and answers his own question (haven't we all done that?). If you read the previous verses in Psalm 42, you'll see that he became discouraged by looking at his own (negative) circumstances. He was trying to figure out what to do. Then, he had a light-bulb moment. He realized that his life is saved, made whole, complete, *shalom*, not by himself but by God.

It's also interesting to note that the Hebrew word for 'health' in the King James Version of Psalm 42:11 is *yĕshuw'ah*, which is also Hebrew for 'Jesus.' **It is Jesus who is our health.**

Health, wholeness, and salvation come from God. We can't have healthy bodies if our souls (hearts and minds) aren't looking to and trusting God.

CHAPTER 1 - WHAT DOES IT MEAN TO BE IN HEALTH?

Proverbs 3:7-8 KJV
Be not wise [skillful, shrewd, learned, prudent] *in thine own eyes: fear* [be in awe of, honor, respect, love] *the LORD, and depart from evil.*

It shall be health to thy navel, and marrow to thy bones [essence, substance, self, life]*.*

Proverbs 3:7-8 Bullinger
Be not wise in thine own eyes: Revere the LORD, and shun and avoid evil.

It shall be healing to thy body, and moistening to thy bones.

Many people try to figure out life for themselves. They pride themselves on being intelligent, savvy, and wise. These verses tell us that isn't the way to be. There are two things prescribed here for health:

1. Revere, honor, trust, be in awe of, love God.
2. Shun and avoid evil.

These are God's ways for health. We can do all the other things like eating clean and reducing toxins, but if we don't do these two things, we won't manifest a healthy body.

By the way, 'navel' (in Proverbs 3:8) refers to the umbilical cord, the method of getting sustenance in the womb, and marrow means "moistening," as Bullinger translated it (above). It refers to a refreshing of the bones (your substance, your body).

To summarize what we've discovered thus far, being in health is a result of a prosperous (nothing missing, nothing broken) soul. We can't have

CHAPTER 1 – WHAT DOES IT MEAN TO BE IN HEALTH?

healthy bodies if our souls (hearts, minds, and emotions) aren't looking to and trusting God.

At the end of this chapter, I'll list more verses for study in this area.

Avoid Evil

In addition to trusting and being in awe of God, we must shun and avoid evil. We must know what evil is if we are to avoid it. So, let's look at what God considers evil.

> *1 John 5:19 NIV*
> *We know that we are children of God, and that the whole world is under the control of the evil one.*

If the whole world is under the control of the Evil One, how do we shun and avoid evil? It's everywhere. It's true that God has given us the victory in Christ Jesus (1 Corinthians 15:57) and that we have overcome the Wicked (Evil) One (1 John 2:13). These are spiritual realities that must come into manifestation in our physical lives. Let's look at some ways this is done.

Guarding the Heart

> *Proverbs 4:23 KJV*
> *Keep thy heart with all diligence; for out of it are the issues of life.*

The word 'keep' in Hebrew is *natsar*, which means "to guard, watch, watch over, keep."

'Diligence' is *mishmar*, meaning "a place of confinement, prison, guard, jail, guard post, watch, observance." *Gesenius' Hebrew-Chaldean Lexicon* translates it, "above all the things which are to be guarded."

The phrase 'out of it are the issues' is one Hebrew word, *towtsa'ah*, meaning "outgoing, border, a going out, extremity, end, source, escape." *Gesenius' Hebrew-Chaldean Lexicon* translates it, "the fountain of life, of happiness."

CHAPTER 1 - WHAT DOES IT MEAN TO BE IN HEALTH?

> *Proverbs 4:23 NLT*
> *Guard your heart above all else, for it determines the course of your life.*

> *Proverbs 4:23 NIV*
> *Above all else, guard your heart, for everything you do flows from it.*

We are to guard what goes into our hearts. What goes into our hearts? Things we see, hear, and think.

What You See

> *Psalm 101:3a KJV*
> *I will set no wicked thing before mine eyes:*

The word 'wicked' is *běliya'al*, which is translated "Belial" 16 times. It means "worthless, good for nothing, unprofitable." We are not to look at things that are worthless, good for nothing, or unprofitable.

> *1 John 2:15-16 KJV*
> *Love not the world, neither the things that are in the world. If any man love the world, the love of the Father is not in him.*
>
> *For all that is in the world, the lust of the flesh, and the lust of the eyes, and the pride of life, is not of the Father, but is of the world.*

Because the whole world is under the control of the Evil One (also known as the Devil and Satan), we must take care what we allow ourselves to look at. Are you watching TV shows, movies, YouTube videos, video games, etc., that portray evil (violence, murder, rape, lying, scamming/conning others, adultery, pornography (or other sexually suggestive things), etc.)? Are you reading newspapers, magazines, books, or websites filled with these things?

Proverbs 6 has a list of seven things that are an abomination to God. Do a word search on 'abomination' to find out what God considers evil. We are not only to avoid doing these things, we are to avoid, shun, watching these things being done.

CHAPTER 1 – WHAT DOES IT MEAN TO BE IN HEALTH?

What You Hear

> *Mark 4:24 KJV*
> *And he said unto them, Take heed what ye hear: with what measure ye mete, it shall be measured to you: and unto you that hear* [Hear what?] *shall more be given.*

Let's look at the context.

> *Mark 4:13-25 KJV*
> *And he said unto them, Know ye not this parable? and how then will ye know all parables?*
>
> *The sower soweth the word.*
>
> *And these are they by the way side, where the word is sown; but when they have heard, Satan cometh immediately, and taketh away the word that was sown in their hearts.*
>
> *And these are they likewise which are sown on stony ground; who, when they have heard the word, immediately receive it with gladness;*
>
> *And have no root in themselves, and so endure but for a time: afterward, when affliction or persecution ariseth for the word's sake, immediately they are offended.*
>
> *And these are they which are sown among thorns; such as hear the word,*
>
> *And the cares of this world, and the deceitfulness of riches, and the lusts of other things entering in, choke the word, and it becometh unfruitful.*
>
> *And these are they which are sown on good ground; such as hear the word, and receive it, and bring forth fruit, some thirtyfold, some sixty, and some an hundred.*
>
> *And he said unto them, Is a candle brought to be put under a bushel, or under a bed? and not to be set on a candlestick?*

CHAPTER 1 - WHAT DOES IT MEAN TO BE IN HEALTH?

For there is nothing hid, which shall not be manifested; neither was any thing kept secret, but that it should come abroad.

If any man have ears to hear, let him hear. [Hear what?]

And he said unto them, Take heed what ye hear: with what measure ye mete, it shall be measured to you: and unto you that hear [Hear what?] *shall more be given.*

For he that hath, to him shall be given: and he that hath not, from him shall be taken even that which he hath.

The context is hearing the Word of God.

What are you hearing? Are you listening to talk radio that causes you to become riled up, angry, jingoistic, emotionally disturbed, or filled with hatred for others? Are you listening to music that degrades women, promotes violence, adultery, lying, cheating? Do you listen to your friends or co-workers talk about these things? What about people who are talking about disrespecting God and others, or being self-sufficient instead of being God-sufficient (2 Corinthians 3:5)? We are to avoid, shun, evil. We don't even listen to it.

What You Think

> 2 Corinthians 10:5 KJV
> *Casting down imaginations, and every high thing that exalteth itself against the knowledge of God, and bringing into captivity every thought to the obedience of Christ;*
>
> 2 Corinthians 10:5 NIV
> *We demolish arguments and every pretension that sets itself up against the knowledge of God, and we take captive every thought to make it obedient to Christ.*

If what you're seeing, hearing, and thinking is causing you to be angry, fearful, or confused, none of which are from God, you must see, hear, and think something else instead.

CHAPTER 1 – WHAT DOES IT MEAN TO BE IN HEALTH?

> *Philippians 4:6-9 KJV*
> *Be careful* [anxious, worried] *for nothing; but in every thing by prayer and supplication with thanksgiving let your requests be made known unto God.*
>
> *And the peace of God, which passeth all understanding, shall keep your hearts and minds through Christ Jesus.*
>
> *Finally, brethren, whatsoever things are true, whatsoever things are honest, whatsoever things are just, whatsoever things are pure, whatsoever things are lovely, whatsoever things are of good report; if there be any virtue, and if there be any praise, think on these things.*
>
> *Those things, which ye have both learned, and received, and heard, and seen in me, do: and the God of peace shall be with you.*

Look at verse 7: "And the peace of God, which passeth all understanding, shall keep your hearts and minds through Christ Jesus."

'Keep' is *phroureō*, meaning "to guard, protect by a military guard, either to prevent hostile invasion or to keep the inhabitants of a besieged city from fleeing." *Thayer's Greek Lexicon* says, "by watching and guarding to preserve one for the attainment of something."

What to Think About

What should we be thinking in order to avoid evil?

> *Philippians 4:8 KJV*
> *Finally, brethren, whatsoever things are true, whatsoever things are honest, whatsoever things are just, whatsoever things are pure, whatsoever things are lovely, whatsoever things are of good report; if there be any virtue, and if there be any praise, think on these things.*

'Think' is *logizomai*, which means "to consider, take account, weigh on, meditate on a thing with a view to obtaining it." We don't think just any thought that pops into our minds. We make a conscious decision regarding what we will think about.

We are to fill our thoughts with things that are:

1. True – *alēthēs* = true, truly, truth

   John 17:17 KJV
   Sanctify them through thy truth: thy word is truth.

   Think about God and His Word, how everything He says is true.

2. Honest – *semnos* = august (respected and impressive), venerable (accorded a great deal of respect, especially because of age, wisdom, or character), reverend (worthy of reverence: revered)

   Deuteronomy 5:27-29 KJV
   [Moses is recounting what the children of Israel had said to him] Go thou near, and hear all that the LORD our God shall say: and speak thou unto us all that the LORD our God shall speak unto thee; and we will hear it, and do it.

   And the LORD heard the voice of your [Israel's] words, when ye spake unto me [Moses]; and the LORD said unto me, I have heard the voice of the words of this people, which they have spoken unto thee: they have well said all that they have spoken.

   [Moses is recounting what God told him about Israel] O that there were such an heart in them [Israel], that they would fear [be in awe of] me [God], and keep all my commandments always, that it might be well with them, and with their children for ever!

   The word for 'fear me' means "to stand in awe of, be awed." If you're afraid of something, you're admitting that it's greater than you and worthy to be held above you. So, anything we fear other than God, we are saying it's greater than God in our life.

   Think about God and His Word, His complete trustworthiness.

CHAPTER 1 – WHAT DOES IT MEAN TO BE IN HEALTH?

3. Just – *dikaios* = righteous

   What is righteousness? It's to be fully accepted by God. Who is righteous?

   > *John 17:25 KJV*
   > [Jesus is praying] *O righteous Father, the world hath not known thee: but I have known thee, and these have known that thou hast sent me.*

   > *Acts 3:14 KJV*
   > *But ye denied the Holy One and the Just* [just means righteous]*, and desired a murderer to be granted unto you;*

   > *Romans 5:19 KJV*
   > *For as by one man's disobedience many were made sinners, so by the obedience of one shall many be made righteous.*

   Think about God's righteousness, Jesus Christ's righteousness, your righteousness (your acceptance by God) because of Christ.

4. Pure – *hagnos* = pure from every fault, immaculate

   > *2 Corinthians 11:2 KJV*
   > *For I am jealous over you with godly jealousy: for I have espoused you to one husband, that I may present you as a chaste virgin to Christ.*

   > *Ephesians 1:4 KJV*
   > *According as he hath chosen us in him before the foundation of the world, that we should be holy and without blame before him in love:*

   > *James 3:17 KJV*
   > *But the wisdom that is from above is first pure, then peaceable, gentle, and easy to be intreated, full of mercy and good fruits, without partiality, and without hypocrisy.*

   Think about God and His Word. Think about who He has made you in Christ.

CHAPTER 1 - WHAT DOES IT MEAN TO BE IN HEALTH?

5. Lovely – *prosphilēs* = acceptable, pleasing – only usage in Bible

    Ephesians 1:6 KJV
    [We, God's children are] *To the praise of the glory of his grace, wherein he hath made us accepted in the beloved.*

    Accepted – *charitoō* = to pursue with grace, compass with favor; to honor with blessings

    Who is the beloved?

    Matthew 3:17 KJV
    "And lo a voice from heaven, saying, This is my beloved Son, in whom I am well pleased."

    Think about who you are in Christ. Think about how God has accepted you because of Christ.

6. Good report – *euphēmos* = things spoken in a kindly spirit, with goodwill toward others – only usage in Bible. This is regarding the things we speak about and how we say them. Let's look at what it isn't, that is, what not to speak:

    Matthew 7:1-2 KJV
    Judge not, that ye be not judged.

    For with what judgment ye judge, ye shall be judged: and with what measure ye mete, it shall be measured to you again.

    This is the same phrase used regarding what we hear, now being used regarding what we say and what we think in judgment of others.

    Ephesians 4:29 KJV
    Let no corrupt communication proceed out of your mouth, but that which is good to the use of edifying, that it may minister grace unto the hearers.

    Ephesians 5:4 KJV
    Neither filthiness, nor foolish talking, nor jesting, which are not convenient: but rather giving of thanks.

CHAPTER 1 – WHAT DOES IT MEAN TO BE IN HEALTH?

Filthiness – *aischrotēs* = obscenity, filthiness, baseness, dishonor. Only usage in the Bible.

Foolish talking – *mōrologia* – only usage in Bible. To learn about what a fool speaks of, see Proverbs. Foolishness is the opposite of wisdom.

Jesting – *eutrapelia* – only usage in the Bible. Means ready at repartee (sarcasm); witticism in a vulgar sense. Crude or coarse joking. Sarcasm can be traced back to the Greek verb *sarkazein*, which initially meant "to tear flesh like a dog." Even today, sarcasm is often described as sharp, cutting, or wounding, reminiscent of the original meaning of the Greek word.

Convenient – *anēkō* = fitting

These are the only usages of these words in the Bible, so they should arrest our attention and stand out to us.

Do and speak the opposite of these things.

> *Psalm 141:13 KJV*
> *Set a watch, O LORD, before my mouth; keep the door of my lips.*

Here is one verse on what to speak:

> *Ephesians 4:15 KJV*
> *But speaking the truth in love, may grow up into him in all things, which is the head, even Christ:*

I used to be very sarcastic. Then, I learned that it's a defense mechanism to protect oneself. The idea is that I'll say something sharp and biting to you before you can say it to me. This isn't loving or kind.

Think about and speak things that are kind, loving, encouraging, and nonjudgmental.

7. Virtue – *aretē* = any particular moral excellence, as modesty, purity

> *2 Peter 1:3 KJV*
> *According as his divine power hath given unto us all things that*

CHAPTER 1 - WHAT DOES IT MEAN TO BE IN HEALTH?

pertain unto life and godliness, through the knowledge of him that hath called us to glory and virtue:

2 Peter 1:5 KJV
And beside this, giving all diligence, add to your faith virtue; and to virtue knowledge;

Think about things that are morally excellent and pure.

8. Praise – *epainos* = approbation (approval or praise), commendation, praise

   Ephesians 1:12 KJV
   That we should be to the praise of his glory, who first trusted in Christ.

   Ephesians 1: 14 KJV
   Which is the earnest of our inheritance until the redemption of the purchased possession, unto the praise of his glory.

   Philippians 1:11 KJV
   Being filled with the fruits of righteousness, which are by Jesus Christ, unto the glory and praise of God.

   It's God who gets our praise.

So, what do we think about? The Word of God; God Himself; Jesus Christ; things that are righteous (Christ in you); things that are without fault (you in Christ); the fact that you're pleasing to God because of Christ and are therefore honored with blessings; things that are done in a kind spirit with goodwill toward others; things that are morally excellent; things that bring praise to God.

Thinking about anything other than God and His Word is completely useless and unprofitable. Yes, you have to think about what to buy at the grocery store (ask God) and which gas station to stop at (ask God). Do you see a pattern here?

CHAPTER 1 – WHAT DOES IT MEAN TO BE IN HEALTH?

These are the things we are to think about, to ponder, to give logical consideration to (*logizomai*). Perhaps they should also be the things we allow ourselves to see and hear.

> *Philippians 4:9 KJV*
> *Those things, which ye have both learned, and received, and heard, and seen in me [Paul], do: and the God of peace shall be with you.*

Actions (what you do) follow thoughts (what you have seen and heard). What we see and hear become our thoughts. Our thoughts become our heart beliefs. We guard our hearts by not worrying but by making our requests to God with thanksgiving (Philippians 4:6).

> *Isaiah 55:6-13 KJV*
> *Seek ye the LORD while he may be found, call ye upon him while he is near:*
>
> *Let the wicked forsake his way, and the unrighteous man his thoughts: and let him return unto the LORD and he will have mercy upon him; and to our God, for he will abundantly pardon.*
>
> *For my thoughts are not your thoughts, neither are your ways my ways, saith the LORD.*
>
> *For as the heavens are higher than the earth, so are my ways higher than your ways, and my thoughts than your thoughts.*
>
> *For as the rain cometh down, and the snow from heaven, and returneth not thither, but watereth the earth, and maketh it bring forth and bud, that it may give seed to the sower, and bread to the eater:*
>
> *So shall my word be that goeth forth out of my mouth: it shall not return unto me void, but it shall accomplish that which I please, and it shall prosper in the thing whereto I sent it.*
>
> *For ye shall go out with joy, and be led forth with peace: the mountains and the hills shall break forth before you into singing, and all the trees of the field shall clap their hands.*

CHAPTER 1 - WHAT DOES IT MEAN TO BE IN HEALTH?

Instead of the thorn shall come up the fir tree, and instead of the brier shall come up the myrtle tree: and it shall be to the LORD for a name, for an everlasting sign that shall not be cut off.

Being in health is two-fold. As with most things in life, there's a spiritual component and a physical component. According to scripture, being in health is a result of a prosperous (nothing missing, nothing broken) soul and is based on the promise in 1 Peter 2:24 that we were healed by the stripes (wounds) of Jesus Christ.

When our souls are prospering because we love and trust God and we avoid/shun evil, then we are walking in harmony with God's ways, which are much higher than our ways (Isaiah 55:9). God promises us such abundance, but we must take hold of it.

My prayer for you is that you be in health and prosper, even as your soul prospers.

Here are more verses you can study about the soul prospering.

Psalm 23:3	Psalm 25:1
Psalm 25:12-14	Psalm 25:20
Psalm 33:20-21	Psalm 34:2
Psalm 35:9	Psalm 41:4
Psalm 42:2	Psalm 42:5
Psalm 42:11	Psalm 43:5
Psalm 57:1	Psalm 62:1
Psalm 62:5	Psalm 63:1-8
Psalm 66:8-9	Psalm 66:16
Psalm 71:23	Psalm 84:2
Psalm 86:4-5	Psalm 94:19
Psalm 103:1-6	Psalm 107:8-9

CHAPTER 1 – WHAT DOES IT MEAN TO BE IN HEALTH?

Psalm 116:7-8	Psalm 121:7
Psalm 130:5-6	Psalm 138:3
Psalm 143:5-6	Psalm 143:8
Psalm 139:14	Proverbs 2:10-11
Proverbs 15:32	Proverbs 16:24
Proverbs 18:7	Proverbs 19:2
Proverbs 19:8	Proverbs 19:16
Proverbs 21:23	Proverbs 22:24-25
Proverbs 24:13	Mark 4:23-25
Hebrews 4:12	1 Peter 2:11

CHAPTER 2

GOD'S WAYS VS. MAN'S WAYS

O LORD, I know that the way of man is not in himself: it is not in man that walketh to direct his steps.
Jeremiah 10:23 KJV

Whatever we do in life, we must keep in mind that the Word of God is to have the preeminence. Ever since the fall of Adam, mankind has behaved like a toddler, wanting to do things his own way. The NIV translation of the above verse says, "LORD, I know that people's lives are not their own; it is not for them to direct their steps."

> *Isaiah 55:6-9 KJV*
> *Seek ye the LORD while he may be found, call ye upon him while he is near:*
>
> *Let the wicked forsake his way, and the unrighteous man his thoughts: and let him return unto the LORD, and he will have mercy upon him; and to our God, for he will abundantly pardon.*
>
> *For my thoughts are not your thoughts, neither are your ways my ways, saith the LORD.*
>
> *For as the heavens are higher than the earth, so are my ways higher than your ways, and my thoughts than your thoughts.*
>
> *Ecclesiastes 12:13-14 ESV*
> *The end of the matter; all has been heard. Fear [be in awe of] God and keep his commandments, for this is the whole duty of man.*

CHAPTER 2 – GOD'S WAYS VS. MAN'S WAYS

For God will bring every deed into judgment, with every secret thing, whether good or evil.

Our purpose is to live in harmony with God's ways, which are often different from our own. In this book, we will put aside our thoughts and our ways to search out God's thoughts and ways regarding health.

Proverbs 28:26 NLT
Those who trust their own insight are foolish, but anyone who walks in wisdom is safe.

We have the choice whether to be foolish or wise. No one I know likes to be thought of as a fool.

Psalm 107:17-18 KJV
Fools because of their transgression, and because of their iniquities, are afflicted.

Their soul abhorreth all manner of meat; and they draw near unto the gates of death.

The NRSV of Psalm 107:17 says,

Psalm 107:17 NRSV
Some were sick through their sinful ways, and because of their iniquities endured affliction.

The Bible cuts right to the chase. Nowadays, we call it a 'lifestyle choice,' which includes what we eat. The Bible simply calls it sin.

Jeremiah 7:24 NLT
"But my people would not listen to me. They kept doing whatever they wanted, following the stubborn desires of their evil hearts. They went backward instead of forward.

Romans 14:23b KJV
Whatsoever is not of faith is sin.

Anytime we live according to the stubborn desires of our own hearts, we will be moving in the wrong direction.

CHAPTER 2 – GOD'S WAYS VS. MAN'S WAYS

> *Proverbs 3:5-8 NIV*
> *Trust in the LORD with all your heart and lean not on your own understanding;*
>
> *in all your ways submit to him, and he will make your paths straight.*
>
> *Do not be wise in your own eyes; fear* [be in awe of] *the LORD and shun evil.*
>
> *This will bring health to your body and nourishment to your bones.*

What a tremendous promise from God. He tells us plainly how to manifest health in our bodies: we are to put aside our own understanding of things and submit to His ways. When we make this choice to follow His ways, He will "make our paths straight," which means God will make our way in life agreeable and pleasing to Him.

Many of God's holy ones (saints) erroneously think that they can do whatever they want without consequence. "Oh, I bless my food before I eat, so God will make sure it's healthy." Is this the testimony of God's Word?

> *Luke 4:9-12 KJV*
> *And he* [the Devil] *brought him* [Jesus] *to Jerusalem, and set him on a pinnacle of the temple, and said unto him, If thou be the Son of God, cast thyself down from hence:*
>
> *For it is written, He shall give his angels charge over thee, to keep thee:*
>
> *And in their hands they shall bear thee up, lest at any time thou dash thy foot against a stone.*
>
> *And Jesus answering said unto him, It is said, Thou shalt not tempt the Lord thy God.*

After Jesus' 40 days in the wilderness, he was tempted by the Devil. The Devil suggested that if Jesus were truly the Son of God, he could throw

CHAPTER 2 – GOD'S WAYS VS. MAN'S WAYS

himself off the top of the temple because in Psalm 91:11-12, God promises that His angels will rescue those in need.

In addition to tempting Jesus to question his identity as the Son of God, the Devil not only tempted Jesus to violate one of God's laws (in this case, the law of gravity), he tempted Jesus to expect that God would break that law to rescue him. Jesus responded that to do so was to tempt God. How many times have we saints violated one of God's laws yet expected that we would not suffer the consequences?

> *Galatians 6:7-8 KJV*
> *Be not deceived; God is not mocked: for whatsoever a man soweth, that shall he also reap.*
>
> *For he that soweth to his flesh shall of the flesh reap corruption* [that which perishes]; *but he that soweth to the Spirit shall of the Spirit reap life everlasting.*

Mankind wants to do whatever they want (like a toddler) without consequence. That's not how life works. Our thoughts and ways aren't the same as God's. To truly reap the benefits that God has promised to us, we must live in harmony with His ways. In the following chapters, we will examine God's thoughts and ways regarding health.

CHAPTER 3

GOD'S ORIGINAL EATING PLAN FOR MANKIND

God created a perfect world for His perfect man to live in.

> *Genesis 1:31a NIV*
> *God saw all that he had made, and it was very good.*
>
> *Genesis 1:11 NIV*
> *Then God said, "Let the land produce vegetation: seed-bearing plants and trees on the land that bear fruit with seed in it, according to their various kinds." And it was so.*
>
> *Genesis 1:26 NIV*
> *Then God said, "Let us make mankind in our image, in our likeness, so that they may rule over the fish in the sea and the birds in the sky, over the livestock and all the wild animals, and over all the creatures that move along the ground."*

God provided Adam and Eve with everything they needed for a healthy life in companionship with Him. The spirit of God in them gave them dominion (Genesis 1:26). God provided the best food for them.

> *Genesis 1:29 NIV*
> *Then God said, "**I give you every seed-bearing plant on the face of the whole earth and every tree that has fruit with seed in it. They will be yours for food.**"*

This description includes nuts, grains, legumes, and seeds.

The human digestive system was designed for the way of eating God set out in Genesis 1:29. The length of the digestive tract is a strong indicator of what type of food should be eaten,[1] and the human digestive tract is 12-14 times our shoulder-to-hip (trunk) length, the same as fruit-eating animals. Herbivores, such as cattle, have a gut length 20 times their body length since it takes longer to digest the fiber content in the foods they eat. The shortest tracts are found in meat-eaters such as canines, polar bears, and felines.

There's disagreement among scientists whether to classify humans as herbivores, which includes cows, sheep, deer, rabbits, and squirrels, as frugivores (any type of herbivore or omnivore where fruit is a preferred food type), or as omnivores.

After the Fall: Vegetables

Once man fell (Genesis 3:6), his perfect world fell apart, too. No longer was the earth supplying everything he needed.

> *Genesis 3:17-19 NIV*
> *To Adam he said, "Because you listened to your wife and ate fruit from the tree about which I commanded you, 'You must not eat from it,' "Cursed is the ground because of you; through painful toil you will eat food from it all the days of your life.*
>
> *It will produce thorns and thistles for you, and **you will eat the plants of the field**.*
>
> *By the sweat of your brow you will eat your food until you return to the ground, since from it you were taken; for dust you are and to dust you will return."*

After the fall, God told Adam that he would eat plants. Vegetables are very rich in sulfur and are good cleansers of the digestive tract.[2]

After the Flood: Meat

After the flood of Noah, all plant life on land had been wiped out. The earth itself required time to dry out before Noah and his sons could plant crops. The only things possible to eat were the animals that had been on the ark.

> *Genesis 9:1-4 NIV*
> *Then God blessed Noah and his sons, saying to them, "Be fruitful and increase in number and fill the earth.*

CHAPTER 3 – GOD'S ORIGINAL EATING PLAN FOR MANKIND

The fear [awe] *and dread* [terror] *of you will fall on all the beasts of the earth, and on all the birds in the sky, on every creature that moves along the ground, and on all the fish in the sea; they are given into your hands.*

Everything that lives and moves about will be food for you. **Just as I gave you the green plants, I now give you everything.**

But you must not eat meat that has its lifeblood still in it."

So, now man was an omnivore with a body designed as an herbivore/frugivore. Therefore, God set principles regarding the eating of meat, which we will cover in the next chapter.

CHAPTER 3 – GOD'S ORIGINAL EATING PLAN FOR MANKIND

CHAPTER 4

THE DIETARY LAWS OF THE OLD TESTAMENT

After the fall of Adam, God made a plan to reconcile mankind back to Himself (Genesis 3:15), but until the time that Christ came in the flesh, God in His love provided a way for man to stay healthy. He did this by instituting various dietary laws. The purpose of these laws was not to make life difficult for people or to prevent them from being free to eat whatever they wanted but to keep them healthy. Even though we are no longer bound by the law to earn our righteousness, dietary and sanitary laws are just good, common sense.

> *Romans 10:4 KJV*
> *For Christ is the end of the law for righteousness to every one that believeth.*

God promised that if the children of Israel would obey His laws, they would stay healthy.

> *Exodus 15:26 NIV*
> *He said, "If you listen carefully to the Lord your God and do what is right in his eyes, if you pay attention to his commands and keep all his decrees, I will not bring on you any of the diseases I brought on the Egyptians, for I am the Lord, who heals you."*

Today, our healing is based on the finished work of Jesus Christ.

> *1 Peter 2:24 NIV*
> *"He himself bore our sins" in his body on the cross, so that we might die to sins and live for righteousness; "by his wounds you have been healed."*

In Genesis 7:2, God made a distinction between clean and unclean animals while giving instructions to Noah about the animals that were to enter the ark, so the concept of clean/unclean predates Mosaic law.

> *Genesis 7:2 NIV*
> *Take with you seven pairs of every kind of clean animal, a male*

CHAPTER 4 – THE DIETARY LAWS OF THE OLD TESTAMENT

and its mate, and one pair of every kind of unclean animal, a male and its mate,

Our healing is a spiritual reality in Christ. Let's continue to look at the advice God has for maintaining our bodies. Here are some of the main dietary guidelines God provided in Leviticus 11 and Deuteronomy 14:

Can Eat (Clean)

- Cud-chewing animals with split hooves: cows, ox, bison, caribou, giraffe, moose, reindeer, sheep/lamb, goats, ibex, deer, gazelle, roe deer, antelope, etc.
- Birds: chicken, turkey, pheasant, dove, duck, goose, quail, sparrow
- Marine life with fins and scales
- Any kind of locust, katydid, cricket, or grasshopper

Do Not Eat (Unclean)

- Animals that eat other animals (scavengers, carrion eaters)
- Mammals such as all cats, dogs, wolves, bears, horses, camels, elephants, gorillas, groundhogs, hippopotamuses, kangaroos, llamas, monkeys, raccoons, weasels, coney (dassie; a type of rodent), hare (rabbit), etc.
- All insects besides those mentioned above
- Swine: pigs, boars, peccaries (pork and bacon)
- All reptiles and amphibians
- Birds: eagle, vulture, kite, raven, gull, owl, stork, heron, cormorant, osprey, hoopoe, flamingo, parrot, crow, cuckoo, penguin, roadrunner, bat (not a bird but listed with them)
- Marine life without fins and scales (such as shellfish – crab, shrimp, lobster, oysters, mussels, clams; also, octopus, squid, shark, whales, catfish, eel, dolphins, marlin, sturgeon (including caviar), swordfish, etc.)

CHAPTER 4 – THE DIETARY LAWS OF THE OLD TESTAMENT

- "Any creature that moves along the ground, whether it moves on its belly or walks on all fours or on many feet," such as moles, mice, weasels, opossum, squirrels, worms, snails, slugs, centipedes, millipedes, etc.

A common denominator of many of the animals God designates as unclean is that they routinely eat things that could sicken or kill human beings. Nutritionist David Meinz observes:

"Could it be that God, in His wisdom, created certain creatures whose sole purpose is to clean up after the others? Their entire 'calling' may be to act exclusively as the sanitation workers of our ecology. God may simply be telling us that it's better for us believers not to consume the meat of these trash collectors." [1]
David Meinz

Simply put, God tells us not to eat these foods because they aren't healthy for human consumption. Many of these animals carry toxins that are stored in their flesh. Rabbits digest their own excrement.[2] Pigs have high levels of bacteria, such as Campylobacter and salmonella.[3] Shellfish are scavengers, eating refuse.[4]

There are many, many types of meat we can choose from (clean list). So, instead of focusing on what we *can't* have, let's thank God for what He has provided for us.

35

CHAPTER 4 – THE DIETARY LAWS OF THE OLD TESTAMENT

CHAPTER 5

FREEDOM IN CHRIST OR LICENSE TO SIN?

Many Christians point to these verses to argue that we are no longer bound to dietary laws.

> *Acts 10:15 NIV*
> The voice spoke to him a second time, "Do not call anything impure that God has made clean."
>
> *Galatians 5:1 KJV*
> Stand fast therefore in the liberty wherewith Christ hath made us free, and be not entangled again with the yoke of bondage.
>
> *Romans 14:14 NIV*
> I [Paul] am convinced, being fully persuaded in the Lord Jesus, that nothing is unclean in itself. But if anyone regards something as unclean, then for that person it is unclean.
>
> *Matthew 15:11 NIV*
> What goes into someone's mouth does not defile them, but what comes out of their mouth, that is what defiles them."
>
> *1 Timothy 4:3-5 NIV*
> They forbid people to marry and order them to abstain from certain foods, which God created to be received with thanksgiving by those who believe and who know the truth.
>
> For everything God created is good, and nothing is to be rejected if it is received with thanksgiving,
>
> because it is consecrated by the word of God and prayer.

Our redemption in Christ frees us from needing to keep the law in order to earn our righteousness. Christ earned our righteousness for us. That does not negate the godly principles of the law.

CHAPTER 5 - FREEDOM IN CHRIST OR LICENSE TO SIN?

> *Romans 10:4 KJV*
> *For Christ is the end of the law for righteousness to every one that believeth.*

> *Romans 7:12 NIV*
> *So then, the law is holy, and the commandment is holy, righteous and good.*

Are the laws that say we're not to steal from or kill others no longer in effect because they're from the Old Testament law? Sadly, I see far too many Christians who think that freedom in Christ means they can do whatever they want without consequence. This is not the testimony of God's Word. The principle of reaping and sowing is always in effect.

> *Galatians 6:7-8 KJV*
> *Be not deceived; God is not mocked: for whatsoever a man soweth, that shall he also reap.*
>
> *For he that soweth to his flesh shall of the flesh reap corruption* [that which perishes]; *but he that soweth to the Spirit shall of the Spirit reap life everlasting.*

In chapter 2, we discussed how the Devil tempted Jesus Christ. Jesus was tempted to prove he was the Son of God by breaking one of God's laws yet expecting that God would break that law Himself to order to save Jesus. **This is the kind of convoluted thinking the Devil specializes in.** Jesus' response was that to do this would be to "tempt the Lord thy God."

Certainly, we as God's people don't want to tempt God, but how many times do we do things that go against godly principles yet expect that God will intervene, rescuing us from reaping what we have sown? So it is with the laws, the principles, that govern how God made our bodies work.

When we live in harmony with God's ways (which are above our own ways), we will reap the benefits. When we live in disharmony with (disregard for) God's ways, we reap the consequences (the breakdown of our bodies).

CHAPTER 5 - FREEDOM IN CHRIST OR LICENSE TO SIN?

John 5:5-9, 14 KJV
And a certain man was there, which had an infirmity thirty and eight years.

When Jesus saw him lie, and knew that he had been now a long time in that case, he saith unto him, Wilt thou be made whole?

The impotent man answered him, Sir, I have no man, when the water is troubled, to put me into the pool: but while I am coming, another steppeth down before me.

Jesus saith unto him, Rise, take up thy bed, and walk.

And immediately the man was made whole, and took up his bed, and walked: and on the same day was the sabbath.

Afterward Jesus findeth him in the temple, and said unto him, Behold, thou art made whole: sin no more, lest a worse thing come unto thee.

This is a fascinating record. After Jesus healed this man, he told him to sin no more, lest a worse thing come upon him. What does this man sinning have to do with his healing?

The word 'sin' here is the Greek word *hamartanō*, which means "to miss the mark or to wander from the path of uprightness and honor." When we sin, we aren't in harmony with God's ways and we reap the consequences. In this case, the consequence this man reaped was an infirmity of 38 years' duration.

When we repent of sin, we turn around and go in the opposite direction; that's the meaning of repentance. In other words, Jesus was telling this man that if he continued to live in disharmony with God's ways, he would end up back in the same situation from which Jesus had just delivered him.

Our freedom in Christ is that we are forever freed from having to try to earn our own righteousness. It's already been done for us in Christ Jesus.

CHAPTER 5 - FREEDOM IN CHRIST OR LICENSE TO SIN?

> 1 Corinthians 10:23 KJV
> All things are lawful for me, but all things are not expedient [profitable]: all things are lawful for me, but all things edify not.

> Galatians 5:13 KJV
> For, brethren, ye have been called unto liberty; only use not liberty for an occasion [a base of operations] to the flesh, but by love serve one another.

Why have I spent all this time on this subject?

> 1 Corinthians 6:19-20 NLT
> Don't you realize that your body is the temple of the Holy Spirit, who lives in you and was given to you by God? You do not belong to yourself,
>
> for God bought you with a high price. So you must honor God with your body.

YOU are a beautiful, marvelous, perfect masterpiece, gloriously created by an awesome, loving Father. Honor your temple by nourishing your body with the foods God provided for us.

For more information, see the following:

http://AmazingDiscoveries.org/C-deception-diet_unclean_clean_law_Bible

http://AmazingDiscoveries.org/C-deception-diet_unclean_clean_New_Testament

PART 2

A SPIRITUAL ATTACK IS UNDERWAY

There's something going on that most of us aren't paying attention to. The current medical/health care and food systems are not designed to help us. The church is under attack.

CHAPTER 6

HEALTH CARE OR SICK CARE?

The origins of the current health care crisis in the U.S. started centuries ago. There's something going on that most of us aren't paying attention to. The current medical/health care system isn't designed to make us well. Let's look at the origins of health care.

God's Plan for Health

When God formed, made, and created Adam and Eve, He placed them in a perfect paradise and gave them dominion over everything else on earth. There was no need for healing or health care; their bodies were perfect.

Once man decided to disobey God, God's first response was to clean up the mess by promising to send a redeemer.

> *Genesis 3:14-15 KJV*
> *And the LORD God said unto the serpent, Because thou hast done this, thou art cursed above all cattle, and above every beast of the field; upon thy belly shalt thou go, and dust shalt thou eat all the days of thy life:*
>
> *And I will put enmity* [hatred, hostility] *between thee and the woman, and between thy seed and her seed; it shall bruise thy head, and thou shalt bruise his heel.*

This Redeemer would also provide health and wholeness to whosoever would believe on him. Psalm 42:11 shows us where health comes from.

> *Psalm 42:11 KJV*
> *Why art thou cast down, O my soul? and why art thou disquieted within me? hope thou in God: for I shall yet praise him, who is the health of my countenance and my God.*

The Hebrew word for 'health' in this verse is *yĕshuw'ah*, which is also Hebrew for 'Jesus.' It's Jesus who is our health.

CHAPTER 6 – HEALTH CARE OR SICK CARE?

The first use of 'be in health' is in Genesis 43:28 where it's translated 'in good health.' The Hebrew word is *shalom*. You may be familiar with this word. It means not only peace (quiet, tranquility, contentment), but also completeness, soundness (in body), welfare (health and prosperity), and friendship. It means to be whole (also called saved). I've heard it described as 'nothing missing, nothing broken.'

Even before Jesus Christ was born, God provided health for His people.

> *Psalm 103:3 KJV*
> Who forgiveth all thine iniquities; who healeth all thy diseases;

The children of Israel looked forward to the Christ. We look back on his accomplishments. Our healing is a done deal. The price has been paid.

> *Isaiah 53:5 KJV*
> *But he was wounded for our transgressions, he was bruised for our iniquities: the chastisement of our peace was upon him; and with his stripes we are healed.*

> *1 Peter 2:24 NASB*
> *and He Himself bore our sins in His body on the cross, so that we might die to sin and live to righteousness; for by His wounds you were healed.*

The Health Benefits of Plants

God also provided for health and wellness through plants. People have used herbs, spices, and the essential oils of plants for thousands of years for medicinal, cosmetic, religious, and embalming purposes. Essential oils are also used to positively affect the emotions and to elevate spirituality because of how they affect the limbic system (the seat of emotions). Essential oils support body systems. Many people today use them in place of toxic household cleaners and beauty products.

<u>What are Essential Oils?</u>

Just as the life of the flesh is in the blood (Leviticus 17:11), the life of the plant is in its essential oil. It's the lifeblood of plants. What happens when you peel an orange? Lots of tiny drops of oil come bursting out. Those are essential oils.

Essential oils are non-fatty oils that are distilled from the roots, bark, leaves, flowers, peels, and seeds of bushes, plants, shrubs, flowers, fruit, and trees.

More specific information on essential oils and how I use them as part of the Be in Health lifestyle is in chapter 29.

Health Care in the Early Church

Before the Middle Ages, providing health care to the masses was the responsibility of the church. Local church leaders fulfilled the role of healer, getting their information directly from the guidance of God.

> *Mark 6:13 KJV*
> *And they cast out many devils, and anointed* [massaged] *with oil many that were sick, and healed them.*
>
> *James 5:14 KJV*
> *Is any sick among you? Let him call for the elders of the church; and let them pray over him, anointing* [massaging] *him with oil in the name of the lord:*

Let's take a moment to discuss secular health care during this time. Hippocrates (born c. 460 BC in Greece) is considered 'the father of western medicine.' He based his medical practice on observations and on the study of the human body. So, there were Gentile pagans who were practicing 'healing arts.'

In the scriptures, the "beloved physician" Luke, who wrote both the gospel of Luke and the Book of Acts, was a Gentile (pagan) convert to Christianity who accompanied the apostle Paul on many of his travels. The 'job' of physician/doctor was common among the Gentile pagans but not among the children of Israel or the first-century church.

CHAPTER 6 – HEALTH CARE OR SICK CARE?

The Origin of Doctors

During medieval times, the responsibility for health care started to drift away from the church and into the hands of specialists called doctors. 'Doctor' is an academic title that originates from the Latin word of the same spelling. The word originally meant "to teach." In medieval times, a doctor was someone who was licensed to teach at a university.[1]

All physicians are doctors, but not all doctors are physicians. Doctor refers to a person with a certain level of academic education in any field. Physicians have a doctorate level education in medicine. Medical Doctors (M.D.) are called "doctor" much more often than, say, Doctors of English Literature, but it would be completely correct to refer to the latter as "doctor," as well.[2] We use the terms physician and doctor interchangeably.

The term 'physician' is at least 900 years old, meaning a specialist in internal medicine. Today, we call them 'internists.' They were different from surgeons.[3] (More on this later.)

12th century Italy saw the emergence of universities and the first medical schools. Medieval physicians analyzed symptoms, examined excreta, and made their diagnoses. Then they might prescribe diet, rest, sleep, exercise, or baths, or they could administer emetics and purgatives. They routinely used herbs and spices in their practice.

In contrast, surgeons would treat fractures and dislocations, repair hernias, and perform amputations and a few other operations. Some of them prescribed opium, mandragora (a nightshade; see chapter 14), or alcohol to deaden the pain. Childbirth was left to midwives, who relied on folklore and tradition.[4]

Have you ever wondered where the word 'medicine' comes from? It has nothing to do with health. Through banking and commerce, the Medici family rose to become one of the most important houses in Florence, Italy. Their influence declined by the late 14th century but later resurged through the 18th century.[5]

CHAPTER 6 – HEALTH CARE OR SICK CARE?

The Medici family financed the works of Michelangelo, Leonardo da Vinci, and Galileo and invented the field of accounting with the general ledger. The family was in power for many centuries and their influence on society is still felt today. We get the word 'medicine' from the Medici family.

During this time, doctors were divided into two social classes, physicians and barber surgeons.[6] The barber surgeon, which was the lower-class doctor and the most common, cared for soldiers during and after battle. In this era, surgery was seldom conducted by physicians, but instead by barber surgeons who, because they used razors in their trade, were called upon for numerous tasks ranging from cutting hair to amputating limbs to tooth extractions. They believed in bloodletting and using leeches. The physician class of doctors didn't believe in surgery; they chose academia instead and served the wealthy. The physicians practiced 'medicine.'

The Black Death, also known as the Great Plague or simply Plague, was one of the most devastating pandemics in human history, resulting in the deaths of an estimated 75 to 200 million people in Eurasia and peaking in Europe from 1347 to 1351.[7]

Many physicians died from the Plague. (I discuss in chapter 29 why many barber surgeons didn't succumb.) With the scarcity of physicians (plus the fact that the remaining ones didn't do surgery), people increasingly relied on the barber surgeons for medical procedures.

Physicians and the upper class regarded the barber surgeons as 'quacks.' They were not scientifically trained in universities, but nonetheless, they were effective.

Few traces of the barbers' links with the surgical side of the medical profession remain.[8] The modern striped barber's pole harkens back to the bloodstained towels that would hang outside the offices of these barber surgeons.[9] Another vestige is the use of leeches. Surprisingly, the use of leeches (just like the barber surgeons used) has been approved by the FDA as a medical device.[10]

CHAPTER 6 – HEALTH CARE OR SICK CARE?

Paracelsus

Medical intervention using chemicals started earlier than most people think. In the early 16th century, Paracelsus pioneered the use of chemicals and minerals in medicine.[11] He rejected book knowledge, calling for experimental research, with heavy doses of mysticism, alchemy, and magic mixed in. He rejected the miracles that the church espoused and looked for cures in nature instead.[12]

Paracelsus,[13] born Theophrastus von Hohenheim (1493-1541), was a Swiss-German physician, alchemist, and astrologer. He is credited with being the 'father of toxicology,' which is the study of the safety and biological effects of drugs, chemicals, agents, and other substances on living organisms. The purpose of toxicology is to develop methods to determine harmful effects, the dosages that cause those effects, and safe exposure limits. This is important to remember as we continue our discussion.

Paracelsus came from a family of medical professionals. He himself worked as a military (barber) surgeon. By 1527, he was a licensed physician teaching at the University of Basel in Basel, Switzerland.

Astrology was a very important part of Paracelsus' medicine and he was a practicing astrologer, as were many of the university-trained physicians working in Europe at the time.[14]

Paracelsus extended his interest in chemistry and biology to what is now considered toxicology. He clearly expounded the concept of dose response in his *Third Defense*, where he stated that "**Solely the dose determines that a thing is not a poison.**" (*Sola dosis facit venenum,* "Only the dose makes the poison.")[15] He used this argument to defend his use of inorganic (not alive) substances in medicine since others frequently criticized his use of chemical agents as too toxic to have therapeutic benefit.[16]

Paracelsus was especially venerated by the German Rosicrucians, who regarded him as a prophet and developed a systematic study of his writings, which is sometimes called Paracelsianism.[17]

CHAPTER 6 – HEALTH CARE OR SICK CARE?

Rosicrucianism is a spiritual and cultural movement that arose in Europe in the early 17th century. The Encyclopedia Britannica says that "Rosicrucian teachings are a combination of occultism and other religious beliefs and practices, including Hermeticism, Jewish mysticism, and Christian Gnosticism. The central feature of Rosicrucianism is the belief that its members possess secret wisdom that was handed down to them from ancient times." [18]

The Nazis may have been inspired by German Rosicrucianism.[19] In his 1985 book *The Occult Roots of Nazism: The Ariosophists of Austria and Germany, 1890-1935*, historian Nicholas Goodrick-Clarke makes a serious attempt to identify these ideological origins. The book "demonstrates the way in which Nazism was influenced by powerful occult and millenarian sects that thrived in Germany and Austria at the turn of the 20th century. Their ideas and symbols filtered through to nationalist-racist groups associated with the infant Nazi party and their fantasies were played out with terrifying consequences in the Third Reich." [20]

Paracelsus is a highly controversial figure in the history of medicine, with most experts hailing him as a 'father of modern medicine' for shaking off religious orthodoxy and inspiring many researchers; others say he was a mystic more than a scientist and downplay his importance.[21]

Paracelsus' argument that "**Solely the dose determines that a thing is not a poison**" plays a critical role in today's medicine, which we will discuss later in this chapter.

A Dual System of Medicine Emerges

As we skip ahead to the 1800s in Europe, a dual system of medicine evolved. There was a new breed of doctor that went to universities and became more scientific and evidence-focused. As more and more people began to trust this new type of doctor, the abdication of health care by the church was nearly complete.

In this dual system of medicine, there were the aforementioned university-trained physicians on one side and an older breed of rural

CHAPTER 6 – HEALTH CARE OR SICK CARE?

doctors that relied on traditional medicine on the other. The latter were seen as primitive and not up-to-date on the new ideas of where sickness comes from. They didn't go to the university to learn their trade, they learned it from experience and they didn't use sophisticated tools to make people well. Many of these older practitioners considered the laws of nature and of God to be their licensing authorities.

This dual system led to a class war in medicine. On one side were those who believed in scientific evidence of disease such as germs. The other side relied on letting God/nature heal and used herbalism to help alleviate symptoms. This class warfare in the delivering of health care goes on to this day.

The Battle Against Germs

In 1889, Thomas Eakins painted *The Agnew Clinic*,[22] which depicted a surgery being performed in a medical amphitheater with an audience of onlookers. (Notice that the words used are similar to those used in the entertainment arts: perform, theater, audience.) The effect of *The Agnew Clinic* painting on medicine at the time can't be overstated. This paragraph is taken from the *American Medical Association Journal of Ethics*:

> *Shortly after the Agnew painting, the Flexner report (1910) led to the closure of a large number of borderline medical educational institutions and the restructuring of medical education around laboratory science. Coupled with William Osler's 1892 textbook of medicine and Walter Reed's observation of the spread of malaria by mosquitoes during the construction of the Panama Canal, the value of cleanliness and antisepsis was firmly fixed as the core of medical science.*[23]

The medical profession became obsessed with cleanliness. Joseph Lister[24] (1827-1912), considered the 'father of modern surgery' and after whom Listerine® is named, is the one who started the push to eliminate all germs. Lister wanted to find a way to sterilize wounds without using heat. He developed a theory that patients were being killed by germs.

He theorized that if germs could be killed or prevented, no infection would occur.

Lister reasoned that a chemical could be used to destroy the micro-organisms that cause infection. When he tried this on a patient using carbolic acid (now call phenol, an impure form of coal tar), the wound did heal, however, the patient received chemical burns. So, he diluted the carbolic acid on the second application and no chemical burn occurred. Remember what Paracelsus said, "**Solely the dose determines that a thing is not a poison.**"

20th Century Health Care

The 1900s is when mainstream medicine became state-sponsored. Doctors went to government-approved schools and received a license from the government to practice their trade.

The aforementioned Flexnor Report,[25] which was underwritten by the Carnegie Foundation,[26] called for American medical schools to enact higher standards, among other things. Many schools closed and the ones that remained became focused on teaching new doctors to manage patient care through pharmaceutical drugs and surgery. This focus remains today.

A 2016 article[27] by two medical students at UC Irvine states,

> Medical students are subjected to a barrage of advertising that inevitably leads to a physician-industry connection that can be harmful to our health care system.
>
> Medical students' exposure to pharmaceutical marketing begins early,[28] growing in frequency throughout their training. Students receive gifts[29] such as free meals, textbooks, pocket texts, small trinkets, and even drug samples.
>
> Forty to 100 percent of medical students report exposure[30] to the pharmaceutical industry,[31] with clinical students[32] being more likely than preclinical students to report exposure.
>
> The number of students recalling over 20 exposures to marketing

rose from 33.3 percent to nearly 72 percent[33] as students entered their clinical training. Pharmaceutical companies, recognizing the formative nature of the clinical years of medical education, seek to form relationships with medical students years before they are ready to independently practice medicine.

> **"One of the first duties of the physician is to educate the masses not to take medicine."**
> **Sir William Osler,**
> **Father of Modern Medicine**

A 2014 report from One Green Planet[34] reveals the following:

- Over 50 percent of Americans are on a prescription drug right now.

- Around 50 percent of doctors admit to prescribing drugs they don't believe will work.

- The typical medical student receives only 19.6 contact hours of nutrition education.

According to a 2015 article in *The Boston Globe*, "Federal law allows pharmaceutical and medical device companies to funnel millions of dollars a year, without disclosure, to doctors who teach continuing education programs. The conduits for the money are independent companies that sponsor medical lectures for doctors. Since 2011, drug industry payments to these outside companies have risen 25 percent, to $311 million in 2014." [35]

The Creation of Cancer

In her 2018 medical research paper called *Cancer; an induced disease of the twentieth century! Induction of tolerance, increased entropy and 'Dark*

CHAPTER 6 – HEALTH CARE OR SICK CARE?

Energy': loss of biorhythms (Anabolism v. Catabolism), author Dr. Mahin Khatami, Ph.D., of the National Cancer Institute, states in her abstract:

> American health status ranks last among other developed nations while America invests the highest amount of resources for healthcare. In this perspective, we present evidence that **cancer is an induced disease of the twentieth century**, facilitated by a great deception of cancer/medical establishment for huge corporate profits. Unlike popularized opinions that cancer is 100, 200 or 1000 diseases, we demonstrate that cancer is only one disease; the severe disturbances in biorhythms [frequencies] *(differential bioenergetics) or loss of balance in Yin and Yang of effective immunity. Cancer projects that are promoted and funded by decision makers are reductionist approaches, wrong and unethical and resulted in the loss of millions of precious lives and financial toxicity to society. Public vaccination with pathogen-specific vaccines (e.g., flu, hepatitis, HPV, meningitis, measles) weakens, not promotes, immunity. Results of irresponsible projects on cancer sciences or vaccines are an increased population of drug-dependent sick society.*[36]

To understand more about frequency, see chapter 29.

Health Care?

Let's take a moment to discuss the difference between medicine and health care. Doctors don't deliver health to their patients, they deliver medical care. We don't have a health care system, we have a medical care system, that is, a symptom management system. I call it 'sick care.'

20th and 21st-century medicine is about managing patient care through pharmaceutical drugs and surgery. Yes, there are many, many individual medical practitioners who truly care about their patients and want the best outcomes for them. Unfortunately, they, along with their patients, are caught up in a system controlled by the pharmaceutical industry.

CHAPTER 6 – HEALTH CARE OR SICK CARE?

How did we get to this place where we stopped going to God for our healing and instead go to doctors to get drugs and/or surgery to cure our diseases?

(A side note on cures: The definition of 'cure' is "to relieve the symptoms of a disease or condition." I was surprised to learn this because I thought that curing something meant it was gone, over, done. So, when the medical profession talks about a cure, it means managing the symptoms. Remember that the next time a solicitor asks for a donation to 'find a cure.')

An interesting development during the 20th century is that state-sponsored medicine became known as 'traditional' or allopathic medicine and the healing arts (chiropractic, homeopathy, essential oils, herbalism, etc.) became known as 'alternative' medicine. Quite a switch from just a century earlier.

German Influence

Our current system of health care is greatly influenced by Germany. In the early 20th century, Germany wanted to become the greatest world power. That meant they needed the world's greatest army. And for that, they needed a strong industrial complex.

In the late 1800s, Germany had discovered that the industrial waste from making synthetic dyes was poisonous and therefore would make effective military weapons.[37]

After Germany first used poisonous gases during World War I, the Allies quickly realized the Germans had a military advantage. So, the Allies raced to get their own synthetic dye industries so that they, too, could have the waste material to make weapons of war.[38]

The most common weapons made from industrial waste were chlorine gas, phosgene, and mustard gas. The latter two were most effective because they worked so slowly that the victims didn't know when or where they had been poisoned. Indeed, many didn't know they had been poisoned because their symptoms indicated pneumonia or a pox.[39]

CHAPTER 6 – HEALTH CARE OR SICK CARE?

"Solely the dose determines that a thing is not a poison."

Eugenics

The Germans' egos had been bruised by their defeat in World War I and they wanted to prove that their people were superior to others. For that to happen, anyone they considered imperfect (the disabled, Jews, Catholics, Gypsies, Slavs, people of color) had to be eliminated.

The German government believed that Charles Darwin's studies on natural selection ('survival of the fittest') would help them bring this about. This led to the rise of eugenics (the science of improving a human population by controlled breeding to increase the occurrence of desirable inherited characteristics) and ultimately, the Holocaust.[40]

The Holocaust was the end result of the Nazi government taking eugenic principles to the extreme, seeing it as a way to get rid of the people that were deemed 'inferior.'[41] It didn't start with the Jews, who made up less than 1% of the German population in 1933.[42]

It started with eliminating disabled German children[43] because the German government believed it wasn't fair for the healthy and strong to have to support the weak and frail who couldn't contribute to society.[44] It escalated to adults who were mentally frail and disabled, then expanded to ethnic groups.

The idea for gas chambers at the concentration camps came from psychiatric hospitals.[45] Once the methods of mass asphyxiation were perfected, gas chambers at the hospitals were disassembled, transported, and then rebuilt at the concentration camps. The doctors and the nurses trained to use this 'medical equipment' went with the machinery.

Methods of killing included injections of morphine, tablets, and gassing with cyanide or chemical warfare agents. It was common to have the poisons administered slowly over several days or weeks so that the cause of death could be disguised as pneumonia, bronchitis, or some other complication induced by the injections.

CHAPTER 6 – HEALTH CARE OR SICK CARE?

A Crackdown on Natural Healing Arts

Because the Nazis wanted all Germans to be like-minded with the same attitudes, values, and mentalities, naturopathic healers were barred from using occult methods such as dowsing rods or pendula to diagnose or treat diseases.[46]

Chiropractors were barred from treating cancer. Natural doctors were still allowed to treat cancer using recognized methods such as homeopathy, natural herbs, and physical therapy (massage). In his book *The Nazi War on Cancer*, Robert N. Proctor states,

> *The most commonly expressed concern was that people would squander their money or health on useless remedies, but the campaign must also be understood as **a move by medical professionals to consolidate their power over the healing arts**. Quack medicine (by definition) was considered ineffective medicine and ineffective medicine was regarded as a drag on German economics and fighting power.*[47]

The Germans did not want anyone involved in supernatural healing, which includes healing from God through Christ.

Operation Paperclip

After World War II, the U.S. covertly started Operation Paperclip.[48] It was a secret program of the Joint Intelligence Objectives Agency (JIOA) largely carried out by Special Agents of Army CIC, in which more than 1,600 German scientists, engineers, and technicians, such as Wernher von Braun and his V-2 rocket team, were recruited in post-Nazi Germany and taken to the U.S. for government employment, primarily between 1945 and 1959. Many were former members, and some were former leaders, of the Nazi Party.

The primary purpose for Operation Paperclip was U.S. military advantage in the cold war and the space race with the Soviet Union. The Soviet Union was more aggressive in forcibly recruiting (at gunpoint) more than 2,200 German specialists – a total of more than 6,000 people including family members.[49]

CHAPTER 6 – HEALTH CARE OR SICK CARE?

War criminals who had engineered eugenics and the Holocaust were now working for the U.S. government and influencing policy. What do you think happened?

Use of Industrial Waste

IG Farben

IG Farben [50] was a German chemical and pharmaceutical industry conglomerate. The company was formed in 1925 from a number of major synthetic dye and chemical companies that had been working together closely since World War I. During its heyday, IG Farben was both the largest company in Europe overall and the largest chemical and pharmaceutical company in the world.

According to Wikipedia, "IG Farben scientists made fundamental contributions to all areas of chemistry and the pharmaceutical industry. Due to the company's entanglement with the Nazi regime, it was considered by the Allies to be too morally corrupt to be allowed to continue to exist after the war. The Soviet Union seized most of IG Farben's assets located in the Soviet occupation zone as part of their reparation payments."

"In the western occupation zone, however, the idea of destroying the company was very quickly abandoned as the policy of denazification evolved, in part due to the need for productive industry to support reconstruction, and in part because of the company's large entanglement with American companies, notably with the successors of Standard Oil which IG Farben was modeled after and which had itself been broken up into several companies."

"In the late 1940s, IG Farben was being rebuilt in the western zones and continued doing business. In 1951, the company was split into its original constituent companies. The four largest quickly bought the smaller ones. Today Agfa, BASF, and Bayer AG remain, Hoechst having in 1999 spun off its chemical business as Celanese AG before merging with Rhône-Poulenc to form Aventis, which later merged with Sanofi-Synthélabo to

CHAPTER 6 – HEALTH CARE OR SICK CARE?

form Sanofi." [51] See Chapter 41 for more information on Bayer AG's 2018 purchase of Monsanto Company.

<u>Current Uses of Industrial Waste</u>

Today in the U.S., coal tar waste is used in products such as soap and shampoo. It's also used as medicine ("**Solely the dose determines that a thing is not a poison**").[52] Side effects include skin irritation, sun sensitivity, allergic reactions, and skin discoloration. It's unclear if use during pregnancy is safe for the baby and use during breastfeeding is not typically recommended. The use of coal tar in cosmetic products is banned in Canada and the European Union.

Petroleum waste byproducts are turned into fertilizer, floor coverings, perfume, insecticide, petroleum jelly, soap, and vitamin capsules.[53]

Synthetic dyes are used in food[54] and personal care products.[55]

Why can't you taste or smell the chemicals that are used in these products? If you could smell or taste the poisons, you wouldn't use those products, so artificial fragrances are used to mask the odors.

> **"Honest doctors can no longer practice honest medicine. We have a complete health care system failure and an epidemic of misinformed doctors and misinformed and harmed patients."**
> Dr. Aseem Malhotra, April 12, 2018,
> European Parliament, Brussels

Our Current System

Modern American medicine is a government-sanctioned method of using surgery and poison ("**Solely the dose determines that a thing is**

CHAPTER 6 – HEALTH CARE OR SICK CARE?

not a poison.") instead of traditional methods of being in tune with God and nature. Natural healers are ridiculed, called 'quacks.'

When we allowed the laws of nature and of God to be cast aside, horrible things started to happen. Medicine changed. It was no longer an agent of health.

We study disease and look for 'cures.' We manage symptoms with varying results. Once caught up in this system, very few manage to escape.

What are Drugs Doing to Us?

Today, most medicines are produced through chemical means. Scientists isolate the chemicals in plants that 'cure' certain ailments. Over time, they're able to create those substances artificially and use them to produce medicines.[56] The reason for this is that a plant can't be patented but a chemical process can.

The human body does not recognize these chemicals isolated from their original plant sources and considers them poisonous. As Paracelsus said, **"Solely the dose determines that a thing is not a poison."** The FDA requires testing of drugs to determine dosages. If test subjects have horrible reactions or die, then they know that the recommended dosage needs to be less than what caused those reactions.

The current system of medicine is set up for us to start taking these chemical substances at an early age. Have you ever experienced what the drug industry calls 'side effects?' That happens when your body can't handle the chemicals in the drug. In reality, you have exceeded the poisoning dose.

Prescription drugs kill over 100,000 people in the U.S. every year.[57] These are people who went to their doctor and trusted they were getting something that would alleviate their symptoms. Instead, they died.

Poison 'Control'

Chemicals in household and personal care products became widely available after World War II because the industrial waste was no longer

CHAPTER 6 – HEALTH CARE OR SICK CARE?

being used for weapons of war. They had to do something with it. After the war a proliferation of drugs and chemicals became available, and the first victims of 'accidental' poisonings were children. The first poison control center was opened in Chicago in 1953. The American Association of Poison Control Centers was founded in 1958. Today, there are 55 centers operating in the U.S.

In 2016, the 55 U.S. poison control centers [58] provided telephone guidance for nearly 2,159,000 human poison exposures. That's about:

- 6.6 poison exposures/1000 population
- 41.3 poison exposures in children younger than 6 years/1000 children
- 1 poison exposure is reported to U.S. poison control centers every 14.6 seconds

Why does our society passively accept this?

> "When poison becomes a habit, it ceases to injure: it makes your soul gradually acquainted with death."
> Saib Tabrizi, Poet

The FDA monitors food and drugs because our current food and medicines are chemical-laden. Real, whole food and plant medicine are not. But we, as a society, are addicted to this lifestyle, which leads to disease, disability, and death.

Note: Do NOT stop taking any prescription medications without consulting your doctor.

Drugs Contribute to Nutritional Deficiencies

Pharmaceutics — Open Access Journal says,

CHAPTER 6 – HEALTH CARE OR SICK CARE?

The long-term use of prescription and over-the-counter drugs can induce subclinical and <u>clinically relevant</u> micronutrient deficiencies, which may develop gradually over months or even years. Given the large number of medications currently available, the number of research studies examining potential drug-nutrient interactions is quite limited. A comprehensive, updated review of the potential drug-nutrient interactions with the chronic use of the most often prescribed medications for commonly diagnosed conditions among the general U.S. adult population is presented.[59]

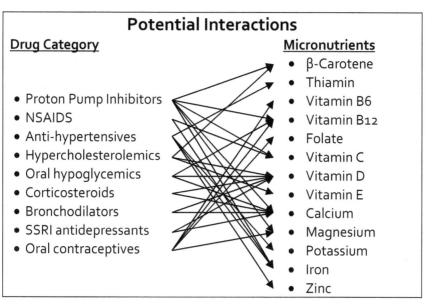

Take Control of Your Health

Thank you for taking the time to read this lengthy but extremely important chapter. If we want to reclaim our health, we have to know what is opposing us.

This information can be overwhelming. And scary. There's something going on that most of us aren't paying attention to. Do you think this giant industrial complex profits more from a healthy populace or from

CHAPTER 6 – HEALTH CARE OR SICK CARE?

sick and weak people who depend on it? It counts on our ignorance to succeed. You are no longer ignorant.

Now you're beginning to see why we're sick. The next chapter will continue your education.

In the Introduction, I said that my parents "were both miserable in their final years. And I have their genes. But, I also knew that I could turn off those destructive genes with different choices. I already had the biggest factor for health: my spiritual relationship with my Father God. The other factors within my control were my food choices and toxin exposure."

You see, genetics is only 10% of our destiny.[60] Environment (food and drink, drugs taken, exposure to air/water pollution, cleaning products, products we put on/in our bodies, etc.) is 90% of whether one gets sick or stays healthy.

I have genes that predispose me to certain sicknesses. I've turned them off by my environmental choices. The rest of this book will show you exactly how I did it.

CHAPTER 7

THE CHURCH UNDER ASSAULT

The health and well-being of the church are under assault in the United States of America. To this end, our food supply has been poisoned.

The Spiritual Battle

According to the Word of God, we are in a spiritual battle.

> *Ephesians 6:12 KJV*
> *For we wrestle not against flesh and blood, but against principalities, against powers, against the rulers of the darkness of this world, against spiritual wickedness in high places.*

We need to look at things from a spiritual viewpoint. Things may seem a certain way on the surface, but we need to look behind the scenes to see the spiritual reality of what is happening.

> *John 10:10 KJV*
> *The thief cometh not, but for to steal, and to kill, and to destroy: I am come that they might have life, and that they might have it more abundantly.*

The Evil One wants to steal our health from us, he wants to kill us and destroy us. We cannot afford to ignore this.

> *2 Corinthians 2:11 KJV*
> *Lest Satan should get an advantage of us: for we are not ignorant of his devices.*

God encourages us to understand the Evil One's devices (ways, methods of operation). Having this knowledge will take away his advantage.

> *1 Peter 5:8 APNT*
> *Be watchful and remember, because your enemy, Satan, roars as a lion and walks about and seeks who he may swallow. Therefore, stand against him, being steadfast in faith and know*

CHAPTER 7 – THE CHURCH UNDER ASSAULT

> *that these sufferings also happen to your brothers who are in the world.*

I don't write this to frighten you, but to encourage you to be vigilant. God has given us the victory in Christ, but we must take a stand.

> *1 John 4:4 KJV*
> *Ye are of God, little children, and have overcome them* [the spirit of anti-Christ that is already in the world]: *because greater is he that is in you, than he that is in the world.*

> *Ephesians 6:11-13 KJV*
> *Put on the whole armour of God, that ye may be able to stand against the wiles of the devil.*

> *For we wrestle not against flesh and blood, but against principalities, against powers, against the rulers of the darkness of this world, against spiritual wickedness in high places.*

> *Wherefore take unto you the whole armour of God, that ye may be able to withstand in the evil day, and having done all, to stand.*

One of the best ways for the Evil One to take down the church without many people noticing is to kill us off one by one. What better way to accomplish this than through our food and our health care systems, two industries that should be helping people. Yet, these two industries are systematically harming us. Why?

> *1 Timothy 6:10a KJV*
> *For the love of money is the root of all evil:*

"We won't have a cure for disease until we first have a cure for greed."
Dr. Sachin Patel

CHAPTER 7 – THE CHURCH UNDER ASSAULT

Have you ever heard the phrase, 'Follow the money trail?' Doing so will lead you to the truth.

The church today is sick. Diabetes, obesity, and cancer, among other diseases, are rampant. This ought not to be. If any group of people today should be healthy, it should be God's children.

> *3 John 2 KJV*
> *Beloved, I wish above all things that thou mayest prosper and be in health, even as thy soul prospereth.*
>
> *Acts 9:34a KJV*
> *And Peter said unto him, Aeneas, Jesus Christ maketh thee whole:*

The Greek word translated "maketh thee whole" in Acts 9:34 is *iaomai*. It's translated "make whole" only twice while it's translated "heal" 26 times. It's in the present tense. Jesus Christ heals us every single time we need it.

We are God's beloved and He gave His son Jesus Christ as a sacrifice for us so we could be well. So, why are we sickly? The Evil One has lied to us and deceived us into thinking we can do as we please without regard for consequences. But we have seen that we cannot disregard God's ways and still reap His promises (see chapter 2).

What is Happening to Our Food?

The biggest thing that is happening to our food supply in the U.S. is that it's being modified (biologically changed). A GMO (genetically modified organism) is the result of a laboratory process where genes from the DNA of one species are extracted and artificially forced into the genes of an unrelated plant or animal. The foreign genes may come from bacteria, viruses, insects, animals, or even humans.

According to The Non-GMO Project, "This relatively new science creates unstable combinations of plant, animal, bacteria, and viral genes that do not occur in nature or through traditional crossbreeding methods." [1] In

CHAPTER 7 – THE CHURCH UNDER ASSAULT

other words, man is changing the way God made plants and animals into something else entirely.

According to the Institute for Responsible Technology, here are 10 reasons to avoid GMO's.[2]

1. GMO's are not healthy. The American Academy of Environmental Medicine (AAEM) urges doctors to prescribe non-GMO diets for all patients. They cite animal studies showing organ damage, gastrointestinal and immune system disorders, accelerated aging, and infertility.[3]
2. GMO's contaminate forever. They cross-pollinate and their seeds travel on the wind.[4]
3. GMO's increase herbicide use. Because they are designed to be herbicide-tolerant, farmers must spray more and more of Bayer/Monsanto's Roundup® (glyphosate) on them. Roundup® is linked to sterility, hormone disruption, birth defects, and cancer.[5]
4. Genetic engineering creates dangerous side effects from mixing the genes of unrelated species. (Not to mention being explicitly contrary to God's Word; see Genesis 1:11, 12, 21, 24, 25.)
5. Government oversight is dangerously lax. There's a lot of crossover between the agricultural industry and government jobs. For example, Monsanto's former attorney and vice president later served as U.S. Food Safety Czar.[6]
6. The biotech industry uses superficial, rigged research to claim product safety.[7]
7. Independent research and reporting are attacked and suppressed.[8]
8. GMO's cause harm to the environment.[9]
9. GMO's do not increase yields versus sustainable farming.[10]
10. By avoiding GMO's, you contribute to consumer rejection, ultimately forcing them out of our food supply.

CHAPTER 7 – THE CHURCH UNDER ASSAULT

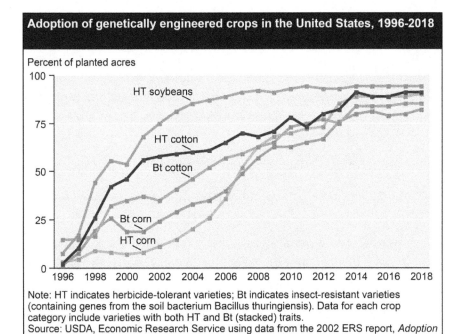

The above graphic from the U.S. Dept. of Agriculture [11] shows the increase in GMO crops in the last 20 years.

The top GMO foods are:[12]

- Alfalfa (used mainly as hay for cattle)
- Apples (GMO apples were introduced to U.S. market in 2017, using the label "Arctic® Apples") [13]
- Canola (approx. 90% of U.S. crop)
- Corn (approx. 93% of U.S. crop)
- Cotton (approx. 94% of U.S. crop)
- Papaya (most of the Hawaiian crop; approximately 988 acres)
- Potatoes (GMO potatoes have been approved by the FDA; they're called White Russett™)
- Soybeans (approx. 94% of U.S. crop)

67

CHAPTER 7 – THE CHURCH UNDER ASSAULT

- Squash (GMO zucchini and yellow summer squash have been commercially available in the U.S. since the mid- to late-'90s) [14]
- Sugar Beets (approx. 95% of U.S. crop)

This is why it's so important to buy organic food. If food is organic, the chances of it being contaminated with GMO's are substantially less, but not zero. (See point 2 above.)

For more information about common GMO ingredients, see Appendix 1.

From a *GMO-Free USA* (a nonprofit organization) Facebook post on June 11, 2018: [15]

> *How to differentiate between USDA organic, the Non-GMO Project Verified butterfly label and so-called "natural" foods... What you need to know:*
>
> *Non-GMO Project Verified does NOT mean organic or pesticide free. Non-GMO Project means conventionally grown from non-GMO seeds and with testing of the supply chain/product to make sure there are no more than nine-tenths of 1% GMO contamination (this is the same standard used in the EU). Conventionally grown non-GMO foods are grown with toxic synthetic agrichemicals, such as Roundup®, dicamba, neonicotinoids, chlorpyrifos, etc.*
>
> *Organics must be grown from organic seeds (which can't be GMO) and without toxic, synthetic pesticides. But it is important to know that there is little testing of organics for potential GMO contamination.*
>
> *So for high-risk ingredients such as corn, soy, sugar, canola, cottonseed oil...* **look for BOTH the USDA organic AND the Non-GMO Project Verified butterfly** *to be sure to avoid toxic synthetic pesticides and GMO contamination. Happy shopping! And by the way... "Natural" is an undefined word in the FDA food world and it should not be taken at face value.*

CHAPTER 7 – THE CHURCH UNDER ASSAULT

What's the Difference?

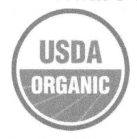 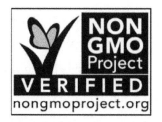

Grown from organic seeds without toxic synthetic pesticides **(little testing for GMO contamination)**

Conventionally grown from non-GMO seeds, tested for potential GMO contamination **(grown with toxic synthetic pesticides)**

To avoid both GMO's and toxic synthetic pesticides, LOOK FOR BOTH USDA ORGANIC AND THE NON-GMO PROJECT VERIFIED LOGO WHEN THERE ARE HIGH-RISK INGREDIENTS DERIVED FROM CORN, SOY, SUGAR, CANOLA, COTTONSEED OIL.

A group of 94 scientists recently published a study that strongly suggests that glyphosate (the active ingredient in Roundup®) is a carcinogen,[16] meaning it causes cancer. Glyphosate is in our water and in our food. It's been found in umbilical cord blood[17] and breast milk.[18] We don't yet know the complete ramifications of Roundup® use. How does it damage DNA and what happens when that damaged DNA is passed down to our children? By choosing organic **and** non-GMO foods, we can help protect ourselves and our families from this poison.

What is Organic Food?

The USDA regulates organic food in America. The process to become USDA-certified organic is lengthy and expensive.[19] That's why many smaller farmers don't bother with the process even though they don't use pesticides, GMO seeds, or other harmful products on their plants/soil. You may run into these farmers at local farmers markets.

Organic produce and other ingredients are grown without the use of pesticides, synthetic fertilizers, sewage sludge, genetically modified organisms (GMOs), or ionizing radiation. Animals that produce meat, poultry, eggs, and dairy products do not take antibiotics or growth hormones.[20]

According to Organic.org, "The USDA has identified for three categories of labeling organic products:

- 100% Organic: Made with 100% organic ingredients
- Organic: Made with at least 95% organic ingredients
- Made with Organic Ingredients: Made with a minimum of 70% organic ingredients with strict restrictions on the remaining 30% including no GMOs (genetically modified organisms)
- Products with less than 70% organic ingredients may list organically produced ingredients on the side panel of the package but may not make any organic claims on the front of the package." [21]

Mycotoxins

Another little-known problem in the U.S. food supply is the presence of mycotoxins.[22] Mycotoxins form from yeast and fungi that develop on foods grown in microbe-deficient soils, which are more the norm than the exception these days. In 1936, yes, over 80 years ago, the U.S. Senate was presented with the results of a scientific study [23] it had commissioned on the mineral content of our food. The results demonstrated that many human ills could be attributed to the fact that American soil no longer provided the plants with the mineral elements that are so essential to human nourishment and nutritional health. Things haven't improved since then.

Mycotoxins can lead to nervous system damage, hormone imbalances, and cancer.[24] Processed, non-organic foods, in general, tend to be prone to mycotoxin formation.

Food Additives

Not only is American food a mycotoxin nightmare, it's also a chemical nightmare. This is because of all the additives, preservatives, and

CHAPTER 7 – THE CHURCH UNDER ASSAULT

colorful food dyes used in much of what you'll find on grocery store shelves today. There are a number of common food chemicals used in the U.S. that are banned[25] elsewhere due to their questionable safety profile. They include:

- rBGH/rBST artificial growth hormones added to milk
- Antibiotics in meat, poultry, and fish
- Propylene glycol in food and alcohol
- Arsenic in chicken and rice

Other links to check out:

- Is it Gluten Intolerance or Are We Being Poisoned?[26]
- Our Unsafe Food Supply is Killing Us[27]
- 12 Ways to Rid the Planet of GMO's and Bayer/Monsanto's Roundup®[28]

What Can We Do About This?

The best way to avoid GMO's, mycotoxins, and chemicals in food is to eat real, whole, organic, non-processed food. In chapter 25, I list the specific ways I do this.

What will changing your diet do? Three button mushrooms per day can reduce breast cancer rates by 64%.[29] Drinking green tea daily reduces breast cancer rates by 89%.[30] Turmeric helps in preventing breast cancer and Alzheimer's disease.[31] The list goes on and on.

It's also important to let your elected representatives know how you feel about having real, whole, nutritious food available to you. Many of them are working against our health interests[32] in favor of their own monetary interests. Organizations like Environmental Working Group (http://EWG.org) help keep these issues in the forefront and are a good source of consumer information.

What about the cost of healthy food? That's a reasonable question and I cover it in chapter 45.

CHAPTER 7 – THE CHURCH UNDER ASSAULT

Did you know that many obese people are actually malnourished?[33] When we eat foods with no nutritional value, the stomach will signal that it's full, but the cells aren't getting the nutrition they need, so they keep signaling us to eat more. So, we eat and eat, we gain weight, and our bodies are starving for real nutrition. If we're always hungry, our bodies aren't getting the nourishment they need. With healthy food, we will eat less because our cells will be satisfied, saving money in the long run.

The bottom line is that the church is sick and tired and as such, we are distracted from our main mission. And as long as that remains the case, the Evil One can say, "Mission accomplished."

**And he said unto them, Go ye into all the world, and preach the gospel to every creature.
Mark 16:15 KJV**

CHAPTER 8

HEALING IS IN CHRIST

As sons of God, we must keep the Word of God in our minds if we are to successfully stand against the Evil One. We are to put off the thoughts from the world and put on the mind of Christ.

> *1 Corinthians 2:16 KJV*
> *For who hath known the mind of the Lord, that he may instruct him? But we have the mind of Christ.*
>
> *Colossians 3:9 KJV*
> *Lie not one to another, seeing that ye have put off the old man with his deeds;*

What thoughts are we to put off? Thoughts of sickness, hopelessness, despair. Thoughts that we will never get better. Thoughts that we're not worth it, we're undeserving. All of these are lies.

Instead, we are to put on the mind of Christ. We are to think the way Christ thought.

> *Ephesians 2:24 KJV*
> *And that ye put on the new man, which after God is created in righteousness and true holiness.*

How did Christ think? Did he think he was the Son of God? Did he think he was victorious? Did he think that God loved him and wanted only the best for him? Of course, he did.

That's what you're going to think, too. You're going to claim the healing that God has already given you in Christ. Each day, every time a thought that contradicts God's Word comes into your mind, replace it with one of these scriptures.

We must put off before we can put on. We must replace the old thoughts with new ones or the old ones will come back. You can find more information on what to think about in chapter 1.

CHAPTER 8 – HEALING IS IN CHRIST

Ephesians 6:12 KJV
For we wrestle not against flesh and blood, but against principalities, against powers, against the rulers of the darkness of this world, against spiritual wickedness in high places.

2 Corinthians 10:5 NIV
We demolish arguments and every pretension that sets itself up against the knowledge of God, and we take captive every thought to make it obedient to Christ.

Nahum 1:7,9b KJV
The LORD is good, a stronghold in the day of trouble; and He knows those who trust in Him.

He will make an utter end of it. Affliction will not rise up a second time.

Psalm 103:2-3 KJV
Bless the LORD, O my soul, and forget not all his benefits:

Who forgiveth all thine iniquities; who healeth all thy diseases;

Psalm 119:50 NIV
My comfort in my suffering is this: Your promise preserves my life.

Psalm 30:2 KJV
O LORD my God, I cried unto thee, and thou hast healed me.

Isaiah 54:17 KJV
No weapon that is formed against thee shall prosper; and every tongue that shall rise against thee in judgment thou shalt condemn. This is the heritage of the servants of the LORD, and their righteousness is of me, saith the LORD.

Ezekiel 34:16 KJV
I will seek that which was lost, and bring again that which was driven away, and will bind up that which was broken, and will strengthen that which was sick.

CHAPTER 8 – HEALING IS IN CHRIST

Isaiah 58:8 NIV
Then your light will break forth like the dawn, and your healing will quickly appear; then your righteousness will go before you, and the glory of the LORD will be your rear guard.

Jeremiah 33:6 KJV
Behold, I will bring it health and cure, and I will cure them, and will reveal unto them the abundance of peace and truth.

Isaiah 53:4-5 KJV
Surely He hath borne our griefs [Hebrew: sicknesses] *and carried our sorrows* [Hebrew: pains] *yet we did esteem Him stricken, smitten of God and afflicted.*

But He was wounded for our transgressions, He was bruised for our iniquities; the chastisement of [that purchased] *our peace was upon Him; and by His stripes we are healed.*

Jeremiah 30:17 KJV
For I will restore health unto you, and I will heal you of your wounds, saith the Lord.

1 Peter 2:24 KJV
Who his own self bare our sins in his own body on the tree, that we, being dead to sins, should live unto righteousness: by whose stripes ye were healed.

Acts 5:16 KJV
Also a multitude gathered from the surrounding cities to Jerusalem, bringing sick people and those who were tormented by unclean spirits, and they were all healed.

Romans 8:11 NIV
And if the Spirit of him who raised Jesus from the dead is living in you, he who raised Christ from the dead will also give life to your mortal bodies because of his Spirit who lives in you.

Hebrews 7:25 AMP
Therefore He is able also to save to the uttermost [completely,

> *perfectly, finally, and for all time and eternity] those who come to God through Him, since He is always living to make petition to God and intercede with Him and intervene for them.*
>
> *Acts 13:38-39 KJV*
> *Be it known unto you therefore, men and brethren, that through this man is preached unto you the forgiveness of sins:*
>
> *And by him all that believe are justified from all things, from which ye could not be justified by the law of Moses.*
>
> *Deuteronomy 11:21 KJV*
> *That your days may be multiplied, and the days of your children, in the land which the LORD sware unto your fathers to give them, as the days of heaven upon the earth.*
>
> *Deuteronomy 7:15 KJV*
> *And the LORD will take away from you all sickness, and will afflict you with none of the terrible diseases of Egypt which you have known, but will lay them on all those who hate you.*
>
> *Romans 8:32 KJV*
> *He that spared not his own Son, but delivered him up for us all, how shall he not with him also freely give us all things?*

Everything in life has both a physical and a spiritual component. The Be in Health lifestyle addresses both.

PART 3

WHAT I WAS EATING MADE ME SICK

"When diet is wrong, medicine is of no use. When diet is correct, medicine is of no need."
Ayurvedic Proverb

CHAPTER 9

WHY I AVOID PROCESSED FOOD

I talk a lot about eating real, whole food instead of processed food. Why do I avoid processed food? In this chapter, I'll show you how I decided to give up processed food, which processed foods can be healthy, and why eating real, whole food is best.

What is Processed Food?

A simple definition of processed food is any food that is manipulated into another form other than its original real, whole form. For example, an apple is a real, whole food; applesauce is a processed food. A steak is real, whole food; bacon is processed food. Raw milk is real, whole food; cheese is a processed food.

A note about raw food: raw food can refer to any food that isn't processed or changed in any way before eating. For example, raw honey is unpasteurized, as are raw milk products, juices, and nuts. Raw nuts/seeds aren't roasted or salted. Raw vegetables and fruits are uncooked.

Processed Meats

I mentioned that bacon is a processed food. For various biblical and scientific reasons, I don't eat bacon (see chapter 15). In our society, we eat many types of processed meats. Just visit the deli department of a local grocery store and look at all the varieties.

Processed meat is meat that has been preserved by salting, drying, curing, smoking, or canning. Because of the ways by which they're processed, these meats are considered unhealthy.[1] (Note that chemical processing and mechanical processing aren't the same thing.)

Most people like processed meats because they're salty and they're convenient. Some of the problems with processed meat include:

- Many of these meats have sodium nitrite added, which "can damage cells and also morph into molecules that cause cancer."[2]
- The EPA says that smoking meat can potentially form polycyclic aromatic hydrocarbons (PAHs).[3]
- Heterocyclic amines (HCAs) can form when meats/fish are cooked at high temperatures.[4] The website Cancer.gov says that in laboratory experiments, "HCAs and PAHs [see bullet point above] have been found to be mutagenic — that is, they cause changes in DNA that may increase the risk of cancer."[5]
- Many processed meats have very high levels of sodium chloride (table salt).[6] Over-consumption of sodium "can lead to high blood pressure which in turn leads to an increased risk of heart attack and stroke."[7]

For these reasons, I avoid ALL commercially processed meats.

Are Some Processed Foods Healthy?

I mentioned above that there's a difference between chemically and mechanically processed food. Let's go back to the example of applesauce. I make applesauce at home in my crock pot. After the apples are cooked down, I have applesauce. This is a mechanically processed food. What happens if I add other ingredients to the applesauce, like sugar, stevia, high fructose corn syrup, or other sweeteners; cinnamon, nutmeg, or other flavors; or added vitamins (like ascorbic acid)? I now have a chemically processed food.

I add organic stevia and cinnamon to my homemade applesauce (see recipe in chapter 50). Because I process this food myself and I know what all the ingredients are and where they came from, I have confidence in my processed food. If a friend or someone I trust offers me their homemade processed food (soup is a good example), I simply find out what ingredients they used before I decide if I want to eat it.

CHAPTER 9 - WHY I AVOID PROCESSED FOOD

Reading Labels

What happens when you don't know the people who processed the food, as is the case with grocery store processed food? Do you automatically trust that the big corporations that processed those foods have used the finest organic and non-GMO ingredients and least harmful processing methods? I don't. Big corporations have one motivation, and it's not my well-being. Even smaller companies known for organic processed foods may have been sold to larger corporations,[8] yet they kept the same label, leading people to believe that nothing has changed.

Labels like 'gluten-free,' 'non-GMO,' and 'organic' mean very little. When looking to purchase a processed food, I read the label carefully. Sometimes I even need to visit the company's website to get full ingredient disclosure.

There are some apps that can make this process easier. See chapter 48.

Remember, labels don't tell the whole story. Laws in this area are lax. I've found that if a 'food' has ingredients, it's best to avoid it.

Give Up Processed Food?

For many, many generations, our ancestors ate only the food they or their close neighbors grew and raised. They ate real, whole foods. In contrast, our modern culture is one that runs on speed and convenience. If something isn't fast and easy, we don't want it. If quality suffers at the hands of speed and ease, so be it.

The desire for speed and convenience has led to the rise of fast food, which isn't known for its quality (see chapter 16). Our grocery stores are filled with aisle after aisle of canned, boxed, bottled, and frozen foods, all designed to give us speed and convenience. After all, if we can throw a box into the microwave and have dinner ready in less than 10 minutes, who cares if we're sacrificing a little quality? Turns out, we have reason to care.

This speed + convenience mentality has led to many of the health problems now plaguing western society. Diet-related illnesses are on the

CHAPTER 9 – WHY I AVOID PROCESSED FOOD

rise.[9] Hypertension, heart disease, cancer, diabetes, and obesity are all directly related to diet quality.[10] Heart disease is currently the number one killer of both men and women in the United States.[11] The risk of heart attack and stroke[12] can be lessened with proper diet.

Eat Real, Whole Food

I've found it's much easier and healthier to eat real, whole foods. When I first made the switch, I dreaded the thought of it. Where would I find the time to prepare my own food, three times a day? Wouldn't it be expensive to cook at home exclusively?

Turns out, the anticipation was scarier than the reality. I discovered I had plenty of time; time I had previously frittered away on social media and television. Now, I spend even more time with my husband because we prepare meals together.

Expensive? No, actually, it's much cheaper. My husband and I don't miss eating out because the food at home is so much better than anything at a restaurant. When we added up the cost of fast food, restaurant food, sodas, alcohol, stops at the convenience store (see why they call it that?), the donut shop, and Starbucks®, we realized that we could eat real, whole, healthy food for much less cost than 'convenient,' fast processed food. (More about this in chapter 45.)

I challenge you to prove this for yourself.

CHAPTER 10

WHEAT: THE STAFF OF LIFE

The 'staff of life' is an expression referring to a food that is a staple of a culture; something that everyone relies on and eats regularly. For many in the western world, this means wheat. Wheat has come under scrutiny lately because of gluten. So, what's the deal with gluten?

Wheat is nutritious, concentrated, easily stored and transported, and is easily processed into various types of food. Wheat contains gluten protein, which enables a leavened dough to rise by forming minute gas cells that hold carbon dioxide during fermentation. This process produces a light textured bread.

Gluten is a part of wheat that was originally beneficial. So, why do so many people today seem to have problems with it? To put it simply, today's wheat has far more gluten in it than in the past. Wheat today just isn't the same as it was 50 years ago.

How Man Changed Wheat

This is because of two things: first, in the 1870s, a new type of processing was invented. The modern steel roller mill was faster and more efficient than the older stone-grinding method. It could separate the component parts of wheat, producing a whiter wheat devoid of the bran, germ, shorts, and red dog mill streams that are richest in proteins, vitamins, lipids, and minerals.[1]

Second, in the mid-1900s, a different kind of wheat was introduced in the United States. Norman Borlaug led initiatives that "involved the development of high-yielding varieties of cereal grains, expansion of irrigation infrastructure, modernization of management techniques, distribution of hybridized seeds, synthetic fertilizers, and pesticides to farmers."[2]

CHAPTER 10 – WHEAT: THE STAFF OF LIFE

According to GrainStorm.com,

> *For 10,000 years, we cultivated wheat, stored it, milled it and consumed it. The system worked, and it nourished civilization. Then, in the industrial era, we changed things.*
>
> *First, we invented mechanical technologies to turn wheat into barren white flour. Then, we invented chemical and genetic technologies to make it resistant to pests, drought, and blight, and [make it] easier to harvest, dramatically increasing yield per acre. And, while we were tweaking genetics, we also figured out how to increase glutens for better 'baking properties' (fluffier results).* [3]

Reactions to Gluten

A true wheat allergy is fairly uncommon and is characterized by itching, sneezing, and wheezing immediately after consuming wheat. In this case, see a doctor. Wheat intolerance (sensitivity) is more common and manifests in symptoms like bloating, cramps, and diarrhea.

Coeliac disease, also spelled celiac disease, or gluten intolerance, is a common autoimmune disorder where the intestines can't absorb the gluten found in wheat, barley, rye, and oats. This condition has become more prevalent in recent years. Those diagnosed with this condition are usually advised to follow a gluten-free diet.[4]

Alternatives to Gluten

There are some wheat alternatives available. Einkorn wheat is genetically different from today's modern wheat. It differs from modern wheat in these ways:[5]

- Most modern wheat is a hybrid of many different grains and grasses.
- Einkorn has 14 chromosomes, whereas modern wheat has 42 chromosomes, which changes the gluten structure.

- Einkorn is considered more nutritious than modern wheat, based on the higher level of protein, essential fatty acids, phosphorous, potassium, pyridoxine, and beta-carotene.

Because of its ancient origins, einkorn is known by many names around the world: *Triticum monococcum* (Latin, scientific name), einkorn (German), small spelt (Italian), farro piccolo (Italian), engrain (French), le petit épautre (French), tiphe (Greek), siyez (Turkish), and sifon (Hebrew).

Please note that einkorn wheat does contain a small amount of gluten,[6] so if you have coeliac disease, follow your doctor's recommendations. There are many gluten-free flours on the market, such as almond flour, coconut flour, cassava flour, etc.

Einkorn has a different kind of gluten compared with modern wheat because it does not contain the D genome, only the A genome.[7] This is significant because the most popular test for detecting the presence of gluten is based on the presence of the D genome, so it will not fail an ELISA test.

If you have trouble finding einkorn wheat flour, contact me at Carol@3Jn2Wellness.com.

Why I Don't Eat Grains

I had an interesting, yet frustrating, discussion on Facebook. I made the simple statement that I'm grain-free. Someone replied, "You eat no grains at all?" (I thought that's what I said, but...) I replied, "No grains at all." The same person responded, "So, no rice, no nothing?" Still not sure what I had been unclear about, I replied, "No." Again, the same person came back with, "So, no quinoa or amaranth either?" Again, I said, "No grains." Fortunately, it ended there. Apparently, not eating any grains is a foreign concept to some. So, I'm going to explain to you why I don't eat grains.

First, let's define what grains are. They're the small, hard, edible seeds of grass-like plants.[8] Within the classification of grains, there are two subgroups, cereals (like wheat, barley, rye, oats, corn, and rice) and legumes (beans, soybeans, carob, peas, lentils, and peanuts). Legumes

CHAPTER 10 – WHEAT: THE STAFF OF LIFE

don't contain gluten; for this reason, I differentiate them from cereal grains like wheat.

The most common varieties of cereal grains eaten around the world are wheat, rice, corn, and oats. Many civilizations use one or more of these grains as the staple of their diet.

Cereal grains are popular because once harvested, they keep for much longer than other staple foods like tubers (sweet potatoes, cassava) and starchy fruits (plantains, breadfruit), thus making them easier to transport.

Cereal grains have three main parts: the bran, which is the hard, outer layer or shell; the germ, which is the reproductive part that germinates to grow into a plant (it's the embryo of the seed); and the endosperm, the part of the seed that surrounds the germ and contains oils and protein, which is the part of the seed that is ground into flour.

Whole Grain vs. Refined Grain

You may have heard the phrase 'whole grain.'[9] It refers to all three of the seed parts being intact. Refined grains have the bran and/or the germ mechanically removed (processed), leaving just the starchy endosperm.

The nutritional value of wheat depends on the form in which it's eaten. The most commonly used form of wheat in American wheat products is called 60% extraction.[10] That means that 40% of the original grain is removed and only 60% is left. Unfortunately, the 40% that is removed are the most nutritious parts – the bran and the germ. In addition, hybridized wheat contains twice the amount of gluten.[11]

Is the Problem Gluten or Glyphosate?

According to EcoWatch, "18.9 billion pounds [of glyphosate] have been used globally since its introduction in 1974, making it the most widely and heavily applied weed-killer in the history of chemical agriculture. Significantly, 74 percent of all glyphosate sprayed on crops since the mid-1970s was applied in just the last 10 years, as the cultivation of GMO corn and soybeans expanded in the U.S. and globally."[12]

CHAPTER 10 - WHEAT: THE STAFF OF LIFE

Glyphosate is often sprayed on crops right before harvest when there's been a particularly rainy season and the crop is very wet. In this application, it's used as a desiccant (drying agent) to speed up harvest time. "Desiccation [the drying of crops using glyphosate] is done primarily in years where conditions are wet, and the crop is slow to dry down," says Joel Ransom, an agronomist at North Dakota State University.

A group of 94 scientists recently published a study that strongly suggests that glyphosate (the active ingredient in Roundup®) is a carcinogen,[13] meaning it causes cancer. Glyphosate is in our water and in our food. It's been found in umbilical cord blood[14] and breast milk.[15] We don't yet know the complete ramifications of Roundup® use.

Spraying crops with glyphosate/Roundup® is not done by all farmers in the U.S. every harvest. However, the products made from crops sprayed with glyphosate aren't labeled as such, so how do we know what we are buying? The phrase, "Better safe than sorry," comes to mind.

Grains, Leaky Gut, and Autoimmune Disorders

Gluten, the protein found in some cereal grains, isn't found in all grains, but it's in some of the most common: wheat, barley, rye, and oat, as well as in hybrid grains like spelt, Khorasan, emmer, einkorn, triticale, and Kamut. Some cereal grain products contain excessive amounts of gluten, which is used to produce a light, fluffy, chewy texture. For this reason, many manufacturers add additional gluten to their products.[16]

Coeliac disease is a common autoimmune disorder where the intestines can't absorb the gluten found in wheat, barley, rye, and oats. This condition has become more prevalent in recent years. Those diagnosed with this condition are usually advised to follow a gluten-free diet.

Gluten can trigger systemwide inflammation, even in those without coeliac disease.[17] This inflammation can cause weight gain, diabetes, other autoimmune disorders, and many chronic illnesses.

Please note that millet, sorghum, amaranth, buckwheat, and quinoa are naturally gluten-free.

CHAPTER 10 – WHEAT: THE STAFF OF LIFE

Eating the wrong types of foods (typically called a Standard American Diet, or SAD) can lead to leaky gut syndrome, which is a condition where the lining of the small intestines becomes permeable, and undigested proteins (like gluten) and other endotoxins can escape into the bloodstream.[18] When this happens, the immune system thinks these molecules are foreign invaders and mounts an attack against them, resulting in a chronic inflammatory response. This leads to autoimmune disorder.

Because I have multiple autoimmune disorders (actually multiple symptoms/manifestations of the same disorder), my gut needs to heal. For this reason, I choose to avoid foods that are difficult to digest, like legumes (which, although they're grains, I'm differentiating from cereal grains, which I will simply call grains), and foods that may contain gluten or other proteins (like the casein protein found in dairy products) that could trigger even more inflammatory responses and autoimmune manifestations. I've found that since I no longer fill up on nutrient-deficient grains, I eat more healthy produce, lean grass-fed meat, and healthy fats.

CHAPTER 11

DAIRY PRODUCTS: YEA OR NAY?

Because of God's goodness and His love for us, He laid out dietary principles (see chapter 4), things that we should and should not consider as 'food.' One area of interest is dairy products. The word 'cheese,' or curdled milk, appears twice in the King James Version.

> *2 Samuel 17:27-29 KJV*
> *And it came to pass, when David was come to Mahanaim, that Shobi the son of Nahash of Rabbah of the children of Ammon, and Machir the son of Ammiel of Lodebar, and Barzillai the Gileadite of Rogelim,*
>
> *Brought beds, and basons, and earthen vessels, and wheat, and barley, and flour, and parched corn* [grain; corn is a new world food and wasn't around in the Bible lands during this time], *and beans, and lentiles, and parched pulse,*
>
> *And honey, and butter, and sheep, and cheese of kine* [cattle], *for David, and for the people that were with him, to eat: for they said, The people is hungry, and weary, and thirsty, in the wilderness.*

In this section, King David's son Absalom had risen up against his father. As David and his men were on the move, three men from the children of Ammon and Gilead (pagan Gentiles), brought food, including cheese and other items, for them to eat.

> *Job 10:10 KJV*
> *Hast thou not poured me out as milk, and curdled me like cheese?*

In this section, Job is complaining to God about his life, saying that God had "curdled me like cheese." Most likely, he was referring to curdled milk, since there are no other references to cheese being food prior to Job (Job was written before 2 Samuel).

CHAPTER 11 – DAIRY PRODUCTS: YEA OR NAY?

Only once in the KJV is cheese used in reference to food, albeit food of pagan Gentiles. There is no record of God's people eating cheese. Butter, however, is referred to 10 times in the KJV as food for the children of Israel.

Cow's Milk, Goat's Milk, and Sheep's Milk

Here are some references to milk as food.

> *Genesis 18:7-8 KJV*
> And Abraham ran unto the herd, and fetcht a calf tender and good, and gave it unto a young man; and he hasted to dress it.
>
> And he took butter, and milk, and the calf which he had dressed, and set it before them; and he stood by them under the tree, and they did eat.
>
> *Deuteronomy 32:14 KJV*
> Butter of kine, and milk of sheep, with fat of lambs, and rams of the breed of Bashan, and goats, with the fat of kidneys of wheat; and thou didst drink the pure blood of the grape.
>
> *Judges 4:19 KJV*
> And he said unto her, give me, I pray thee, a little water to drink; for I am thirsty. And she opened a bottle of milk, and gave him drink, and covered him.
>
> *Judges 5:25 KJV*
> He asked water, and she gave him milk; she brought forth butter in a lordly dish.
>
> *Proverbs 27:27 KJV*
> And thou shalt have goats' milk enough for thy food, for the food of thy household, and for the maintenance for thy maidens.
>
> *Song of Solomon 5:1 KJV*
> I am come into my garden, my sister, my spouse: I have gathered my myrrh with my spice; I have eaten my honeycomb with my honey; I have drunk my wine with my milk: eat, O friends; drink, yea, drink abundantly, O beloved.

CHAPTER 11 - DAIRY PRODUCTS: YEA OR NAY?

> *Isaiah 55:11 KJV*
> *Ho, every one that thirsteth, come ye to the waters, and he that hath no money; come ye, buy, and eat; yea, come, buy wine and milk without money and without price.*

> *Ezekiel 25:4 KJV*
> *Behold, therefore I will deliver thee to the men of the east for a possession, and they shall set their palaces in thee, and make their dwellings in thee: they shall eat thy fruit, and they shall drink thy milk.*

In the book *Everyday Life in Old Testament Times*, E.W. Heaton writes about beverages used by the Israelites:

> *Since water was scarce and not very palatable, a good deal of milk was drunk. It came from goats and sheep. Hebrew has a word for fresh milk, but in the climate of Palestine, it cannot have been used as much as another term meaning sour milk or curds. As soon as the fresh milk was put into the goat-skin bottle, it thickened slightly and went sour. All the better, it was thought, for quenching the thirst.*[1]

Keep in mind that the above verses refer to milk in its natural, God-given, raw, unadulterated state. Clean raw milk from grass-fed, pasture raised sheep and goats provides many wonderful health-promoting nutrients.[2] The pasteurized cow's milk we have today is something else entirely.

The Land of Milk and Honey

The first mentions of a "land flowing with milk and honey" are in Exodus chapter 3.

> *Exodus 3:8 KJV*
> *And I am come down to deliver them out of the hand of the Egyptians, and to bring them up out of that land unto a good land and a large, unto a land flowing with milk and honey; unto the place of the Canaanites, and the Hittites, and the Amorites, and the Perizzites, and the Hivites, and the Jebusites.*

CHAPTER 11 – DAIRY PRODUCTS: YEA OR NAY?

> *Exodus 3:17 KJV*
> *And I have said, I will bring you up out of the affliction of Egypt unto the land of the Canaanites, and the Hittites, and the Amorites, and the Perizzites, and the Hivites, and the Jebusites, unto a land flowing with milk and honey.*

The promised land, which was said to be "flowing with milk and honey," is set in contrast to the afflictions the Israelites suffered under the hand of the Egyptians. This is the figure of speech *synecdoche* or transfer. It's the exchange of one idea for another associated idea. According to E.W. Bullinger's *Figures of Speech Used in the Bible*,[3] "honey is put for whatever is sweet and delicious."

The milk denotes fertility of the land, a giving of nourishment from a mother. The phrase "the land of milk and honey" is figurative, not literal.

Why Do We Think Cow's Milk is Healthy?

In 1993, an advertising company developed the "got milk? ™" campaign. It became the most successful commodity advertisement in history and still runs to this day. It has been incredibly influential in the way a generation of parents feeds their children. It seemed to validate the idea (around for even more generations) that humans need cow's milk and other dairy products for essential health. But does science validate this sentiment? Why do we think cow's milk is healthy for human consumption?

The History of Human Milk Consumption

Milk is the source of primary nutrition for baby mammals, whose mothers produce the milk their offspring need. This food provides the baby with all the nutrients it requires. Once the baby can digest more adult forms of food, weaning takes place and the baby never again drinks its mother's milk for the rest of its life. This leads us to two questions.

First, why did humans start consuming the milk of other mammals and, second, why do humans keep consuming the milk of other mammals?

CHAPTER 11 - DAIRY PRODUCTS: YEA OR NAY?

Scientists have discovered that milking cattle for human consumption began in central Europe.[4] I've seen dates put at between 6,000 to 12,000 years ago.

In addition to being less contaminated than water, cow's milk also provided a calorie- and protein-rich food source that wasn't dependent on seasonal crops and weather changes. However, it was usually second-choice after drinks like ales, beer, hard cider, and other alcoholic beverages.

These are logical reasons why humans started drinking the milk of other mammals. The answer to the second question, why do humans keep consuming the milk of other mammals, especially when other safe beverages (like clean water) are available, is more complicated.

Why We Keep Drinking Cow's Milk

By the late 1800s, conditions among milking operations were becoming less sanitary, leading to fewer people drinking milk. Louis Pasteur conducted the first pasteurization tests in 1862 and he is credited with revolutionizing the safety of cow's milk and, in turn, the ability to store and distribute milk well beyond the farm. Commercial pasteurization machines were introduced in 1895.[5]

Later, as the temperance movement spread, groups advocated serving milk instead of alcohol. In the 1920s in the United States, producers of agricultural products, including milk, formed associations to promote their products. Eventually, cow's milk became a staple of the Standard American Diet (SAD).

Does Milk Really "Do a Body Good?"

The dairy industry has convinced many Americans that cow's milk is good for them. But, is it really? In 2013, Care2 put out this information:[6]

- The USDA tells American kids to drink 3 servings of milk per day.
- Per capita, the U.S. drinks 9 times more milk than China.
- The average U.S. yearly dairy consumption is 593 lb.

CHAPTER 11 – DAIRY PRODUCTS: YEA OR NAY?

- Compare that to the U.S. yearly vegetable consumption of 428 lb.
- 4% of adults have food allergies.
- Cow's milk is the #1 cause of food allergies among infants and children.
- 33% of American adults are lactose intolerant.
- 75% of African-American, Mexican-American, and Jewish adults are lactose intolerant.
- 90% of Asian-Americans are lactose intolerant.
- Only 40% of adults maintain the ability to digest lactose after childhood.
- The average amount of time until the effects of lactose intolerance occur after dairy intake is 30 minutes.
- Only 13.1% of American adults don't drink cow's milk.
- That's 62,200,000 people regularly drinking cow's milk who can't digest it properly (nearly the entire populations of California and Texas combined).
- In 1970, one cow produced 9,700 pounds of milk per year.
- In 2013, one cow produced 19,000 pounds of milk per year. How are cows producing more milk?
- Cows doped on growth hormones produce 10 pounds more milk per year.
- The growth hormones end up in the milk that humans drink.
- The growth hormones contain IFG-1 (Insulin Growth Factor 1), which humans already have.
- Increased IFG-1 is linked to early puberty in girls.
- Men with increased levels of IFG-1 are four times more likely to get prostate cancer.

CHAPTER 11 - DAIRY PRODUCTS: YEA OR NAY?

- Ounce for ounce, milk has the same calorie count as soda.
- In a study of 20 countries, high milk consumption meant higher rates of Type 1 diabetes and heart disease.
- One serving of 2% milk has the same saturated fat count as a serving of French fries.
- Women who increase their lactose intake to equal to one glass of milk per day are 13% more likely to get ovarian cancer.

The Autoimmune Connection

The connection between dairy products and autoimmune disorder is beta-casein. Beta-casein is a protein that is found in milk and there are two types: A1 and A2.[7] Most people who are intolerant of cow's milk are sensitive to A1 beta-casein and lack the ability to digest it. A1 beta-casein is highly inflammatory for many people, which can lead to leaky gut syndrome.[8]

The Problem with Modern Dairy Products

If milk (and its sub-products butter, cheese, sour cream, yogurt, and kefir) is so nutritious, as the advertisements would have us believe, why does it cause digestive problems for so many people?

Why are people who grew up elsewhere in the world consuming dairy products with no problem suddenly unable to digest American dairy products? The answer is that most dairy products sold in the U.S. come from cows with A1 beta-casein.

Whether milk has A1 or A2 beta-casein depends on what breed of cow it comes from. Milk from breeds of cows that originated in northern Europe is generally high in A1 beta-casein. A1 milk comes from breeds like Holstein, Friesian, Ayrshire, and British Shorthorn.

People with dairy sensitives may want to switch to A2 dairy products. Milk that is high in A2 beta-casein is mainly found in breeds that originated in the Channel Islands and Southern France. This includes breeds like Guernsey, Jersey, Charolais, and Limousin.

CHAPTER 11 – DAIRY PRODUCTS: YEA OR NAY?

Unfortunately, there's no way to know if dairy products like milk or cheese are from A1 or A2 cows unless it's specifically labeled as such, it's best to assume that it's A1 and should be avoided unless labeled otherwise.

Goat's milk and sheep's milk contain much less or no A1 beta-casein,[9] therefore, they should be preferred over cow's milk/cheese. Milk products from goats and sheep are available in specialty/health stores. You may need to ask for it.

I've found Pecorino-Romano cheese (made from sheep's milk) from Italy to be a good substitute for parmesan when making pesto.

Another problem with modern dairy products is pasteurization, which alters the chemical structure of food, makes fats rancid, destroys nutrients, and results in the formation of free radicals in the body.[10] Pasteurization (which is the heating of food to 280° F) isn't just for dairy products; it's used on commercially produced fruit juices, vinegar, sauerkraut, eggs, and nuts, as well.[11]

Those who wish to keep dairy in their diet may want to consider raw dairy products (including raw goat and sheep products). Another option is to switch to coconut milk products, which aren't dairy and aren't pasteurized. This is my personal choice.

CHAPTER 12

SOY: FRIEND OR FOE?

Soy has been promoted as a health food since the 1990s when the FDA warned that eating too much red meat was a heart attack in the making. (This has been debunked; see chapter 35.) Instead of meat, many health-conscious people turned to soy in the form of tofu, tempeh, soy milk, miso, etc. to get their protein.

Since then, it's become quite the controversial food. So, is soy a friend or a foe? The answer is... it depends. It depends on which reports and studies one chooses to believe.

History of Soy

The following information from the North Carolina Soybean Producers Association is quite illuminating.

> Soybeans originated in Southeast Asia and were first domesticated by Chinese farmers around 1100 BC. By the first century AD, soybeans were grown in Japan and many other countries.
>
> Soybean seed from China was planted by a colonist in the British colony of Georgia in 1765. Benjamin Franklin sent some soybean seeds to a friend to plant in his garden in 1770.
>
> By 1851, soybean seeds were distributed to farmers in Illinois and the corn belt states. This seed was a gift from a crew member rescued from a Japanese fishing boat in the Pacific Ocean in 1850. In the 1870s, soybeans increased in popularity with farmers who began to plant them as forage for their livestock.
>
> In 1904, the famous American chemist, George Washington Carver [of peanut fame] discovered that soybeans were a valuable source of protein and oil. Henry Ford discovered that he could make plastics parts for cars from soybeans. By 1935, Ford was using one bushel of soybeans for every car he manufactured.

CHAPTER 12 – SOY: FRIEND OR FOE?

> *It wasn't until the 1940s that soybean farming really took off in America. Soybean production in China, the major supplier at that time, was halted by World War II and internal revolution. When the United States entered the war, the steep increase in demand for oils, lubricants, plastics, and other products greatly increased the demand for soybeans. United States farmers produced the needed soybeans.*
>
> *Following World War II, the United States experienced a period of increasing prosperity. Demand for meat consumption increased as people's diets improved. Livestock producers found that soybean meal was the preferred source of protein at an affordable cost. Chickens, turkeys, cattle, and hogs were fed diets containing tens of millions of tons of soybean meal each year. This increase in the use of soybean meal for livestock feed began in the 1950s and soybean meal has been the preferred choice ever since.*
>
> *One of the great scientific advances in agriculture was the improvement of the soybean in the 1990s to withstand herbicides. This meant that farmers could control weeds without killing the soybean plant. Today, 31 U.S. states have a soybean production industry.* [1]

The scientific advancement of the 1990s mentioned above is the invention of the genetically modified soybean, also called a Roundup® Ready Soybean, which was introduced to the U.S. market in 1998 by Monsanto.[2] In 2014, 94% of the U.S. soy crop was genetically engineered (GMO).[3] I discuss GMO foods in more detail in chapter 7.

98% of the soy produced in the U.S. is for animal feed.[4] You are not only what you eat, but also what the thing you eat, ate.

Reasons to Consume Soy Products

Some reasons why soy might be beneficial.[5]

- Soy probably doesn't raise breast cancer risk, and it might even lower the risk of some cancers.[6,7]

CHAPTER 12 – SOY: FRIEND OR FOE?

- Soy might improve fertility and help with hot flashes.[8,9,10,11]
- Soy may protect the heart,[12] but maybe not. The FDA recently announced the claim is temporarily off the table due to "inconsistent findings."[13]

Impact of Soy on Hormones

According to the Global Healing Center, soy upsets hormone balance in five ways:[14]

1. Causes premature menstruation[15]
2. Leads to gynecomastia (male breast enlargement)[16,17]
3. Kills libido[18]
4. May cause infertility[19]
5. Linked to breast cancer[20,21]

One of the controversies concerning soy is its high level of plant estrogens, also called phytoestrogens — compounds that mimic estrogen in the human body. Soy contains two primary phytoestrogens, sometimes called xenoestrogens: genistein and daidzein. Both compounds are known to disrupt the endocrine system in both males and females.[22]

A Loma Linda University review[23] of 14 studies found that soy foods don't affect people with healthy thyroids. However, for people with hyperthyroid, Graves' disease, hypothyroid, or Hashimoto's disease, soy foods have been shown to interfere with the body's absorption of thyroid medication.[24]

Other Problems with Soy

94% of all soybeans produced in the U.S. are GMO (see chapter 7). Reading labels is extremely important when consuming soy products.

Natto, miso, traditional soy sauce, and tempeh are all processed foods derived from fermented soybeans. Such foods came into being across

CHAPTER 12 – SOY: FRIEND OR FOE?

China about 2,000 years ago when people began using different methods to remove not-so-healthy antinutrients.[25]

According to Dr. Joseph Mercola, D.O., "Antinutrients are elements and compounds in soy foods such as lectins, saponins, soyatoxins, phytates (which prevent the absorption of certain minerals), oxalates, protease inhibitors, estrogens (which can block the hormone estrogen and disrupt endocrine function), and goitrogens (interfering with thyroid function), as well as a blood clot-inhibiting substance called hemagglutinin." [26]

Fermented vs. Unfermented Soy

Bacteria convert sugars and starch into lactic acid in a process called lactofermentation. Dr. Mercola says that "fermented foods help improve gut health by 'reseeding' the gut with beneficial bacteria. The fermentation process also boosts the nutritional content of the food, producing essential amino acids, short-chain fatty acids, beneficial enzymes, certain nutrients, and increases the bioavailability of minerals."[27]

The fermentation process takes time and effort, but it 'deactivates' many of the antinutrients in soy that act as toxins in the body. These soy foods are not fermented; therefore, I avoid them:

- TVP or textured soy protein
- Soy cheese, soy ice cream, soy milk, and soy yogurt
- Soybean oil
- Soy infant formula[28]
- Edamame (an immature soybean)

I choose to eat organic/non-GMO whenever possible, avoid all soy products, and avoid foods that are heavily processed.

CHAPTER 13

THE ADVANTAGES OF COCONUT MILK

I grew up drinking cow's milk every day. There was always a gallon or two in the refrigerator, and we drank it for breakfast, lunch, dinner, and with snacks. My parents and I never associated my perennial allergies with milk. After all, I had been tested for allergies and milk never came up.

My dad used a low-fat powdered milk (which I thought was gross), but the thought of other types of milk never occurred to me (other than my trip to Egypt at age 16 where I was presented with buffalo milk, but that's another story).

For the past several years I've been using full-fat coconut milk instead of cow's milk. What are the advantages of using coconut milk over cow's milk?

What is Coconut Milk?

Coconut milk is the liquid that comes from the grated meat of a mature coconut. The decadent taste gives the impression of an unhealthy food, but it's actually a very healthy food.

What's the difference between coconut milk and coconut water? Coconut water is the liquid that pours out when you crack open an immature coconut. It's higher in sugar and certain electrolytes than coconut milk, while the milk is higher in healthy saturated fatty acids (from coconut oil) and calories.[1]

Coconut milk is very popular in Thai and other southeast Asian cuisines.

One cup of full-fat coconut milk has 552 calories, 8 grams of naturally occurring sugar, and 57.2 grams total fat. Those who want fewer calories and fat can opt for low-fat coconut milk.

Many people think of coconut as a superfood. Here are 5 great advantages of coconut milk.

CHAPTER 13 – THE ADVANTAGES OF COCONUT MILK

Dairy Free

Coconut milk is a great choice for those who want to stay dairy free. It has no whey or casein protein and no lactose.

Vegan Friendly

Although the FDA classifies coconut as a tree nut, botanically, coconut is a drupe, which is a stone fruit like a peach. This makes it ideal for those allergic to nut-based milk, as well as for vegans and vegetarians. Coconut allergies are relatively rare, but they do exist.

Nutrient-Rich

Coconuts are very nutritious. They're rich in fiber, as well as vitamins B1, B3, B5, B6, C, and E. The minerals in one cup of coconut milk include calcium (38.4 mg), iron (15.6 mg), magnesium (88.8 mg), phosphorus (240 mg), potassium (631 mg), selenium (14.9 mcg), and sodium (36 mg).[2]

The medium-chain triglyceride (MCT) fatty acids found in coconut milk increase energy and result in greater loss of fat (adipose tissue) compared with long-chain fatty acids.[3]

Heart Health

Coconut milk is high in saturated fat (50.7 g per cup), which for many years has been demonized. According to Dr. Mary G. Enig, Ph.D., FACN, approximately 50% of the fatty acids in coconut fat are lauric acid. Lauric acid is a medium-chain fatty acid, which has the additional beneficial function of being formed into monolaurin in the human or animal body.[4]

Lauric acid has antibacterial and antiviral properties. According to many studies, lauric acid is a protective type of fatty acid linked with improved cholesterol levels and heart health.[5]

Digestive Health

Coconut milk provides nourishment to the digestive lining because of its electrolytes and healthy fats, which improve gut health and prevent

CHAPTER 13 – THE ADVANTAGES OF COCONUT MILK

conditions like IBS (Irritable Bowel Syndrome).[6] Drinking coconut milk instead of cow's milk can help decrease diarrhea, abdominal pain, gas, and bloating from lactose intolerance.

Choosing Coconut Milk

Be sure to look for cans that are BPA-free or choose coconut milk in a carton. Choose a brand that contains only coconut and water; avoid extraneous ingredients like carrageenan. Recipes for making coconut milk yourself can be found online. I include my recipe for Coconut Milk Kefir in chapter 50.

For the above reasons, plus the fact that it's delicious, I consume coconut milk daily.

CHAPTER 13 – THE ADVANTAGES OF COCONUT MILK

CHAPTER 14

AVOIDING NIGHTSHADES

Most people think that any and all vegetables are good to eat. After all, they're better than junk food (which is true). But, for those with food sensitivities, allergies, autoimmune disorders, inflammatory bowel disease (IBS), or leaky gut syndrome, there's a certain group of plants that can contribute to symptoms. These symptoms can range from digestive issues to inflammation. Let's find out what nightshades are and why avoiding them can help.

Meet the Solanaceae Family

These plants are part of the botanical family *Solanaceae*, also known as nightshades:

- Tomatoes
- White potatoes (<u>not</u> sweet potatoes)
- Eggplant
- Okra
- Peppers (includes bell peppers, chili peppers, cayenne, paprika, pimento, etc.)
- Tomatillos
- Sorrel
- Gooseberries
- Ground cherries
- Pepino melons
- Tobacco
- Capsicum

CHAPTER 14 – AVOIDING NIGHTSHADES

Most nightshades (there are over 2,000 species in this family) are completely healthy for most people, but I've found avoiding them to be helpful for the following reasons.

Alkaloids

Alkaloids are a group of naturally occurring chemical compounds that mostly contain basic nitrogen atoms. The following alkaloids are found in most nightshade vegetables:

- Solanine/Tomatine
- Capsaicin
- Nicotine

Solanine/Tomatine

Solanine is a glycoalkaloid poison found in potatoes, tomatoes, and eggplants. It can occur naturally in any part of the plant, including the leaves, fruit, and tubers.[1] Solanine seems to be more concentrated in the green parts of the plant like leaves, green spots on potatoes and tomatoes (fried green tomatoes), and sprouts growing out of potatoes. (Solanine is primarily found in potatoes; the tomato counterpart is tomatine.)

Solanine and other nightshade steroidal alkaloids can irritate the gastrointestinal system and act as acetylcholinesterase inhibitors, affecting neurotransmitters.[2] Symptoms of solanine poisoning include nausea, diarrhea, vomiting, stomach cramps, burning of the throat, cardiac dysrhythmia, nightmares, headache, dizziness, itching, eczema, thyroid problems, inflammation, and pain in the joints. In more severe cases, hallucinations, loss of sensation, paralysis, fever, jaundice, dilated pupils, hypothermia, and death have been reported. Symptoms usually occur 8 to 12 hours after ingestion but may occur as rapidly as 10 minutes after eating high-solanine foods.[3]

Capsaicin

According to Dr. Josh Axe, D.N.M., D.C., C.N.S.,[4] capsaicin is the active ingredient in hot peppers. Most people know it for its anti-inflammatory

CHAPTER 14 – AVOIDING NIGHTSHADES

properties, but as an alkaloid, it's one of the strongest substances in food and herbs. Anyone who has eaten a hot pepper like a habanero or a jalapeno can attest to the fire and irritation they cause. If your lips burn after a bite of too-hot salsa, that's capsaicin at work.

Capsaicin's irritant properties cause a release of substance P, which is a neuropeptide that plays a role in the communication of pain messages.[5] After the initial irritation of contact with capsaicin and the release of substance P, there's a period of deadened sensation. You may have noticed that the third and fourth bites of salsa aren't as hot as the first.[6] This reaction chain is why capsaicin is often used topically as an analgesic for osteoarthritis.[7]

Nicotine

The alkaloid nicotine is found in all nightshade vegetables, not just tobacco. Nicotine is a highly addictive substance, which may explain why some people are addicted to French fries and ketchup.[8]

Nightshade Allergy and Sensitivities

Keep in mind that nightshades include quite deadly plants as well as generally safe vegetables. Not all of the above compounds are present in every nightshade plant, and even when they're present, not all are strong enough to feel immediate effects.

A true nightshade allergy, like any food or environmental allergy, should be taken seriously. However, it may not be easy to pinpoint. While many allergens like tree nuts and dairy are easy to single out, nightshade vegetables aren't readily associated with one another. Anyone exhibiting any of the symptoms listed above may want to have food allergy testing done or eliminate nightshades in the Food Reintroduction Challenge (chapter 27).

Those exhibiting apparent sensitivities to nightshade vegetables often have similar complaints as gluten sensitivity reactions. Irritable bowel disorders and other gastrointestinal issues, heartburn, nerve sensitization, and joint pain are commonly associated with nightshade vegetable sensitivity.[9]

CHAPTER 14 – AVOIDING NIGHTSHADES

Studies

A 2002 study monitored the gut permeability of mice to determine how nightshades would affect irritable bowel syndrome or irritable bowel disease (IBS or IBD). Using potatoes which contain glycoalkaloids, they found that existing IBD was aggravated, or even served as a catalyst for symptoms for the mice that were predisposed to having IBD.[10]

There's no direct evidence that nightshade vegetables cause arthritis or that their elimination will relieve symptoms.[11] However, there's anecdotal evidence that would suggest that some people have experienced a decrease in symptoms when nightshades are eliminated. People with nightshade sensitivity frequently have joint pain. Therefore, doing the Food Reintroduction Challenge with nightshades might benefit those experiencing joint pain.

Heartburn or reflux can be a reaction in those with nightshade sensitivity. Because it can irritate the lining of the esophagus and stomach, capsaicin is tied to acid reflux and heartburn.[12] Most individuals can limit the amount of capsaicin they ingest to minimize this discomfort, but a true sensitivity will require its elimination.

Avoiding Nightshades

When attempting to eliminate nightshade vegetables to confirm sensitivity, it's important to be thorough. As I mentioned, there are over 2,000 species of nightshade plants. Note that blueberries, goji berries, and huckleberries all include similar alkaloids. They're not nightshades, but it may be important to eliminate them at the same time. Be cautious of anything that might contain potato starch as a thickener or filler, including medications and baking powders; even envelope glue can contain potato starch.

I've found that eliminating nightshades has reduced inflammation. Others may find similar results.

CHAPTER 15

JUST SAY NO TO BACON

I don't eat bacon. The primary reason is found in the Bible.

> *Leviticus 11:7 KJV*
> *And the swine, though he divide the hoof, and be clovenfooted, yet he cheweth not the cud; he is unclean to you.*
>
> *Deuteronomy 14: 8 KJV*
> *And the swine, because it divideth the hoof, yet cheweth not the cud, it is unclean unto you: ye shall not eat of their flesh, nor touch their dead carcase.*

What Does the Bible Say?

For the Israelites, following God's laws was about more than obedience. It was about showing God that they loved and respected Him. They understood that God knew what was best for them. This showed they knew that God wasn't being mean or punitive, but rather He was expressing His love for them by helping them avoid things that could potentially harm them. After all, they didn't know anything about microbes or pathogens. But God did.

Swine is also known as pig, hog, pork, bacon, sausage, lard, ham, pepperoni, gelatin, etc. Further, the connection between swine and pagan worship became so strong that the prophet Isaiah compared the sacrificial offering of pig's blood with murder; both are called "abominations" in Isaiah 66:3.

Modern Science

One of the benefits of living in a modern society is that we have sanitary living conditions. We have regulations that help keep us healthy (just as the Israelites had God's laws). Because of this, many people are lulled into a false sense that everything they eat is healthy. After all, why would companies be allowed to sell products that are unhealthy? Do I really have to answer that?

CHAPTER 15 – JUST SAY NO TO BACON

One of the biggest problems with swine/pigs is their digestive system. A pig digests what it has eaten in about four hours. This doesn't allow time for the excess toxins to be processed, so these toxins are stored in the muscles and fatty tissues of the pig. This is the part that is eaten. When one consumes pork, one also consumes all the toxins that the pig couldn't digest.

In 2015, the World Health Organization (WHO) said there's sufficient evidence that processed meats cause colorectal cancer. This puts bacon, hot dogs, and sausages into the WHO's Group 1 category, the same as substances like tobacco and asbestos.[1]

Pigs carry a variety of parasites in their bodies. This is one reason why experts recommend that pork and bacon be cooked thoroughly, even though this thorough cooking may not kill all the parasites. Pigs are primary carriers of trichinella tapeworm (which causes trichinosis), Hepatitis E virus (HEV), PRRS, Nipah virus, Menangle virus, and viruses in the family *Paramyxoviridae*.[2]

Could it be that for the above reasons God told us not to eat pork?

Another problem with modern pork is the conditions under which the pigs are raised. Today, 97% of pigs in the United States are raised in factory farms.[3] This means that these pigs never live a healthy life of fresh air and wide-open pastures. These pigs are fed a steady diet of harmful drugs to keep the pig breathing as producers make pigs grow faster and fatter. These drugs, like drug-resistant antibiotics, stay in the flesh of the pig and we eat them.

Bottom Line

As Christians today, we are free to eat whatever we want (Romans 14:14, Matthew 15:11, 1 Timothy 4:3-5). But just because we are free to do something doesn't make it a good idea.

> *1 Corinthians 10:23 KJV*
> *All things are lawful for me, but all things are not expedient [profitable]: all things are lawful for me, but all things edify not.*

CHAPTER 15 – JUST SAY NO TO BACON

Galatians 5:13 KJV
For, brethren, ye have been called unto liberty; only use not liberty for an occasion [a base of operations] *to the flesh, but by love serve one another.*

I try to eat foods that will nourish, strengthen, and sustain my body for a long, satisfying life. Bacon is not one of those foods. I acknowledge that the smell and taste of bacon are delicious. What's not so delicious is what it does to my body.

CHAPTER 15 – JUST SAY NO TO BACON

CHAPTER 16

THE DANGERS OF FAST FOOD

For many, many generations, our ancestors ate only the food they or their close neighbors grew and raised. They ate real, whole foods. In contrast, our modern culture is one that runs on speed and convenience. If something isn't fast and easy, we don't want it. If quality suffers at the hands of speed and ease, so be it.

The desire for speed and convenience has led to the rise of fast food, which isn't known for its quality. Fast food isn't just food that comes from a building on the corner with a drive-thru. True, that's what most of us think of when someone says, 'fast food.' However, our grocery stores are filled with aisle after aisle of canned, boxed, bottled, and frozen processed foods, all designed to give us speed and convenience. After all, if you can throw a box into the microwave and have dinner ready in less than 10 minutes, who cares if you're sacrificing a little quality? Turns out, we all have reason to care.

Lack of Nutrition

The problems with fast food, whether from the drive-thru or from the grocery store, are two-fold. Number one is what's in it and number two is what's not in it.

Most fast foods lack nutritional balance. They're very heavy on simple carbohydrates and protein (a hamburger on a bun with a side of French fries). There are very few fresh vegetables and healthy fats to balance this.

The U.S. Department of Agriculture designed a Healthy Eating Index (HEI) [1] to compare nutritional content. It's designed to measure nutritional values on a scale of 1 (bad) to 100 (best). Researchers looked at eight fast-food restaurants – McDonald's, Burger King, Wendy's, Taco Bell, Kentucky Fried Chicken (KFC), Arby's, Jack in the Box, and Dairy Queen – using data from 1997 to 2010. According to the latest figures, from 2010, the average score for these fast-food restaurants was just 48 out of 100. For comparison, the average American's diet score is (a low) 55 out of 100.

Fast-foods tend to have high amounts of sugar, unhealthy fat, and salt. GMO and non-organic ingredients are common in fast food. Studies show that organ damage, gastrointestinal and immune system disorders, accelerated aging, and infertility can result from consuming GMO food.[2]

A group of 94 scientists recently published a study that strongly suggests that glyphosate (the active ingredient in Roundup®) is a carcinogen, meaning it causes cancer.[3] Glyphosate is in our water and in our food. It's been found in umbilical cord blood.[4] We don't yet know the complete ramifications of this. By choosing organic and non-GMO foods, we can help protect ourselves and our families from this poison.

Health Problems

This speed + convenience mentality has led to many of the health problems now plaguing western society. In addition to low nutritional value, the high fat, calorie, and sodium content of fast food[5] can lead to a variety of health problems.

Diet-related illnesses are on the rise.[6] Hypertension, heart disease, cancer, diabetes, and obesity are all directly related to diet quality.[7] Heart disease is currently the number one killer of both men and women in the United States.[8] The risk of heart attack and stroke[9] can be lessened with a healthful diet.

Fast food can lead to vitamin deficiencies. Nutrients like calcium, vitamin D, potassium, and fiber are not abundant in fast food.

High Cost

The average American eats 4.2 commercially-prepared meals per week.[10] In other words, as a nation, we eat out between four and five times a week, on average. This number equates to 18.2 meals in an average month eaten outside the home.[11] Studies show that most people choose fast food for convenience. But, is it really all that convenient?

CHAPTER 16 – THE DANGERS OF FAST FOOD

Is it convenient to be malnourished? Did you know that many obese people are actually malnourished? [12] When we eat foods with no nutritional value, the stomach will signal that it's full, but the cells aren't getting the nutrition they need, so they keep signaling us to eat more. So, we eat and eat, we gain weight, and our bodies are starving for real nutrition. If we're always hungry, our bodies aren't getting the nourishment they need. With healthy food, we will eat less because our cells will be satisfied, saving money in the long run.

Is it convenient to be sick? Are hypertension, heart disease, cancer, diabetes, and obesity convenient? Is the cost of being sick (doctor/hospital visits, medications, time off work) less than the cost of fast food?

I've found it's much easier and healthier to eat real, whole foods. Before I made the switch, I dreaded the thought of it. Where would I find the time to prepare my own food, three times a day? Wouldn't it be expensive to cook at home exclusively?

Turns out, the anticipation was scarier than the reality. I discovered I had plenty of time; time I had previously frittered away on social media and television. Now, I spend even more time with my husband because we prepare meals together.

Expensive? No, actually, it's much cheaper. My husband and I don't miss eating out because the food at home is so much better than anything at a restaurant. When we added up the cost of fast food, restaurant food, sodas, alcohol, stops at the convenience store (see why they call it that?), the donut shop, and Starbucks®, we realized that we could eat real, whole, healthy food for much less cost than 'convenient,' fast processed food. (More about this in chapter 45.)

I challenge you to prove this for yourself.

CHAPTER 16 – THE DANGERS OF FAST FOOD

PART 4

UNDERSTANDING LEAKY GUT

"Just because you're not sick doesn't mean you're healthy."
Unknown

CHAPTER 17

"ALL DISEASE BEGINS IN THE GUT"

Hippocrates, the 'father of western medicine,' spoke these words over 2,000 years ago. Certainly, some diseases, like genetic diseases, don't start in the gut, but for just about everything else, the gut is where it all begins.

The reason for this is the different gut bacteria residing in our digestive tracts, as well as the integrity of the gut lining.[1] According to numerous studies, the lining of the small intestine (the gut) can become porous so that unwanted bacterial products called endotoxins, as well as undigested proteins, can sometimes leak through the lining and enter the bloodstream.[2]

This is called leaky gut syndrome (so-called because there are many symptoms and no two people manifest it the same way). For many years, the traditional medical community did not recognize this disease, but now it's known to them as intestinal permeability.[3]

When these molecules enter the bloodstream, the immune system thinks they're foreign invaders and mounts an attack against them, resulting in a chronic inflammatory response.[4]

Here are a couple more Hippocrates quotes.

"Make a habit of two things: to help, or at least to do no harm."

"Natural forces within us are the true healers of disease."

CHAPTER 17 – "ALL DISEASE BEGINS IN THE GUT"

Causes of Leaky Gut Syndrome

- Processed food
- Gluten
- Cow's dairy (A1 beta-casein)
- Sugar
- Unsprouted grains
- GMO foods
- Not enough probiotics and fiber
- Hydrogenated oils
- Prescription drugs, OTC pain relievers, birth control pills, antibiotics, and steroids (these cause bacterial imbalance by killing the natural good bacteria in the gut)
- Chronic stress
- Inflammation
- Yeast (or candida)
- Lack of zinc

According to research published in the *International Journal of Gastroenterology and Hepatology 2006*,[5] leaky gut syndrome may cause Hashimoto's Thyroiditis, rheumatoid arthritis, fibromyalgia, psoriasis, multiple sclerosis, lupus, depression, and anxiety, among others.

8 Symptoms of Leaky Gut Syndrome

People who suffer from any of the following symptoms may have leaky gut syndrome. More symptoms increase the likelihood. Based on the prevalence of these symptoms, leaky gut syndrome can be considered an epidemic today.[6]

CHAPTER 17 – "ALL DISEASE BEGINS IN THE GUT"

- Food sensitives or allergies (especially gluten and dairy)
- Inflammatory bowel disease (IBS, Crohn's, bloating, gas, chronic diarrhea/constipation)
- Autoimmune disorders (rheumatoid arthritis, fibromyalgia, lupus, multiple sclerosis, etc.)
- Thyroid problems (Hashimoto's Disease, Graves' Disease, hypothyroid, hyperthyroid)
- Adrenal fatigue, candida, or a slow metabolism
- Malabsorption (of vitamin B12 and magnesium, among others)
- Inflammatory skin conditions (acne, psoriasis, eczema)
- Mood issues (anxiety, depression)

Please note that digestive upset is not normal. God designed the digestive system to function without disruption or pain. Bloating, heaviness, gas, reflux, heartburn, difficulty in eliminating, etc., are the body's responses to foods the body can't handle. I found that when I changed what I eat, digestive upset became a thing of the past.

In part 7, I will talk about how I restored my health from leaky gut syndrome.

CHAPTER 17 – "ALL DISEASE BEGINS IN THE GUT"

CHAPTER 18

YOUR GUT: YOUR SECOND BRAIN

Have you ever had butterflies in your tummy before a big event? Or felt a queasy feeling in your stomach when things weren't quite right? Or relied on your 'gut instinct' when making an important decision?

Why do we feel things emotionally in our gut? Scientists have learned that we have a second brain, called the enteric brain. It's located in the gut and it affects our mood. Time to meet your gut, your second brain.

The Enteric Brain

The enteric nervous system (ENS) consists of more than 100 million nerve cells lining your gastrointestinal tract (this is more cells than your spinal cord has). Because of this vast number of nerve cells, we can 'feel' what is happening in our gut. The ENS communicates with your head brain in ways scientists are only beginning to understand.

According to Dr. Jay Pasricha, M.D., director of the Johns Hopkins Center for Neurogastroenterology (a newly emerging field), the enteric brain's main role is "controlling digestion, from swallowing to the release of enzymes that break down food to the control of blood flow that helps with nutrient absorption to elimination. The enteric nervous system doesn't seem capable of thought as we know it, but it communicates back and forth with our big brain — with profound results." [1]

The Head Brain – Gut Brain Connection

"For decades, researchers and doctors thought that anxiety and depression contributed to these problems. But our studies and others show that it may also be the other way around," Pasricha says. Researchers are finding evidence that irritation in the gastrointestinal system may send signals to the central nervous system (CNS) that trigger mood changes.[2] It's not all in your head, it's in your gut.

Things that are happening in the gastrointestinal (digestive) system, like leaky gut syndrome, will affect the central nervous system. Those

CHAPTER 18 – YOUR GUT: YOUR SECOND BRAIN

feelings we talked about that we experience in our gut start in the gut and can affect our mental state, as well as whether we develop certain diseases.

Scientists have learned that around 90% of the fibers in the vagus nerve (the 10th cranial nerve which is part of the involuntary nervous system) carry information from the gut to the brain and not the other way around.

According to Dr. Rosalyn M. King, Ed.D., professor of psychology, Northern Virginia Community College, [3] "As light is shed on the circuitry between the two brains, researchers are beginning to understand why people act and feel the way they do. When the central brain encounters a frightening situation, it releases stress hormones that prepare the body to fight or flee. The stomach contains many sensory nerves that are stimulated by this chemical surge – hence the 'butterflies.'"

On the battlefield, the higher brain tells the gut brain to shut down. Fear also causes the vagus nerve to 'turn up the volume' on serotonin circuits in the gut. Thus over-stimulated, the gut goes into higher gear and diarrhea results.

Similarly, people sometimes 'choke' with emotion. When nerves in the esophagus are highly stimulated, people have trouble swallowing. Even the so-called 'Maalox moment' of advertising can be explained by the interaction of the two brains, according to Dr. Jackie D. Wood, Ph.D., chairman of the department of physiology at Ohio State University. "Stress signals from the head's brain can alter nerve function between the stomach and esophagus, resulting in heartburn." [4]

In cases of extreme stress, Dr. Wood says that "the higher brain seems to protect the gut by sending signals to immunological mast cells in the plexus (a network of nerves or vessels in the body). The mast cells secrete histamine, prostaglandin, and other agents that help produce inflammation. This is protective. By inflaming the gut, the brain is priming the gut for surveillance. If the barrier breaks, then the gut is ready to do repairs. Unfortunately, the chemicals that get released also cause diarrhea and cramping." [5]

You Are What You Eat

Our entire being is affected by what we eat (after all, 'you are what you eat'). UCLA's Dr. Emeran Mayer, M.D., Ph.D.,[6] is doing work on how the trillions of bacteria in the gut 'communicate' with enteric nervous system cells. The head brain affects the gut brain as much as the gut brain affects the head brain.

Everything we consume becomes a part of our cells. If we eat real, whole food that the body recognizes, the body can pull nutrients from the food and use them to build, maintain, and support the body. The body doesn't recognize fake, junk food, so the body will attempt to eliminate as much of it as possible. Whatever can't be eliminated or assimilated is stored wherever the body can put it. In many cases, this leads to autoimmune disorders.

CHAPTER 18 – YOUR GUT: YOUR SECOND BRAIN

PART 5

DEALING WITH AUTOIMMUNE DISORDERS

> "Let food be thy medicine and
> medicine be thy food."
> Hippocrates

CHAPTER 19

WHY DOES THE BODY ATTACK ITSELF?

What do lupus, Sjogren's syndrome, Hashimoto's thyroiditis, Graves' disease, rheumatoid arthritis, juvenile (type 1) diabetes, fibromyalgia, multiple sclerosis, irritable bowel syndrome, psoriasis, and asthma have in common? They're all autoimmune disorders. According to Wikipedia,[1] autoimmunity is "the system of immune responses of an organism against its own healthy cells and tissues." Why would the body attack itself?

In order to understand autoimmunity, we need to understand how the immune system works. In a healthy person, the immune system will launch an attack on foreign invaders (bacteria, viruses, etc.) to protect the body from disease.

There are, however, people whose immune systems don't work properly. Instead of attacking foreign invaders, the immune system attacks healthy tissue. Why does this happen?

"All Disease Begins in the Gut"

Hippocrates said that all disease begins in the gut. Certainly, some diseases, like genetic diseases, don't start in the gut, but for just about everything else, the gut is where it all begins.

The reason for this is the different gut bacteria[2] residing in our digestive tracts, as well as the integrity of the gut lining. According to numerous studies, the lining of the small intestine can become porous and unwanted bacterial products called endotoxins[3] can sometimes leak through the lining and enter the bloodstream.

Additionally, undigested proteins can also leak out into the bloodstream. Proteins that many people can't digest such as gluten (from grains) and casein (from dairy products) can end up in the bloodstream.

CHAPTER 19 - WHY DOES THE BODY ATTACK ITSELF?

This is called leaky gut syndrome. For many years, the traditional medical community did not recognize this disease, but now it's known to them as intestinal permeability.[4]

Autoimmune Disorder Begins

Once these 'foreign' objects enter the bloodstream, the body chooses to store them in an organ, gland, or other tissue. When enough of these foreign particles are stored in the same area, the immune system takes notice and mounts an attack[5] against them and the organ/gland/tissue in which they reside.

If, for example, these foreign invaders are stored in the thyroid (a gland), the immune system attacks the thyroid. Then we have symptoms of thyroid disease and we call it Hashimoto's disease (hypothyroid) or Graves' disease (hyperthyroid).

If the invaders are stored in the fascia (a system of connective tissue), the symptoms are called fibromyalgia. If the symptoms manifest themselves in a rash, it's called psoriasis or eczema.

If autoimmunity is left unchecked, multiple glands/organs/systems will be filled with foreign invaders and attacked by the immune system, which then manifests in many different autoimmune disorders.

It can take years of attacks before one recognizes what is happening. For myself, the attacks have spread to my thyroid (Hashimoto's), fascia (fibromyalgia), skin (psoriasis and eczema), and lungs (asthma), among others.

What Causes Leaky Gut Syndrome?

See a list of causes of leaky gut syndrome in chapter 17.

According to research published in the *International Journal of Gastroenterology and Hepatology 2006*,[6] leaky gut syndrome may cause Hashimoto's Thyroiditis, rheumatoid arthritis, fibromyalgia, psoriasis, multiple sclerosis, lupus, depression, and anxiety.

CHAPTER 19 - WHY DOES THE BODY ATTACK ITSELF?

How to Restore the Gut

The traditional medicinal answer to autoimmunity is to prescribe immunosuppressants, such as steroids. Unfortunately, while suppressing the immune system may lead to some relief of symptoms, it can also leave one open to other infections. Suppressing the entire immune system indefinitely is not a good idea.

Fortunately, there is a way to restore the gut that is simple and inexpensive. It does, however, require a change of mindset. It required me to change what I eat.

This is the simplest, yet the most difficult, part. I eat real food. Whole food. Non-processed food. Food without additives. A list of what I ate (and still eat) to regain (and maintain) my health is in chapter 24.

It's simple because this food doesn't come in boxes or cans. It comes from the farmer and the rancher, the fisher and the gatherer. This food comes in a rainbow of colors. It's full of flavor and nutrients that the body recognizes.

It was difficult because I didn't grow up eating real food and I wasn't used to it. My taste buds had been impaired by sugar and processed foods, so real food didn't taste good (until my body purged the sugar; then real food was delicious).

Processed foods are more readily available, and our culture likes to eat on the go. When we go out or visit with others, they usually offer processed, sugary foods. So, it did take a resolve to change the way I eat.

In chapter 50 are some recipes that I like; however, I've found that keeping it simple is best. For breakfast, I make my Super Restoring Smoothie. For lunch, I usually have a baked sweet potato (with ghee, Himalayan pink salt, Ceylon cinnamon, and some walnuts or pecans) and a mug of bone broth. For dinner, I'll pick a protein and a veggie (e.g., salmon and asparagus; scrambled eggs and zucchini; taco salad). My go-to snack is homemade applesauce or a nut mix of raw, unsalted walnuts, pistachios, and macadamia nuts.

CHAPTER 19 - WHY DOES THE BODY ATTACK ITSELF?

What I Avoid

The list of what not to eat grows as new, fake foods come on the market seemingly daily. Here are the top foods I avoid:

- Sugar
- Cow's Dairy (A1)
- Grains
- Legumes (including peanuts and peanut oil)
- Shellfish
- Pork
- Nightshades
- GMO food[7] like corn
- Food additives like flavorings, colorings, MSG[8], etc.
- Pasteurized food[9]
- Soy products
- Processed food
- Vegetable oils (canola, corn, sunflower, cottonseed, palm, rapeseed)
- Anything I'm allergic to or intolerant of (see chapter 26)

Why I Changed What I Eat

I never connected how I felt to what I ate, yet food is fuel for the body. You wouldn't put water in your car's fuel tank and expect it to run properly, would you? Our bodies were made to withstand a lot of punishment, but at some point, they can't handle any more abuse and they break down. Just because you're not sick doesn't mean you're healthy.

Most food sold in the U.S. is unhealthy, and the government is making it more difficult[10] for citizens to know what's in the food we eat. In fact,

CHAPTER 19 - WHY DOES THE BODY ATTACK ITSELF?

because of the National Bioengineered Food Disclosure Standard (otherwise known as the DARK Act, for Deny Americans the Right to Know) that became U.S. law in 2016, the USDA in 2018 announced these ways that food producers can now label their GMO food:

- QR codes that must be scanned by the consumer with a smartphone.
- Text messages. The consumer must initiate the process by texting the company then wait for their reply.
- Symbols such as smiley faces that contain the letters "BE" (for bioengineered) instead of GMO or GE.

Changing what I eat was one of the things I did to restore my health from leaky gut syndrome, and thus, autoimmune disorder.

CHAPTER 19 - WHY DOES THE BODY ATTACK ITSELF?

CHAPTER 20

SPIRITUAL REASONS THE BODY ATTACKS ITSELF

Many of the people I work with struggle with autoimmune disorders like Hashimoto's thyroiditis, fibromyalgia, lupus, rheumatoid arthritis, multiple sclerosis, asthma, psoriasis, IBS, vitiligo, coeliac disease, etc. From a physical perspective, we know that leaky gut syndrome is usually the culprit, leading the immune system to attack the body (see chapter 19).

However, there's often an underlying spiritual cause to what we see in the physical realm. Sometimes we need to pull back the curtain and expose the darkness to light. Why is the body attacking itself? The most common spiritual reason for this is self-hate, not loving oneself as one should.

Having an Autoimmune Disorder Sucks

I know. Usually, there's more than one manifestation. Myself, I've suffered from asthma, fibromyalgia, Hashimoto's, IBS (irritable bowel syndrome), and psoriasis, (among others). My immune system was attacking many different parts of my body. One cause, many manifestations.

Why Isn't What I'm Doing Working?

I was doing my best to restore health to my body. I made all the changes I knew I should; I changed my diet, reduced toxins in my body and my environment, and added supplements and essential oils to my routine. I checked with my doctor to make sure there were no underlying health problems like anemia or diabetes. I saw great improvements, I felt better, I lost some weight. But I still didn't feel 100% healthy.

Time to look at the spiritual causes of sickness. Time to check in with my heavenly Father and get His guidance. What is seen on the surface is the manifestation of something much deeper. Usually, when there's a chronic symptom that doesn't go away when healing has been ministered in the name of Jesus Christ, there's a spiritual cause (meaning either a devil spirit – usually a spirit of infirmity – is causing the problem, or one's thoughts/emotions are preventing healing from being received).

What Am I Telling My Body?

It has been said that health is a mirror of one's relationship with oneself. In other words, the body will reflect the messages it's being sent. How do I feel about myself? What messages am I sending to my body?

Am I looking in the mirror and thinking how much I hate my nose, or my thighs, or some other body part? Do I berate myself for my failings, real or perceived? How does my body respond after years of being told I hate it?

These responses are understood by a new field of science called epigenetics. Epigenetics is the study of changes in organisms caused by modification of gene expression rather than alteration of the genetic code itself.

For example, two people have leaky gut syndrome, which is very prevalent in our society due to the foods we eat and the medicines we take. One of these people develops an autoimmune disorder while the other doesn't. The difference between the two is not the physical presence of leaky gut syndrome, but rather how other factors flip a switch, so to speak, that turns on the autoimmune response.

Spiritual Causes of Autoimmune Disorders

If the problem is simply the presence of a devil spirit, it's easily removed in the name of Jesus Christ. No condemnation is necessary in this situation; just take spiritual control and demand that it leave. It must obey the name of Jesus Christ.

Ask God to make you aware of the thoughts you have that are contributing to self-hate (rejection, condemnation, fear, self-righteousness, judgment (of yourself and others), self-unforgiveness, self-resentment, etc.). He will certainly bring them to your attention, so

CHAPTER 20 – SPIRITUAL REASONS THE BODY ATTACKS ITSELF

you can cut off the thought process and start thinking loving thoughts about yourself instead.

> *2 Corinthians 10:3-5 ESV*
> *For though we walk in the flesh, we are not waging war according to the flesh.*
>
> *For the weapons of our warfare are not of the flesh but have divine power to destroy strongholds.*
>
> *We destroy arguments and every lofty opinion raised against the knowledge of God, and take every thought captive to obey Christ,*

Strongholds are thought patterns that are entrenched. They're things you've been thinking for a very long time and they've worn a groove in your mind so that they tend to replay themselves without much prompting.

Our thoughts and our emotions are very much intertwined. There's a way to change your response to memories that in the past may have brought up negative emotions. You can find more information about this in chapter 29.

Who Are You in Christ?

We are to examine our every thought to make sure they line up with what God says. What does God say about you? His is the only opinion that counts. You are in Christ; you are as Christ to God and in this world. Fill your mind with scriptures that keep your thoughts focused on this. Here are some scriptures to get you started.

> *1 John 3:1 NIV*
> *See what great love the Father has lavished on us, that we should be called children of God! And that is what we are! The reason the world does not know us is that it did not know him.*
>
> *Ephesians 1:5 NIV*
> *He [God] predestined us for adoption to sonship through Jesus Christ, in accordance with his pleasure and will*

CHAPTER 20 – SPIRITUAL REASONS THE BODY ATTACKS ITSELF

Galatians 4:6-7 NIV
Because you are his sons, God sent the Spirit of his Son into our hearts, the Spirit who calls out, "Abba, Father."

So you are no longer a slave, but God's child; and since you are his child, God has made you also an heir.

Ephesians 1:4 NIV
For he chose us in him before the creation of the world to be holy and blameless in his sight.

Colossians 1:21-22 NIV
Once you were alienated from God and were enemies in your minds because of your evil behavior.

But now he has reconciled you by Christ's physical body through death to present you holy in his sight, without blemish and free from accusation

Romans 5:17 NIV
For if, by the trespass of the one man [Adam], death reigned through that one man, how much more will those who receive God's abundant provision of grace and of the gift of righteousness reign in life through the one man, Jesus Christ!

Romans 12:2 NIV
Do not conform to the pattern of this world, but be transformed by the renewing of your mind. Then you will be able to test and approve what God's will is—his good, pleasing and perfect will.

Renewing your mind to God's Word (replacing worldly thoughts with God's thoughts) allows God to transform you (see chapter 1). This is our daily job. The benefits are priceless. We can be free from autoimmune disorders.

CHAPTER 21

I HURT ALL OVER. DO I HAVE FIBROMYALGIA?

It happened out of the blue. I was newly married and very happy. Yet, shortly after we moved into the new home we built, it hit me like a ton of bricks. Pain. Fatigue. Brain fog (although I didn't know what to call it at the time). All I knew was that I couldn't function like I had the day before. You may be saying the same thing. "I hurt all over. Do I have fibromyalgia?"

Back then, I had never heard of fibromyalgia. Most of the many doctors I visited had never heard of it, either. They told me it was "all in my head." They looked at me like I was crazy.

But, I'm not crazy. I'm an intelligent, spiritually-minded woman with many reasons to live. Yet, here I was, in my mid-30's, feeling like a cross between a newborn baby who needed to sleep all day, and someone bent over with unrelenting pain.

What is Fibromyalgia?

Fibromyalgia, also called fibrositis (inflammation of the fibrous connective tissue called fascia [1]), is an autoimmune disorder that is characterized by widespread muscle pain and tenderness. The pain can be dull and aching or sharp and pointed. Sometimes it was both at the same time. My muscles seemed to be in a constant state of spasm.

The pain made it very difficult to sleep. My husband and I established a routine. I would lie with a pillow under my stomach (since lying on my back made it difficult for me to breathe – asthma – and lying on my side made my hips ache). My husband would place ice packs up and down my back. I would sleep in this position for a couple of hours until the ice packs became warm. Then I would get up for a few hours. Then we would repeat the process. Not the best way to get a restful night of sleep for either of us.

CHAPTER 21 – I HURT ALL OVER. DO I HAVE FIBROMYALGIA?

The third part of my symptoms was a feeling of cognitive dullness. I felt as though there was a veil over my brain. I could read a book and not know what I had read. I had difficulty remembering the simplest things. This is what is referred to as brain fog.

There were other unpleasant symptoms: gastrointestinal issues like irritable bowel syndrome, sensitivity to cold and pain, tingling in the extremities, anxiety, and depression (hey, who wouldn't be depressed if you felt like that all the time?).

Fibromyalgia symptoms can come and go. I could go days or weeks without incapacitating symptoms, then experience a fibro-flare. The triggers for flares can vary by person, but these are some of the most common:[2]

- Physical or psychological stress
- Temperature and/weather changes
- Hormonal changes
- Traveling and/or changes in schedule
- Changes in treatment
- Diet
- Poor sleep (which is kind of an endless loop, in that a symptom of fibromyalgia is poor sleep, which then triggers more symptoms)

Fibromyalgia affects about 3 million new people every year. It can only be diagnosed by a doctor. Medical conditions such as lupus, arthritis, chronic fatigue syndrome, hypothyroidism, Lyme disease, and others must be ruled out. Everyone experiences fibromyalgia in a slightly different way; that is why it's referred to as a syndrome: someone can experience some, many, or all symptoms.

If you're experiencing widespread pain and tenderness for at least three months in all four quadrants of the body, you may have fibromyalgia. When I was finally diagnosed after 5 years, I had tenderness or pain in 13 out of 18 specified tender points when pressure is applied. (To receive the diagnosis, you must have pain or tenderness in at least 11 of the 18 points.)

What Causes Fibromyalgia?

Fibromyalgia is an autoimmune disorder, meaning the body is attacking itself. See chapter 19.

How to Deal with Fibromyalgia

Autoimmune disorders are caused by leaky gut syndrome. See a list of causes of leaky gut syndrome in chapter 17.

As I've mentioned, the traditional medical community's answer to autoimmunity is immunosuppressants, such as steroids. Fortunately, there is a way to restore the gut that is simple and inexpensive. It does, however, require a change of mindset. It required me to change what I eat.

This is the simplest, yet the most difficult, part. I eat real food. Whole food. Non-processed food. Food without additives. See the list of foods I ate to restore my health in chapter 19.

In chapter 50 are some recipes that I like; however, I've found that keeping it simple is best.

The list of what not to eat grows as new, fake foods come on the market seemingly daily. A list of the top foods I avoid is in chapter 19.

Today, I'm mostly free of fibromyalgia symptoms. I can sleep through the night without heat or ice. I don't have to use a TENS (Transcutaneous Electrical Nerve Stimulator) device around the clock anymore. I can exercise without pain or fatigue. The brain fog is gone. I feel like I have my life back.

CHAPTER 21 – I HURT ALL OVER. DO I HAVE FIBROMYALGIA?

CHAPTER 22

THYROID, HORMONES, AND AUTOIMMUNE

The thyroid gland is a butterfly-shaped endocrine gland located in the lower front of the neck. The thyroid's job is to make thyroid hormones, which are secreted into the blood and carried to every cell in the body. Thyroid hormone helps the body use energy, stay warm, and keep other organs working properly.

According to Healthline, [1] the most common thyroid disorders are hyperthyroidism and hypothyroidism.

Hyperthyroidism

Hyperthyroidism happens when the thyroid gland is overactive, producing too much thyroid hormone. Hyperthyroidism affects about 1 percent of women, less in men.

Hyperthyroidism is usually caused by Graves' disease, which is an autoimmune disorder. Graves' disease usually results in an enlarged thyroid.

Symptoms of hyperthyroidism include:

- Restlessness
- Nervousness
- Racing heart
- Irritability
- Increased sweating
- Shaking
- Anxiety
- Trouble sleeping
- Thin skin

- Brittle hair and nails
- Muscle weakness
- Weight loss
- Bulging eyes (in Graves' disease)

Hypothyroidism

Hypothyroidism is the opposite of hyperthyroidism. The thyroid gland is underactive, not producing enough of its hormones. Hypothyroidism is often caused by Hashimoto's disease, an autoimmune disorder. In this case, the thyroid gland is gradually being destroyed. Hypothyroidism is thought to affect up to 9% of the U.S. population, mainly women.

Too little thyroid hormone production leads to symptoms such as:

- Fatigue
- Dry skin
- Increased sensitivity to cold
- Memory problems
- Constipation
- Depression
- Weight gain
- Weakness
- Slow heart rate

Dr. Izabella Wentz, PharmD, says that 95% of those with hypothyroidism may actually have Hashimoto's (an autoimmune disorder).[2]

For years, I suffered from Hashimoto's, although it was just diagnosed recently. For a very long time, I was told that all the blood markers for thyroid disease came back negative. In other words, the fatigue, sensitivity to cold, weight gain, etc. didn't have a physiological cause. ("It's all in your head.") Far too many people suffer like this.

CHAPTER 22 – THYROID, HORMONES, AND AUTOIMMUNE

There are two ways to detect hypothyroidism: blood tests and basal body temperature. I diagnosed myself using the latter. My doctor then reluctantly agreed to put me on thyroid medication and lo and behold, my symptoms lessened considerably.

Dr. Wentz recommends the following be included when blood testing for thyroid function:[3] TSH, Free T4, Free T3, TPO and Tg antibodies, and Reverse T3. Her website, https://ThyroidPharmacist.com, has more information that may be helpful.

An average basal (lowest) body temperature (BBT) between 97.8° and 98.2° Fahrenheit is considered normal. Temperatures from 97.6° to 98.0° Fahrenheit are considered evidence of possible hypothyroidism, and temperatures less than 97.6° can be even more indicative of hypothyroidism.

To use the BBT method, take your temperature every morning <u>before you get out of bed</u> for two weeks and record your temperature. This will give you a pattern that you and your doctor can discuss. You can buy a basal thermometer at most pharmacies. Dr. Alan Christianson, N.M.D., has good information about BBT testing on his website, https://DrChristianson.com.[4]

The Autoimmune Connection

As you know, autoimmune disorder is caused when endotoxins and proteins escape the gut into the bloodstream and are stored in various places in the body. The immune system then starts attacking both these foreign invaders and the healthy tissue where they're residing. In the case of the thyroid, this attack causes the thyroid to lose its ability to make thyroid hormones.

Dr. Wentz says that "Hashimoto's, and the autoimmune process, likely developed 5-10 years prior to the time of diagnosis. In the early stages, the TSH screening test for Hashimoto's often comes up normal [it did for me-CR]. In the later stages of Hashimoto's, the TSH will become elevated, allowing doctors to make a diagnosis of hypothyroidism. Testing for thyroid antibodies can help a person determine that they

CHAPTER 22 – THYROID, HORMONES, AND AUTOIMMUNE

have Hashimoto's and can uncover the condition many years before there is a change in TSH." [5]

Getting the Right Dose

According to Dr. Wentz, "In recent years, The National Academy of Clinical Biochemists indicated that 95% of individuals without thyroid disease have TSH concentrations below 2.5 µIU/L, and a new normal reference range was defined by the American College of Clinical Endocrinologists to be between 0.3- 3.0 µIU/ml in 2012." [6] Unfortunately, most labs haven't recognized these new levels so many patients with thyroid disease aren't getting the proper dosage of their medications.

If you still experience symptoms even though you take thyroid medication, increasing your dosage may help. Talk to your doctor. If it doesn't help, you may want to consider bioidentical hormones.

Bioidentical Hormones

A client of mine I'll call Sue adopted the Be in Health lifestyle, changed the way she eats, and was taking thyroid medication, yet she was still experiencing "fatigue, dry skin, thinning hair, foggy-brain issues, and persistent low-grade depression." She went to a new doctor who told her her thyroid levels were fine but offered no relief for her symptoms.

I was 43 when I began experiencing peri-menopause symptoms. My gynecologist said I was too young, so I suffered for five years with fatigue, anxiety/depression, insomnia, brain fog, vaginal dryness, and lack of libido, even though I was taking thyroid medication. Then a friend recommended I see Dr. Joseph Collins, R.N., N.D., author of *Discover Your Menopause Type: The Exciting New Program That Identifies the 12 Unique Menopause Types & The Best Choices for You.*

Dr. Collins was able to identify my menopause type quickly (even though I was still in peri-menopause) and prescribed bioidentical hormones. These turned out to be a lifesaver for me, my sanity, and probably my marriage. Since then, I've let my clients know about them.

Sue started taking bioidentical hormones. Here's what she says: "In general, I feel much better overall. Less fatigue and discomfort throughout my body. Less physical restlessness. Depression occurs less and less. Libido exists."

History of HRT

The first replacements for progesterone and estrogens (hormone replacement therapy or HRT) hit the U.S. market in the 1960s. Millions of women found relief. Then, in 2002, the results of the *Women's Health Initiative* (WHI) came out. The study, which included over 16,000 postmenopausal women, found the combination of non-bioidentical estrogen and progestin to significantly increase the risk of breast cancer and heart attack.[7] It also found an increased risk of stroke in non-bioidentical estrogen users,[8] among other risks. Women stopped using HRT despite having their symptoms return.

According to *Forever Health*,[9] "Bioidentical hormones, which have the same molecular structure as the hormones produced in the body, have actually been shown to have a protective effect against some diseases, including those whose risk is increased by non-bioidentical hormones. In a study, women who used non-bioidentical estrogen and progestin had a 69% greater risk of developing invasive breast cancer over an eight-year period in comparison with non-HRT users. Those who used bioidentical estrogen and progesterone experienced a similar risk as non-HRT users."[10]

My doctor and I have discussed my use of bioidentical hormones and have concluded that the benefits outweigh the risks for me. For millions of women, they're the missing link. You and God and your doctor can decide together if they're right for you.

CHAPTER 22 – THYROID, HORMONES, AND AUTOIMMUNE

CHAPTER 23

WHAT CAN BE DONE ABOUT IBS

For many people, the very first sign of autoimmune disorder is IBS, irritable bowel syndrome. IBS is characterized by alternating diarrhea and constipation, indigestion, nausea, passing excessive amounts of gas, and other gastrointestinal distress. Because it's a syndrome, you don't have to have all the symptoms to be diagnosed with IBS. As many as 60% of people with IBS also have fibromyalgia. Both are caused by leaky gut syndrome. In this chapter, we'll look at four unsettling symptoms of IBS and what can be done about it.

Many people will tell you that IBS can't be cured and can only be treated with medications. I suffered from IBS for over a decade and it's now gone. I'm going to show you what I did to receive deliverance.

The Underlying Cause

The underlying cause of IBS is leaky gut syndrome. According to numerous studies, the lining of the small intestine can become porous and unwanted bacterial products called endotoxins, [1] as well as undigested proteins, can sometimes leak through the lining and enter the bloodstream. This is called leaky gut syndrome. For many years, the traditional medical community did not recognize this disease, but now it's known to them as intestinal permeability. [2]

When this happens, the immune system thinks these molecules are foreign invaders and mounts an attack[3] against them, resulting in a chronic inflammatory response.

See a list of causes of leaky gut syndrome in chapter 17.

Symptoms

Remember, IBS is a syndrome, so not everyone experiences all of the symptoms. Symptoms may even change over time.

CHAPTER 23 – WHAT CAN BE DONE ABOUT IBS

<u>Frequent Constipation</u>. Constipation can be caused by IBS or by a food or medication so it's advisable to see a doctor to rule out other conditions. Once IBS was diagnosed, I used these supplements to overcome constipation (but not all at the same time).

- One teaspoon of ICP [4] twice per day.
- Flax Seed Oil or Cod Liver Oil. 1 tablespoon of either flax or cod liver oil mixed with carrot juice every day.
- ComforTone, [5] a combination of herbs and essential oils to support digestive health. This was my favorite and the most effective for me.
- AlkaLime[6] to help my body stay in proper pH balance. I continue to use this.

<u>Stomach Distress</u>. Stomach pain, gas, cramps, indigestion, and bloating are common IBS symptoms. I found it helpful to keep a food journal (see chapter 49) to see if any of the foods I was eating were connected to gastrointestinal distress.

<u>Incomplete Bowel Movements</u>. Many people with IBS struggle to move their bowels, even over several days trying to completely empty the bowels. I found a change of diet helped.

<u>Diarrhea</u>. Diarrhea is very common in IBS. Again, make sure you **check with your doctor to rule out any more serious conditions**. I experienced alternating diarrhea and constipation, which made for a not-so-fun roller coaster ride. I avoided dairy products, caffeine, alcohol, and greasy, fatty, and spicy foods, and tried bland foods instead. I stayed away from OTC medications that stop diarrhea. Instead, I used these:

- Bentonite clay. I drank food grade bentonite clay almost every day, 1/2 to 1 teaspoon once per day. I mixed the clay with water in a jar with a lid, so I could shake the clay and make it dissolve, then I drank it right away. I always take bentonite clay a few hours before or after taking medications; bentonite clay binds toxins in the body and will bind medications if taken too close together.

- AlkaLime[7] to help my body stay in proper pH balance.
- L-glutamine powder (5 grams 2x daily). L-glutamine is an amino acid that helps repair the digestive tract, especially important for people with chronic diarrhea.

Spiritual Causes

Remember, there's often an underlying spiritual cause to everything we see in the physical realm. Sometimes we need to pull back the curtain and expose the darkness to light. I discuss the spiritual causes of autoimmune disorder (including IBS) in chapter 20. My road to restoring my body to health began here.

CHAPTER 23 – WHAT CAN BE DONE ABOUT IBS

PART 6

BE IN HEALTH

The best way to restore health to our bodies is to cooperate with God's ways of health, rather than living cross purpose to them.

CHAPTER 24

OVERVIEW OF THE BE IN HEALTH LIFESTYLE

I call the plan I developed to restore my body to health the Be in Health lifestyle. It's not so much about what to do; it's a way of being. It encompasses the body, the soul, and the spirit. Health and wellness, wholeness, means nothing is missing and nothing is broken.

This lifestyle addresses spirit (my relationship with my heavenly Father God and His son Jesus Christ), body (what I eat and the things my body is exposed to), and soul (my thoughts and emotions).

Spirit health is the most important part of anyone's state of being. There are ways to improve spirit health scattered throughout this book. We are to put off the thoughts from the world and put on the mind of Christ. As a child of God, this is the first step toward a state of being in health.

Soul health includes thoughts and emotions. I address thoughts in chapters 1, 2, 5, 8, 9, 16, 20, 29, 40, 41, 43, 51, 52, 53, 54, and 55. Emotions are discussed in chapters 18, 20, 27, 29, 34, 49, 52, and 54.

The body part of the Be in Health lifestyle combines a healthy eating plan for leaky gut syndrome restoration with a Food Reintroduction Challenge, as well as a plan for reducing toxin exposure (Part 7).

Here are some of the benefits I've experienced from this lifestyle:

- Clarity on what was causing my health problems.
- It's a form of gentle detox. I felt lighter, brighter, and sharper as a result.
- People tell me that I'm glowing and look healthier than they've ever seen me.

Implementing the Lifestyle

- I prayed and set my goals for this new lifestyle with God's input. I knew that mental and spiritual changes would be necessary.

CHAPTER 24 – OVERVIEW OF THE BE IN HEALTH LIFESTYLE

- I recommend that readers of this book go through it once to get an overview of the lifestyle so there are no surprises.
- I started using the FMP Journal (chapter 49). I did NOT change anything about the way I was eating for the first five days. I just wrote down everything I ate and drank, how I felt, and I described my bowel movements via the Bristol Stool Chart (chapter 49).
- After five days of journaling, because I was dealing with severe leaky gut syndrome, I started with a 3-day 'fast' of bone broth (also called collagen therapy), cooked vegetables, and raw (unpasteurized), local honey (up to 1 Tbsp. per day). This gave my body a head-start toward health restoration.
- After the 3-day fast, I started eating:
  - Complex carbohydrates: vegetables, low fructose fruits, and raw (unpasteurized), local honey (up to 1 Tbsp. per day). These are the quickest sources of energy.
  - Easily digestible fats: coconut oil, olive oil, and avocado oil
  - Easily digestible protein: wild-caught fish, pasture raised chicken and turkey, and 100% grass-fed and finished beef and lamb
  - Bone broth (see recipe in chapter 50)
  - Probiotic-rich foods (like sauerkraut and kefir)
- I started taking probiotics, digestive enzymes, and other supplements I needed (chapter 28).
- I implemented the colon cleanse (chapter 28).
- I supported my body systems and cleared out negative emotions with essential oils (chapter 29).
- I started reducing my toxin exposure (chapter 41).

PART 7

HOW I RESTORED MY BODY TO HEALTH

"If we could give every individual the right amount of nourishment and exercise, not too little and not too much, we would have found the safest way to health."
Hippocrates

CHAPTER 25

HOW I CHANGED WHAT I EAT

To restore my health, I knew I needed to change what I eat. My digestive system needed to rest. Food doesn't restore health to the body, the body does that itself, which is how God designed it. So, I gave my body the building blocks it needed to repair itself. I ate foods that are easy to digest.

Many people with severe leaky gut syndrome find that starting with a 'fast' of bone broth (also called collagen therapy), cooked vegetables, and raw (unpasteurized), local honey (up to 1 Tbsp. per day) for a few days will give their bodies a head start toward health restoration.

The Be in Health Lifestyle

The Be in Health lifestyle combines a healthy eating plan for leaky gut syndrome restoration with a Food Reintroduction Challenge (chapter 27), as well as a plan for reducing toxin load. A list of some of the benefits I experienced from this lifestyle is in chapter 24.

At least 70% of the immune system is in the lining of the gut. This means that a healthy gut contributes to overall health, and an unhealthy gut leads to a myriad of health problems.

How I Feel Living the Be in Health Lifestyle

- Freed of the symptoms I started with
- Energized
- Sharper in mind and spirit
- Slimmer. When the body is chronically inflamed it stores fat. (That's why that stubborn belly fat never wanted to go away.)
- Radiant; people tell me my eyes and skin glow
- Excited, knowing I've prevented future chronic diseases

CHAPTER 25 – HOW I CHANGED WHAT I EAT

Potential Detox Symptoms

The Be in Health lifestyle is a gentle form of detox. There are two reasons for this:

1. Eliminating processed food led to the elimination of the toxins my body stored from the processed foods I had previously eaten
2. Eliminating food that my body is sensitive to led my body to release the toxins my body stored from previously eating those foods

Some potential detox symptoms include:

- Fatigue (but only in the first 2-3 days)
- Weird dreams
- Body odor
- White coating on the tongue
- Film-like coating on the teeth
- Pimples
- Moodiness
- Nausea
- Poor sleep
- Headaches

For more information on toxin release and how to deal with it, see chapter 44. **If you experience detox symptoms that you're unable to handle, please talk to your doctor.**

What I Eat

A list of what I ate (and still eat) to regain (and maintain) my health is in chapter 24.

CHAPTER 25 – HOW I CHANGED WHAT I EAT

Substitutions

I changed my eating habits by eliminating sugars (chapter 33), dairy (chapter 11), grains and legumes (chapter 10), shellfish (chapter 4), pork (chapter 15), nightshades (chapter 14), and other irritating foods (chapter 27) to alleviate the inflammation and starve out the yeast overgrowth. I found the best way to do this is by making substitutions.

- Instead of sugar, I use stevia or raw (unpasteurized), local honey (up to 1 tablespoon per day). Sugar is the number one enemy of health, contributing to everything from diabetes, obesity, and cancer to tooth decay and cardiovascular disease.

- Instead of processed meat, I eat fresh 100% grass-fed and finished beef and lamb, and pasture raised poultry. (It's helpful to develop a relationship with a local farmer/rancher.)

- Instead of farm-raised fish, I eat wild-caught fish.

- Instead of tilapia, I eat wild-caught salmon. Farm-raised tilapia can cause inflammation and have been found to contain high concentrations of pesticides and antibiotics.[1]

- I don't eat shellfish or pork (see Old Testament dietary principles in chapter 4).

- Instead of gluten-filled flour products, I eat coconut flour and almond flour products I make myself (no store-bought processed foods).

- I buy organic as much as possible, paying attention to The Clean 15 List and The Dirty Dozen List.[2] This saves me money on shopping because I know which foods should always be purchased organic and which I can get non-organic. (Not everyone can afford organic or sustainable food. This article[3] provides good information and guidelines.)

- I drink bone broth every day. **This is probably the most restoring thing I can do for my gut.**

CHAPTER 25 – HOW I CHANGED WHAT I EAT

- Instead of hydrogenated oils like canola oil, I use coconut oil, avocado oil, and olive oil.
- Instead of butter (a dairy product), I use coconut oil or ghee.
- Instead of white potatoes (including French fries), I eat sweet potatoes (sweet potatoes fries are awesome).
- Instead of raw nuts and seeds, I sprout them[4] first by soaking them in purified water overnight, then drying them out in a low oven, then use as normal. (I stay away from peanuts/peanut butter altogether. They're highly allergenic and are susceptible to contaminants like mold and aflatoxin, a known carcinogen.[5])
- Instead of table salt, I use Himalayan pink salt.
- Instead of eating raw food, I eat cooked food. Eating raw food is harder on the digestive system than eating cooked food.[6]
- Instead of coffee or soda, I drink purified water (not tap water) and herbal teas. Bottled water isn't good because it often contains fluoride,[7] a neurotoxin, and the plastic from the bottle can leach[8] into the water.
- Limit alcohol to 1 glass of red or white wine per day (if necessary). I think of alcohol as liquid sugar, making it easier for me to stay away from it.

In other words, I eat fresh, real, whole food instead of dead, processed, GMO food.

Depending on the severity of one's leaky gut syndrome, changes may be noticed fairly quickly. For me, as well as others with severe leaky gut syndrome, it took a year or more for health restoration to be completely manifested. After time, many people are able to go back to conventional dairy and (sprouted) grains, although I don't do it (for reasons listed elsewhere in this book).

CHAPTER 25 – HOW I CHANGED WHAT I EAT

Growing My Own Food

I liked the idea of growing my own food but none of my gardens in the past were successful. I didn't like having to get out in the harsh summer sun and pull weeds. It was rough on my back. Water, weed, water, weed. Then I found the Tower Garden®.

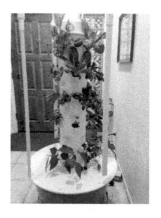

The Tower Garden® is a vertical, aeroponic growing system that allows me to grow up to 20 vegetables, herbs, fruits, and flowers in less than three square feet — indoors or out.

Using aeroponics — the same technology NASA uses — the Tower Garden® grows plants with only water and nutrients rather than soil. Research has found aeroponic systems grow plants three times faster and produce 30% greater yields on average.

Food grown using the Tower Garden® contains far more nutrients than soil-grown food.[9] The fact is the soil in the United States is depleted of minerals. In 1936, yes, over 80 years ago, the U.S. Senate was presented with the results of a scientific study[10] it had commissioned on the mineral content of our food. The results demonstrated that many human ills could be attributed to the fact that American soil no longer provided plants with the mineral elements that are so essential to human nourishment and health. Things haven't improved since then.

I've done two growing seasons so far: summer/fall and winter/spring. For both, I used my Tower Garden® outside. It did well despite the fierce Arizona summer. I've decided to do this coming summer season indoors using a light kit.

I've enjoyed being able to harvest directly from my Tower Garden® into my smoothie or salad. The best crops for me have been various types of lettuce, kale, chard, basil, parsley, mint, scallions, and oregano. I'm looking forward to trying cilantro, spinach, thyme, rosemary, bush beans, and various squashes/zucchini, among others.

CHAPTER 25 – HOW I CHANGED WHAT I EAT

The Tower Garden® is available online at TowerGarden.com. I am not a representative for Tower Garden® or its parent company, Juice Plus+.

Tips for Healthier Cooking

I replaced my non-stick cookware with stainless steel. According to TIBBS (UNC School of Medicine's Training Initiatives in Biomedical & Biological Sciences) Bioscience Blog, "The most common non-stick coating used to coat pots and pans is Teflon™, a chemical mixture of perfluorochemicals (chemicals with lots of fluoride atoms). Developed by the DuPont chemical company in 1938, these chemicals are extremely non-polar, meaning they do a very good job repelling other chemicals. As such, Teflon™ is used as an additive to paints, fabrics, carpets, and clothing. It's also used to treat materials to make them resistant to oils (like the inside of microwave popcorn bags). The primary chemical in Teflon™, polytetrafluoroethylene (PTFE), has a high melting point (327 ºC), making it ideal for cooking applications. However, when heated to temperatures above 350 ºC (662 ºF), PTFE begins to degrade, releasing fine particles and a variety of gaseous compounds that can cause damage to the lungs when inhaled (Waritz, 1975)." [11]

The blog continues, "Numerous case studies in the 1900s have documented flu-like symptoms after inhalation of PTFE fumes by workers in PTFE-using factories and by people overheating non-stick pans in the kitchen. This condition is called polymer fume fever, or 'Teflon™ flu,' and presents with temporary, intense, but not serious symptoms such as fever, shivering, sore throat and coughing (Harris, 1951 & Shumizu, 2012). These cases of Teflon™ flu are due to acute (short-term) exposures to PTFE fumes; no studies have been done looking at the long-term effects of brief, repeated PTFE-fume exposure, as would be the case in cooking using non-stick pans for a lifetime." [12]

Because of this, I felt it's best for me to switch to stainless steel for all my pots and pans.

I heat or reheat food on the stovetop, not in the microwave. According to GlobalHealingCenter.com, "Microwaving cooks the food at very high temperatures in a very short amount of time. This results in a great deal

CHAPTER 25 – HOW I CHANGED WHAT I EAT

of nutrient loss for most foods, especially vegetables." [13] For this reason, I don't cook my food in a microwave. I reheat food by steaming it on the cooktop.

Eating healthy means I can eat until I'm satisfied and not go hungry.

CHAPTER 25 – HOW I CHANGED WHAT I EAT

CHAPTER 26

FOOD ALLERGY OR FOOD INTOLERANCE?

A food allergy is when the immune system engages right after you have consumed, inhaled, or touched a food you're allergic to. The reaction is immediate; it could be a rash, itching, swelling, dizziness, vomiting, teary eyes, tight throat, etc. An IgE test (immunoglobulin E) will tell you what allergies you might have. It's important to stay away from food, pets, and molds that we have an allergy to as they over-stimulate the immune system and can cause inflammation.

If you suspect you have allergies, you can ask your doctor to order an IgE test for you or you can order one for yourself.[1]

Food intolerance symptoms take 30 minutes to 3 days to manifest and the symptoms are varied (see below) and cumulative. While there are blood tests for food intolerances (MRT or Mediator Release Testing, ELISA or Enzyme-Linked Immunosorbent Assay, commonly called IgG testing, and ALCAT or Antigen Leukocyte Antibody Test), you can also test for food intolerances yourself.

Symptoms of Food Intolerance

Here are some symptoms of food intolerance:

- Gastrointestinal (stomach and digestive tract – bloating, diarrhea, gas, irritable bowel, colitis, etc.)
- Metabolic (over- or under-active metabolism causing weight gain or loss)
- Respiratory (lungs and breathing – chronic cough, asthma, sinusitis, bronchitis, etc.)
- Dermatological (skin conditions – acne, eczema, psoriasis, etc.)
- Neurological (nervous system – chronic headaches)
- Mental (behavioral, memory, mood issues, anxiety, depression)

CHAPTER 26 – FOOD ALLERGY OR FOOD INTOLERANCE?

- Musculoskeletal (muscle and bone disorders – stiff joints, arthritis, gout)
- Reproductive (genital and fertility issues – inability to conceive, miscarriage)
- Immune system (autoimmune disorders, allergies, frequent infections, and colds)
- Malabsorption (nutrient deficiencies – anemia, osteoporosis, etc.)

If you're suffering from any of these symptoms, first check with your doctor to rule out any more serious conditions.

I utilized the Be in Health lifestyle to eliminate as many of my symptoms as possible. If you find you're still experiencing symptoms after a few months of following the Be in Health lifestyle, you can ask your doctor to do food allergy testing or you can follow the Be in Health Food Reintroduction Challenge (chapter 27).

The Be in Health lifestyle combines a healthy eating plan to restore gut health with a Food Reintroduction Challenge, as well as a toxin reduction plan. Here are the foods that can cause the most issues:

The Big 5	The Small 5
*Gluten	*Nuts and seeds
*Eggs	*Nightshades
*Dairy	*Citrus fruit
*Corn	*Fructose
*Soy	*Yeast

The Food Reintroduction Challenge is for those whose symptoms' cause has not been identified. The purpose is to eliminate the 5 major known food triggers, as well as the 5 minor known food triggers. Then the trigger foods are added back in a planned manner.

A list of some of the benefits I experienced from this lifestyle is in chapter 24.

CHAPTER 26 – FOOD ALLERGY OR FOOD INTOLERANCE?

At least 70% of our immune system is in the gut lining. This means that a healthy gut contributes to our overall health, and an unhealthy gut can lead to a myriad of health problems. How do you know if you have a food allergy or a food intolerance? Sometimes, it's a process of elimination.

CHAPTER 26 – FOOD ALLERGY OR FOOD INTOLERANCE?

CHAPTER 27

THE FOOD REINTRODUCTION CHALLENGE

I used the Food Reintroduction Challenge when some of my symptoms lingered after changing what I ate, and I didn't know what was causing them. The purpose is to eliminate the 5 major known food triggers, as well as the 5 minor known food triggers, for a period of 2 to 3 weeks. After that, I began adding these foods back into my diet in a planned manner.

A list of some of the benefits I experienced from this lifestyle is in chapter 24.

At least 70% of our immune system is in the gut lining. This means that a healthy gut contributes to our overall health, and an unhealthy gut can lead to a myriad of health problems.

How I Felt on the Food Reintroduction Challenge

- Freed of the symptoms I started with
- Energized
- Sharper in mind and spirit
- Slimmer. When the body is chronically inflamed it stores fat. (That's why that stubborn belly fat never wanted to go away.)
- Radiant; people tell me my eyes and skin glow
- Excited, knowing I've prevented future chronic diseases

Potential Detox Symptoms

The Food Reintroduction Challenge is a gentle form of detox. There are two reasons for this:

1. Eliminating processed food reduces the intake of toxins.
2. Discovering food sensitivities: I eliminated food that my body sees as toxic – food that my body is sensitive to.

CHAPTER 27 – THE FOOD REINTRODUCTION CHALLENGE

As your body detoxes, you might experience some temporary unpleasant symptoms, such as:

- Fatigue (but only in the first 2-3 days)
- Weird dreams
- Body odor
- White coating on the tongue
- Film-like coating on the teeth
- Pimples
- Moodiness
- Nausea
- Poor sleep
- Headaches

For more information on toxin release and how to deal with it, see chapter 44. **If you experience detox symptoms that you're unable to handle, please talk to your doctor.**

Food Reintroduction Challenge Stages

The Food Reintroduction Challenge has three stages:

1. Observe
2. Eliminate
3. Challenge

I call this a Food Reintroduction <u>Challenge</u> because I eliminated 5 food categories all at once. But, it takes no longer than 34-41 days (5-6 weeks) to complete. If you decide to follow the FRC, eliminate any foods that you know you have sensitivities to (e.g., pineapple, nuts, eggs, etc.), or if you had an IgG (food tolerance panel) done, cut out those foods as well.

CHAPTER 27 - THE FOOD REINTRODUCTION CHALLENGE

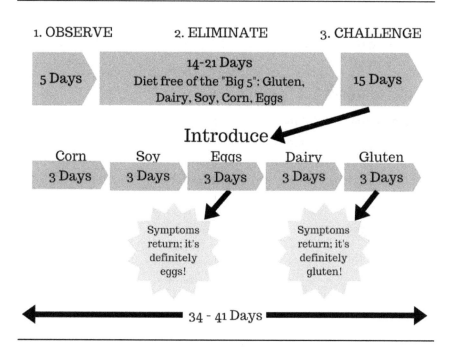

Step 1: Observe

The purpose of this phase was to get a rough idea or an indication of what was making me sick.

I kept my Food-Mood-Poop (FMP) Journal (see chapter 49) for five days detailing what I ate and drank for breakfast, lunch, dinner, and snacks.

I found that the more details about the food I recorded, the better. I wrote down how I felt after I ate certain foods. For example, if I felt bloated or had a headache after a big bowl of pasta, I made note of it.

I found myself getting very tuned in to my body, listening and connecting my symptoms with the food I ate. I did **NOT** change what I ate yet.

This step was very important so that I could:

- Make a connection between the food I eat and how it makes me feel.

CHAPTER 27 – THE FOOD REINTRODUCTION CHALLENGE

- Start seeing what impacts my eating, e.g., emotions, stress, poor chewing, eating too fast, etc.
- Begin to understand how healthfully or unhealthfully I was eating.

Step 2: Eliminate

I cut out all the Big 5's (and whatever else I thought might be a problem for me) at once and kept them out of my diet for the entire 21 days. Those in a rush can complete this step in 14 days, but I found it was better to completely free my body of these food substances and give my body time to adjust.

The Big 5	The Small 5
*Gluten	*Nuts and seeds
*Eggs	*Nightshades
*Dairy	*Citrus fruit
*Corn	*Fructose
*Soy	*Yeast

Step 3: Challenge

After 21 days of eliminating these foods, it was time to see how my body would respond when I re-introduced the foods I had eliminated. I started re-introducing each of the foods, one at a time, three days apart.

I found it was best to introduce food I thought had the most negative effect on me last and the least effect first. A typical sequence looks like this: corn, soy, eggs, dairy, gluten. I chose the progression that was best for me based on my food journal and past experiences with that food. I introduced one food back into my diet and observed how it made me feel.

If I had no reaction the first day, I ate the same food again the next day to see if a reaction occurs. If still no reaction, I ate it again the third day. (Sometimes it takes more than one introduction of the food before the changes become evident.) If after three days of eating this food there were still no changes, I probably don't have a sensitivity to that food.

CHAPTER 27 - THE FOOD REINTRODUCTION CHALLENGE

If I had any reaction of any kind, I stopped eating that food immediately because I now knew that my body doesn't tolerate it.

I repeated this with the rest of the Big 5. This gave me a clear indication of what foods made me sick.

If I had a reaction to a food, I would stop eating that food from now on. I continued testing other foods.

After going through the FRC with the Big 5, I started again with the Small 5 to make sure I got rid of all foods that caused me problems.

Mental Preparation to Start the Food Reintroduction Challenge

- **Reframe**. A sense of anxiety or fear of failure is normal when we start something new. But we know that God is with us and will protect us. I framed the Food Reintroduction Challenge positively:
    - Eliminating these foods will cleanse and soothe my body.
    - It's not forever, it's only for 4 to 6 weeks.
    - My body needs help and I am loving my body by doing this.
    - Even if I have to give up some foods permanently, I will be open to other, new foods.
- **Clean out the kitchen**. I got rid of the foods I was eliminating; out of the house! I enlisted my family members to support me during this testing time (it's similar to a fast). I enjoyed shopping for new, healthful foods.
- **Surround yourself with alternatives**. I came up with a list of snacks and other recipes that I love preparing and eating. I didn't allow myself to feel deprived or confused. I planned ahead so I didn't fall back into bad habits. I reminded myself that if I cheat on the Food Reintroduction Challenge, I need to start all over.

CHAPTER 27 – THE FOOD REINTRODUCTION CHALLENGE

What I Ate on the Food Reintroduction Challenge

I found I could do the Food Reintroduction Challenge very well following the Be in Health eating plan (chapter 25). I replaced cow's milk with coconut milk. I replaced eggs in recipes by combining 1 tablespoon ground flax seed with 3 tablespoons water for each egg replaced. I replaced 1 teaspoon lemon juice in recipes with ½ teaspoon apple cider vinegar.

Completing the Food Reintroduction Challenge

Now I know which foods my body tolerates and which it doesn't. The non-tolerated foods need to be removed from my diet completely. I feel much better when I do. I now have an idea of how to live without them and what foods I can introduce instead so I don't feel deprived.

If I had a very mild reaction to the food, I can keep it in my diet every four to five days, depending on how I feel (I continued using the FMP journal). If the reaction was significant or was something I didn't want to experience at all, I cut the food out completely.

The more one is addicted to a certain food, the more intolerant or sensitive one may be to that food. The good news is that in the process of eliminating the food, the food craving went away. I got to the place where I no longer enjoy a food that I was previously 'addicted' to.

Discovering which specific foods made me feel better and healthier made it easier to give up specific foods that made me sick.

CHAPTER 28

CLEANSING AND MAINTAINING THE COLON

As important as it is to put healthy food into my body, I must also deal with the effects that decades of unhealthy food and prescription medicines have had on my gut. That's why cleansing and maintaining the colon is so important.

There are two steps to this process. The first is to supplement with probiotics, digestive enzymes, and other nutritional supplements.

The second step is to cleanse the colon. After I completed my first successful colon cleanse, I now do a cleanse once a year.

(Note: I use and recommend products from Young Living Essential Oils, for which I'm a distributor. You're not obligated to use these products, but they're the ones I used to help restore and maintain my health, so I can vouch for their effectiveness. If you'd like information on purchasing these products, please contact me at Carol@3Jn2Wellness.com.)

Probiotics

I eat 1 cup of cultured coconut products per day, like coconut milk kefir, which is rich in probiotics. My recipe for Coconut Milk Kefir is in chapter 50. It's very easy to make. I add it to my Super Restoring Smoothie.

According to Dr. Mary Jane Brown, Ph.D., R.D. (UK), probiotics help balance friendly bacteria in the digestive system, can prevent and heal diarrhea, can keep the heart healthy, may reduce the severity of certain allergies and eczema, can help reduce symptoms of IBS, ulcerative colitis, and Crohn's disease, may help boost the immune system, and may help weight loss and loss of belly fat.[1]

I take 50-100 billion units of a probiotic supplement daily. Probiotics can help re-colonize the gut with healthy bacteria, especially when the goal is to restore health to the gut.

CHAPTER 28 – CLEANSING AND MAINTAINING THE COLON

Digestive Enzymes

I take digestive enzymes before each meal. These enzymes improve nutrient absorption and help break down food particles. For acute leaky gut syndrome, digestive enzymes are extremely important, so I don't skip them.

Parasite Cleanse

I've found it very helpful to do a parasite cleanse twice a year. Most people think that in America we don't have parasites, but we do.[2] Parasites live on the things we eat and are unable to digest or pass (especially sugars and starches). These parasites stay in the digestive tract and excrete toxins that make us sick. Let's get rid of the little boogers.

This is the technique I use:

- Take three ParaFree[3] soft gels three times a day with meals for three weeks (9 soft gels per day).
- Stop taking ParaFree for one week.
- Repeat this process twice more (total time 11 weeks)

I haven't found the process to be difficult. I noticed a bit of fatigue and that I had more bowel movements than usual, which in this case is a good thing. If the BM became too loose, I would cut back on the number of soft gels I took until the stools were well formed again.

For Gallbladder Issues

- Spearmint Vitality™ Essential Oil[4] and Peppermint Vitality™ Essential Oil[5] are good for gallbladder support.
- Take a lipase enzyme instead of a full-spectrum digestive enzyme.
- Bile salts in the form of ox bile
- Probiotics

CHAPTER 28 - CLEANSING AND MAINTAINING THE COLON

- Herbs like milk thistle and turmeric

For SIBO

Small Intestine Bacterial Overgrowth (SIBO) is caused by the wrong pH in the stomach and not enough stomach acid.

- Vitamin B12 [6]
- Iron
- One tablespoon of apple cider vinegar before meals
- Hydrochloric acid with pepsin (take with protein). Follow label instructions.
- Cabbage juice (very high in sulfur or vitamin U). I take a supplement called Sulfurzyme.[7]
- Aloe vera juice (1/2 cup 3x daily). Aloe vera is healthful for the digestive system, is supportive of the immune system, and detoxifies the body. I add it to my smoothie each morning.

Nutritional Supplements

As someone wanting to restore their gut to health, I take these supplements.

- Fish oil (1000 mg daily). Fish oil contains the essential fatty acids EPA/DHA which reduce inflammation.[8]
- L-glutamine powder (5 grams 2x daily). L-glutamine is an amino acid that helps repair the digestive tract, especially important for those with chronic diarrhea (take on an empty stomach).[9]

The following essential oils can soothe intestinal inflammation and support the restoration of the gut:

- Ginger Vitality™ Essential Oil [10] (supports digestion). 2 drops internally in a glass of water.
- Peppermint Vitality™ Essential Oil [11] (supports gastrointestinal system comfort and healthy bowel function). Peppermint

essential oil is extremely potent, so use only a small amount. One drop in an 8-ounce glass of water is too much for most people. Take a toothpick and insert it into the essential oil bottle then swirl the toothpick in a glass of water.

- DiGize™ Vitality™ Essential Oil (blend). [12] Add DiGize™ Vitality™ and Peppermint Vitality™ essential oils to water.
- Lemon Vitality™ Essential Oil [13] (helps soothe digestion). Add one drop to water.
- Spearmint Vitality™ Essential Oil [14] (gallbladder stimulant; also helpful for indigestion and bloating). Add one drop to water.
- Mix 3 drops of any of the above essential oils with coconut oil and rub over the abdomen 2x daily.

Cleansing the Colon

According to Dr. LeAnne Deardeuff, D.C., in her book, *Inner Transformations Using Essential Oils*:

The large intestine [colon/gut] is filled with mucous glands, the purpose of which is to coat the chyme [partially digested food] so it can pass over the villi of the large intestine easier, and also protect itself from drugs, heavy metals, and other harmful matter. (The villi, tiny finger-like projections on the inside of the colon, are where the absorption of nutrients takes place.)

Certain unnatural, processed food, like pasteurized milk products, cause these glands to over-produce mucus. Other artificial foods like white flour products, when mixed with this mucus, create a gluey substance that coats the walls of the colon. This coating is then baked on in the 100° oven of the colon. If you have ever made Christmas ornaments or other crafts with your children by mixing white flour and milk, then slow-baking the resulting clay, you know just how hard this substance can become! Not only is it hard like cement but it is virtually immovable so that the peristalsis [a series of wave-like muscle contractions that moves food to different processing stations in the digestive tract] of the colon slows down and practically stops, not

CHAPTER 28 - CLEANSING AND MAINTAINING THE COLON

> *allowing the contents to move forward and leave the colon through the anus.*
>
> *In extreme cases, the colon can become so clogged as a result of poor dietary choices and insufficient fiber and water intake that the colon expands with the mucoid plaque and excess fecal matter to become a megacolon as much as 5 times the colon's normal size, and weighing up to 40 lbs.*[15]

It's for these reasons that it's important to cleanse the colon while changing eating habits. Since I eat at least 3 times a day, it's normal to have 2-3 bowel movements per day. So, that is the goal of this colon cleanse: have 2-3 bowel movements per day that are fast and easy to pass, well-formed, and that float in the toilet. It may take 6 weeks to a year to get there. According to the late Dr. Bernard Jensen, D.C., Ph.D., a leader in the field of herbal cleansing for 50 years,

> *Cleanse until you pass the mucoid plaque* [the lining coating the bowel described earlier]. *It is black and long and holds together in a long tube shape. It consists of all the caked material that had been lining the bowel and was making it difficult for the bowel to function as it was designed to. Once that passes, the bowel automatically begins to function properly. Once that passes, you have achieved your goal.*[16]

Here is Dr. Deardeuff's process for colon cleansing; it's the process I use. It utilizes a product called the Cleansing Trio Kit,[17] which consists of three products: ComforTone, ICP, and Essentialzyme.

- Begin with 1 ComforTone capsule in the morning. The second day, take one in the morning and one in the evening. The third day, take two in the morning and one in the evening, then two in the morning and two in the evening, and so on, building up to a maximum of 10 daily.

- Remember that the goal is 2-3 bowel movements per day that are fast and easy to pass, well-formed, and that float in the toilet. When I reached that goal, I didn't need to add any more capsules daily. I stayed on that level until I passed the mucoid plaque.

CHAPTER 28 – CLEANSING AND MAINTAINING THE COLON

- If I experienced diarrhea during the cleanse, I decreased the number of capsules until my bowels were firm again. If I experienced constipation, I increased the capsules until my bowels were easier to pass or I added magnesium (1/2 to 2 teaspoons of Natural Calm [18] worked well) or Peppermint Vitality™ Essential Oil (a swirl from a toothpick in a glass of water).
- Along with the ComforTone, I took the Essentialzyme digestive enzyme 3 times daily, between meals.
- I drank 3 quarts of water per day.
- When I started having 2-3 good bowel movements daily, I began taking the ICP powder, 1 teaspoon in the morning. I mixed it with water and drank it down quickly. I added ½ teaspoon per day until I reached 1 tablespoon (3 teaspoons) in the morning and 1 tablespoon in the evening. I stayed on ComforTone and Essentialzyme while I was taking the ICP.
- I continued colon cleansing until the mucoid plaque dropped out of the colon. It usually takes between 6 weeks and 18 months. While on the colon cleanse, I take my regular supplements and probiotics, including the ones I mention in this chapter.

If you want information on how to do other organ cleanses after you have finished the colon cleanse, Dr. Deardeuff describes them in her book.

CHAPTER 29

BENEFITS OF ESSENTIAL OILS FOR BODY, SOUL, AND SPIRIT

What are Essential Oils?

Essential oils are non-fatty oils that are distilled from plants, shrubs, flowers, trees, roots, bark, bushes, and seeds. Most essential oils are extracted using steam distillation and are highly concentrated, making them far more potent than dried botanicals or herbs. (For example, 1 drop of peppermint essential oil is equivalent to 28 cups of herbal peppermint tea.)

Essential oils have been used for thousands of years for cosmetic purposes, as well as for their spiritually and emotionally uplifting properties because of how they affect the limbic system (the seat of emotions).[1] They support all body systems.

We've all been exposed to essential oils, sometimes unknowingly. What happens when you peel an orange? Lots of tiny drops of oil come bursting out. Those are essential oils. Have you ever cut into a plant and seen a liquid seep out? That's the plant's essential oil.

Just as Leviticus 17:11 tells us that the life of the flesh is in the blood, the life of the plant is in the essential oil.

Essential oils were mentioned in the *Ebers Papyrus*,[2] an ancient Egyptian list of 877 prescriptions and recipes dating back to 1600 BC.

How Essential Oils Work

There are three main components of essential oils that cause them to be so effective.

Phenols and phenylpropanoids. While they can create conditions where unfriendly viruses and bacteria cannot live, the most important function performed by phenylpropanoids is that they **clean the receptor**

CHAPTER 29 – BENEFITS OF ESSENTIAL OILS

sites on the cells. Without clean receptor sites, cells cannot communicate and the body malfunctions, resulting in sickness.[3]

Phenols and phenylpropanoids are found in clove (90%), cassia (80%), basil (75%), cinnamon (73%), oregano (60%), anise (50%), and peppermint (25%) essential oils.

Sesquiterpenes. According to Dr. David Stewart, Ph.D., in his book, *Healing Oils of the Bible*,

> *Sesquiterpenes seem to work at a subcellular level by affecting membrane fluidity and facilitating oxygen transfer. Sesquiterpenes may also affect the transport of material inside the cell. This allows for access to DNA and RNA which may offer a scientific basis for **"deprogramming or erasing the incorrect information from cellular memory"** often referred to in holistic healing circles.*[4]

Sesquiterpenes are the principal constituents of cedarwood (98%), vetiver (97%), spikenard (93%), sandalwood (aloes) 90%, black pepper (74%), patchouli (71%), myrrh (62%), and ginger (59%). They're also found in galbanum, onycha, and frankincense (8%), which are oils mentioned in the Bible.

Monoterpenes. The most important ability of the monoterpenes is that they can **reprogram miswritten information** in the cellular memory (DNA). With improper coding in cellular memory, cells malfunction and diseases result.[5]

Monoterpenes are found in most essential oils: galbanum (80%), Angelica (73%), hyssop (70%), rose of Sharon (54%), peppermint (45%), Juniper (42%), frankincense (40%), spruce (38%), pine (30%), cypress (28%), and Myrtle (25%).

Essentials oils are absorbed into the body quickly. Within 22 seconds, the molecules reach the brain. Within 2 minutes, they will enter the bloodstream (because essential oil molecules are so small, they can cross the blood-brain barrier), and within 20 minutes they will affect every cell in the body.

CHAPTER 29 – BENEFITS OF ESSENTIAL OILS

These three components in essentials oils are what make them work so quickly and efficiently. They work to support the body, whereas pharmaceuticals are designed to confuse your cells, so you no longer have symptoms. For example, antihistamines block histamine receptors, so you don't sniffle or produce mucus when you have a cold or allergy. In contrast, an oil's constituents will reprogram the cell back to its original state.

Unlike synthetic chemicals, the constituents in different essential oils work in different ways in different people. That's why they're not a substitute for pharmaceuticals.

Biblical References to Essential Oils

What does the Bible say about essential oils? Plants have played a crucial role for man and this was emphasized right from the beginning of the Bible.

> *Genesis 1:29 KJV*
> *And God said, Behold, I have given you every herb bearing seed, which is upon the face of all the earth, and every tree, in the which is the fruit of a tree yielding seed; to you it shall be for meat [food].*

God has always provided for the health and wellness of His people.

> *Ezekiel 47:12 KJV*
> *And by the river upon the bank thereof, on this side and on that side, shall grow all trees for meat [food], whose leaf shall not fade, neither shall the fruit thereof be consumed: it shall bring forth new fruit according to his months, because their waters they issued out of the sanctuary: and the fruit thereof shall be for meat [food], and the leaf thereof for medicine.*

> *Revelation 22:2 KJV*
> *In the midst of the street of it, and on either side of the river, was there the tree of life, which bare twelve manner of fruits, and yielded her fruit every month: and the leaves of the tree were for the healing of the nations.*

CHAPTER 29 – BENEFITS OF ESSENTIAL OILS

Essential oils and the plants they come from are mentioned 1,031 times in the Bible.[6] They're part of God's plan to help mankind stay healthy.

<u>Moses</u>

In the book of Numbers chapter 16, Moses tells the high priest, Aaron, to burn oils as incense to stop a plague.

> *Numbers 16:46-49 KJV*
> *And Moses said unto Aaron, Take a censer, and put fire therein from off the altar, and put on incense, and go quickly unto the congregation, and make an atonement for them: for there is wrath gone out from the LORD; the plague is begun.*
>
> *And Aaron took as Moses commanded, and ran into the midst of the congregation; and, behold, the plague was begun among the people: and he put on incense, and made an atonement for the people.*
>
> *And he stood between the dead and the living; and the plague was stayed.*
>
> *Now they that died in the plague were fourteen thousand and seven hundred, beside them that died about the matter of Korah.*

There are recipes for essential oil blends in the book of Exodus, which we will discuss later in this chapter.

<u>Hyssop</u>

The use of hyssop during both the Passover and the crucifixion of Jesus Christ is not a coincidence.

> *Exodus 12:22 KJV*
> *And ye shall take a bunch of hyssop, and dip it in the blood that is in the basin, and strike the lintel and the two side posts with the blood that is in the basin; and none of you shall go out at the door of his house until the morning.*

When striking the blood-dipped hyssop against the lintel and side posts, the fragrant aroma (essential oil) of the hyssop would be released and mingled with the aroma of the lamb's blood. This distinct fragrance would be one the children of Israel would never forget.

Note that while the symbolism of the blood of the lamb saving the sons of the Israelites has a strong significance for Jews and Christians alike, it's interesting to note that the ancient Hebrews believed that the scent of hyssop would repel evil spirits.[7] Thus, the fragrance of the hyssop was part of the ritual to cause the evil spirit of death to pass over the Israelites that night.

> *Psalm 51:7 KJV*
> *Purge me with hyssop, and I shall be clean: wash me, and I shall be whiter than snow.*

The fragrance of hyssop was considered to be spiritually purifying and an aid in cleansing oneself from sin, immorality, evil thoughts, or bad habits. Psalm 51 was written regarding David's realization of his sin concerning Bathsheba and his repentance of that sin.

> *John 19:28-29 KJV*
> *After this, Jesus knowing that all things were now accomplished, that the scripture might be fulfilled, saith, I thirst.*
>
> *Now there was set a vessel full of vinegar: and they filled a spunge with vinegar, and put it upon hyssop, and put it to his mouth.*

The significance of Jesus Christ accepting the vinegar on the hyssop after he knew that his work was complete is that the Jews present at his crucifixion would be reminded of hyssop's part in the first Passover. Hyssop mingled with blood. Jesus Christ was the true Passover lamb.

<u>Jesus Christ Was Anointed with Essential Oils</u>

Jesus Christ received essential oils at both the beginning and the end of his life. Frankincense and myrrh were presented to him by the Magi.

> *Matthew 2:11 KJV*
> *And when they were come into the house, they saw the young child with Mary his mother, and fell down, and worshipped him:*

CHAPTER 29 – BENEFITS OF ESSENTIAL OILS

and when they had opened their treasures, they presented unto him gifts; gold, and frankincense, and myrrh.

Jesus' head and feet were anointed toward the end of his life with spikenard and myrrh. The cost of the oils (in ointment form) that were used on Jesus is equivalent to $2,000 today. They were usually sealed in alabaster boxes for preservation.[8]

Matthew 26:7 KJV
There came unto him a woman having an alabaster box of very precious ointment, and poured it on his head, as he sat at meat.

Mark 14:3 KJV
And being in Bethany in the house of Simon the leper, as he sat at meat, there came a woman having an alabaster box of ointment of spikenard very precious; and she brake the box, and poured it on his head.

Luke 7:37-38 KJV
And, behold, a woman in the city, which was a sinner, when she knew that Jesus sat at meat in the Pharisee's house, brought an alabaster box of ointment,

And stood at his feet behind him weeping, and began to wash his feet with tears, and did wipe them with the hairs of her head, and kissed his feet, and anointed them with the ointment.

John 12:3 KJV
Then took Mary a pound of ointment of spikenard, very costly, and anointed the feet of Jesus, and wiped his feet with her hair: and the house was filled with the odour of the ointment.

Roman soldiers generally offered wine mixed with myrrh to those being crucified to help reduce pain. Jesus was offered this combination while he hung on the cross, but he refused it, instead choosing to endure the pain of the cross for us.

Mark 15:23 KJV
And they gave him to drink wine mingled with myrrh: but he

CHAPTER 29 – BENEFITS OF ESSENTIAL OILS

received it not.

During his earthly ministry, Jesus sent his disciples to anoint with oils and heal.

> *Mark 6:13 KJV*
> *And they cast out many devils, and anointed with oil many that were sick, and healed them.*

Use of Essential Oils in the Church

What about the use of essential oils in the church today? The only reference is in the book of James.

> *James 5:14 KJV*
> *Is any sick among you? let him call for the elders of the church; and let them pray over him, anointing him with oil in the name of the Lord:*

The Biblical meaning of the word 'anoint' is "to massage or rub." The Hebrew word is *masach*. This is where we get the English word 'massage.'

Is the book of James instruction to the church?

> *James 1:1 KJV*
> *James, a servant of God and of the Lord Jesus Christ, to the twelve tribes which are scattered abroad, greeting.*

The epistle of James was written by Jesus' brother, who was not a believer in Jesus until after his resurrection. He became a pillar of the early church along with Peter and John (see Galatians 2:9). His ministry seemed to be to Judean Christians still actively following Mosaic law.

James was the first epistle to be written, so he and the rest of the church did not yet have the knowledge of the grace of God and who we are in Christ (Romans and Ephesians had not yet been written). The Gentiles had not yet come into the one body of Christ, so, James only knew the Old Testament and Jesus' teachings.

Because the believers to whom James wrote were zealous for the law (Acts 21:20), they were unable to receive information about grace, even

CHAPTER 29 – BENEFITS OF ESSENTIAL OILS

if God had given that revelation to James. James taught them what they could handle.

So, while we can learn a great deal in this section of the epistle of James about how prayer, forgiveness, and healing work, this section isn't doctrine or instruction to the church as we know it from the Pauline epistles.

So, should individual saints today use essential oils? There are many scriptures showing how the Israelites and Jesus and his disciples used them; there are no scriptures telling us to stop using them.

Plague Doctors

In chapter 6, I wrote that many barber surgeons didn't succumb to the Plague while most physicians did. What did the barber surgeons do that saved their lives?

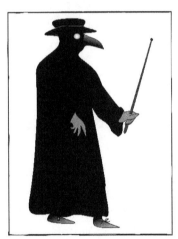

Plague Doctor

In medieval times, barber surgeons were the doctors for the military and the lower classes. People only called on them when they were near death. A visit by one of these doctors was considered a bad omen. It meant death was near. These doctors were considered 'quacks' by the upper classes and university-trained physicians. These 'quack' doctors used salves, herbs, and ointments made from essential oils to treat their patients.

The way these doctors dressed might have had something to do with why people were so afraid of them. They dressed in long, flowing black robes, gloves, and hats. They wore beak-shaped masks that covered their faces[9] (similar to modern gas masks). They filled these masks with herbs and spices.

The purpose of the herbs and spices in the masks was to protect the doctor from breathing in the fumes of sickness from their patients.

CHAPTER 29 – BENEFITS OF ESSENTIAL OILS

During this time, people believed in the miasma theory[10] of illness. This theory said that diseases such as cholera, chlamydia, or the Plague were caused by a miasma (from the ancient Greek word for 'pollution'), a noxious form of 'bad air' also known as 'night air.'

The theory said that the origin of epidemics was due to a miasma emanating from rotting organic matter. The theory was discredited by Paracelsus and was eventually abandoned by most scientists and physicians after 1880, replaced by the germ theory of disease.

When the Plague was raging in Europe, plague doctors[11] successfully protected themselves from this contagious disease. They used herbs, spices, and essential oils based on experiential knowledge of these substances, so they knew which ones to use to protect themselves.

The bacterium *Yersinia pestis*, which results in several forms of plague, is believed to have been the cause of the pandemic of the 14th and 15th centuries. Yet many plague doctors and grave robbers saved their own lives by using these aromatic substances. How do we account for this?

<u>The Miasma Theory</u>

Galen of Pergamon[12] (129 AD – c. 200/c. 216) was a Greek physician, surgeon, and philosopher in the Roman Empire. He made many contributions to medicine that were discredited when people adopted the views of Paracelsus instead. In fact, Paracelsus held a public book burning of Galen's works.[13]

Galen believed the lungs drew *pneuma* (a Greek word translated in the New Testament most often as 'spirit') from the air, which the blood then communicated throughout the body. We get our word 'pneumonia' from this understanding of *pneuma* as 'bad air.'

The miasma theory had many Judeo-Christian overtones. The Bible says that God breathed breath into Adam and he became a living soul. Jesus also breathed on his disciples and told them to receive the holy spirit after his resurrection. When someone dies, we say that they drew their last breath.

CHAPTER 29 – BENEFITS OF ESSENTIAL OILS

> *Job 33:4 KJV*
> *The Spirit of God hath made me, and the breath of the Almighty hath given me life.*

> *Genesis 2:7 KJV*
> *And the LORD God formed man of the dust of the ground, and breathed into his nostrils the breath of life; and man became a living soul.*

> *John 20:22 KJV*
> *And when he had said this, he breathed on them, and saith unto them, Receive ye the Holy Ghost:*

> *1 Kings 17:17 KJV*
> *And it came to pass after these things, that the son of the woman, the mistress of the house, fell sick; and his sickness was so sore, that there was no breath left in him* [he died].

The concept of breath, miasma, does have some merit. If the air we breathe can't make us sick, we wouldn't worry about air quality; we wouldn't try to protect ourselves from inhaling poisons in the air.

The herbal concoctions used by the plague doctors certainly had a fragrance, but their effectiveness went well beyond the aroma alone. Substances can be artificially scented but carry no health benefits. Today, almost everything is scented. Laundry detergent, shampoo, body lotions, even our dishwasher detergents have that 'fresh citrus scent.'

If you will recall from chapter 6, the fragrances in these products are there to disguise the unpleasant odors of the chemicals (industrial waste) used to make these products.

The reason God gave us the senses of smell and taste is to protect us, to let us know that something is poisonous. If you smell sour milk or rotting meat, you wouldn't eat it. If you smelled the chemicals in your cleaning and personal care products, you wouldn't use them. So, the true smell must be masked with something fake. Something that will trick your protective senses of smell and taste into thinking it's not poisonous.

CHAPTER 29 – BENEFITS OF ESSENTIAL OILS

This is something very different from essential oils, which are more than a fragrance mask. Because the scientific and medical communities have told us that 'bad air' (miasma) isn't a valid theory, we have learned to dismiss what we smell. Smell, aroma, has nothing to do with health, they say.

AROMAtherapy vs. AromaTHERAPY

Since we have been convinced that aroma has nothing to do with health, many people today think that essential oils are nothing but perfume, fragrance, a pleasant scent that will mask the bad odors in their homes. That is the 'aroma' part of aromatherapy. I'm more interested in the 'therapy' part.

Drugs are chemical substances that are designed to temporarily stop a body process. (Again, the example, antihistamines block histamine receptors, so you don't sniffle or produce mucus when you have a cold or allergy. The natural process has been stopped.)

Blocking the process of pain can be beneficial if you've been in an accident or had a severe injury. Once you stop taking the drug, the symptoms return if your body hasn't performed its duty to heal itself. (Remember the definition of 'cure.')

Because many of these chemical substances are poisonous, they often have nasty side effects. Whether or not you suffer from the side effects depends on the dose and your body's ability to fight off the poison. ("**Solely the dose determines that a thing is not a poison.**") So, yes, you can have temporary relief. But, remember, drugs only cure, that is, they only alleviate symptoms. They don't heal the body.

Drugs are chemicals that the human body doesn't recognize, and they will weaken the body. The FDA requires that drug manufacturers list all the various ways they will do so (they call them side effects). So, what do you think will happen if you take them long term?

Saying that essential oils stop a natural body process like drugs do isn't true, so the FDA doesn't like it when people say they do. The FDA says I'm legally allowed to say that essential oils can be used to support/enhance a natural body function. In other words, essential oils help the body become stronger and function better.

What's the reason we don't say that essential oils can cure anything? Remember the definition of 'cure.' Drugs cure, that is, they relieve symptoms; essential oils support, enhance, and make stronger.

Because we have been trained from birth by the pharmaceutical industry to take a drug whenever we have a symptom, it has become subconscious for most of us. Many people try to transfer that process to essential oils: experience a symptom, use this essential oil.

I want to teach you how to use essential oils to support your body and emotions, not become a substitute for drugs.

Support Your Body

The concept of using essential oils to support your body and your emotions is unfamiliar to many, but not to the pharmaceutical industry. They know essential oils work. Essential oils were used during World War I to treat injured soldiers.[14]

Have you noticed that essential oils seem to be everywhere these days? Just about every big box store sells cheap, adulterated essential oils. These are pure essential oils that have been mixed with chemicals like alcohol and petroleum or extended with fatty oils or similar, less expensive oils (such as adding lavandin to lavender).

According to the *Journal of Environmental Analytical Chemistry*, "The most adulterated essential oils fall into two categories: high-value oils like sandalwood and rose and the bestselling oils such as lavender, peppermint, citrus oils, wintergreen, oregano, and thyme." [15] The two biggest hints that an oil is adulterated: 1. It's labeled 'Not for Internal Use;' 2. It's inexpensive (cheap).

The use of these fake essential oils will not provide the therapeutic benefits I'm speaking of. They will keep people in the system of sickness. Drug companies aren't in business to help people, they're in business to

CHAPTER 29 – BENEFITS OF ESSENTIAL OILS

make money. More sick people means more money. Healthy people means less money for them.

Can you guess why chronic illness is on the rise?

How Essential Oils Support Your Body

Your cells/tissues/organs, the earth itself, your desk, your phone, your computer, the food you eat, the clothes you wear, your emotions, essential oils, yes, everything has a frequency, which is defined as the rate at which a vibration occurs that constitutes a wave, either in a material (as in sound waves), or in an electromagnetic field (as in radio waves and light), usually measured per second. Frequency is energy, light, and life, which is also a great description of God. Some people refer to frequency as chi or life force.

A substance with a higher frequency can raise a lower frequency due to the principle of resonance[16] – the tendency for two oscillating bodies to lock into phase so that they vibrate in harmony. This principle is key to understanding the effect essential oils can have on our personal electromagnetic frequency.

Because each body system and organ has its own frequency, and each essential oil has its own frequency, each essential oil has an affinity for certain systems/organs. By applying an essential oil with a particular frequency to the human body – through the principle of resonance – the oil's higher frequency will raise the vibratory quality of that individual. Essential oils in the higher frequency ranges tend to influence the emotions.

To understand more about how disruptions in frequency affect health, see chapter 6 about the creation of cancer.

Anointing with Oil

Anointing with oil goes back to Exodus when God told Moses to anoint his brother, Aaron, and Aaron's sons in order to separate them out from the rest of the people as ones God set apart as priests.

CHAPTER 29 – BENEFITS OF ESSENTIAL OILS

> *Exodus 28:41 KJV*
> *And thou shalt put them* [specially made coats] *upon Aaron thy brother, and his sons with him; and shalt anoint them, and consecrate them, and sanctify them, that they may minister unto me in the priest's office.*

> *Exodus 29:7 KJV*
> *Then shalt thou take the anointing oil, and pour it upon his head, and anoint him.*

The anointing was to consecrate and sanctify the person. The Biblical meaning of the word 'anoint' is "to massage or rub." The Hebrew word is *masach*. This is where we get the English word 'massage.'

It's interesting to note that the Hebrew word translated 'messiah' is *mashiyach*, which comes from the root word *masach*. The Messiah is the Anointed One.

'Consecrate' means "to fill one's hand," meaning the priesthood was delivered into Aaron's hand. 'Sanctify' means "to be holy." In other words, God was making sure that all the people knew that Aaron and his sons were special, marked out, anointed, consecrated, holy, as priests who ministered to God. The use of the oil was a physical representation of the spiritual anointing that came from God.

After Aaron and his sons were anointed with oil, they anointed the following with oil:

- The priestly clothing
- The tabernacle and everything in it, including the ark of the testimony, the table and all its vessels, the candlestick and vessels, the altar of incense, the altar of burnt offering and its vessels, and the laver and foot.

Exodus 30:29 says that anything that touches an anointed item would automatically be holy. These items would only be touched by priests and Moses.

This is the essential oil blend that God told Moses to use to anoint Aaron:

CHAPTER 29 – BENEFITS OF ESSENTIAL OILS

Exodus 30:22-25 NLT
Then the LORD said to Moses,

"Collect choice spices—12½ pounds of pure myrrh, 6¼ pounds of fragrant cinnamon, 6¼ pounds of fragrant calamus,

and 12½ pounds of cassia—as measured by the weight of the sanctuary shekel. Also get one gallon of olive oil.

Like a skilled incense maker, blend these ingredients to make a holy anointing oil.

The ratio for the oils is as follows:

- 2 parts myrrh
- 1 part cinnamon
- 1 part calamus (some believe this is cannabis/hemp oil [17])
- 2 parts cassia
- 2.5 parts extra virgin olive oil

God promised His people that one day the yoke and burden they were under (the law) would be lifted from them.

Isaiah 10:27 KJV
And it shall come to pass in that day, that his burden shall be taken away from off thy shoulder, and his yoke from off thy neck, ***and the yoke shall be destroyed because of the anointing****.*

This came to pass with the coming of the Messiah, the Christ, which means "the anointed one." Jesus Christ made this declaration at the opening of his public ministry:

Luke 4:18 APNT
The Spirit of the Lord [is] on me and because of this, he has anointed me to preach to the poor and has sent me to heal the broken-hearted and to preach forgiveness to the captives and sight to the blind and to strengthen the broken with forgiveness.

CHAPTER 29 – BENEFITS OF ESSENTIAL OILS

> *Matthew 11:28-30 KJV*
> *Come unto me, all ye that labour and are heavy laden, and I will give you rest.*
>
> *Take my yoke upon you, and learn of me; for I am meek and lowly in heart: and ye shall find rest unto your souls.*
>
> *For my yoke is easy, and my burden is light.*

The coming of the anointed one, Jesus Christ, forever released God's people from the burden, the yoke, of the law. Righteousness now comes from believing on Jesus Christ, not from doing the works of the law. It's up to us to maintain this freedom.

> *Galatians 5:1 KJV*
> *Stand fast therefore in the liberty wherewith Christ hath made us free, and be not entangled again with the yoke of bondage.*

Today, born-again ones are the royal priesthood.

> *1 Peter 2:9 KJV*
> *But ye are a chosen generation, a royal priesthood, an holy nation, a peculiar people; that ye should shew forth the praises of him who hath called you out of darkness into his marvellous light:*

We have been anointed with holy spirit, which sets us apart from others and marks us out as belonging to God.

> *1 Corinthians 6:11 KJV*
> *And such were some of you: but ye are washed, but ye are sanctified, but ye are justified [made righteous] in the name of the Lord Jesus, and* **by the Spirit of our God.**

> *1 Corinthians 6:19 KJV*
> *What? know ye not that your body is the temple of the Holy Ghost [spirit] which is in you, which ye have of God, and ye are not your own?*

CHAPTER 29 – BENEFITS OF ESSENTIAL OILS

Because of the holy spirit from God that dwells in us, we no longer belong to ourselves. We are bought and paid for by the blood of Jesus Christ. Our bodies are now the temple.

So, now the question is, are we to anoint our temple (body) with the holy anointing oil? There are no scriptures that tell us to do so. There are no scriptures that forbid it. That makes it a personal choice between you and God.

I choose to anoint myself, my house, property, jobs, marriage, bank accounts, etc., using essential oils to help raise my vibrational levels.

Some essential oils to use in anointing are frankincense, myrrh, hyssop, and copaiba. The blend Exodus II™ contains oils similar to the holy anointing oil. It contains olive oil, myrrh, cassia, cinnamon, calamus, Northern Lights black spruce, hyssop, vetiver, and frankincense. There are other blends that may fit specific things you would like to pray about (Forgiveness, Harmony, Transformation, Surrender, Release, Hope, Joy, etc.)

<u>How to Anoint with Oil</u>

I take the essential oil and put one or two drops in my left hand (use the right hand if you're left-handed). Then I rub my hands together several times in a clockwise motion. Then I bring my hands up to my mouth and nose and inhale deeply several times.

Then I touch various parts of my body with my hands (taking special care around the eye area). As I touch each part (head, eyes, ears, hands, heart, feet, etc.), I pray. Some like to use the same prayer each time (you can find many online), but I prefer to pray as God puts things on my heart. I will go around my home and anoint objects and pray over them. We can also pray for and anoint others in this manner.

You are a priest who ministers to God (by prayer, worship, singing). Our service to God is then extended to others when our love for Him overflows. We carry the message that the Christ, the anointing, breaks all yokes and bondage.

CHAPTER 29 – BENEFITS OF ESSENTIAL OILS

> *John 8:32 KJV*
> *And ye shall know the truth, and the truth shall make you free.*

Got Emotions?

Many times, the emotions we feel are the result of patterns that have developed throughout our lives. Sometimes they come from memories belonging to an ancestor that were passed down to us genetically.[18]

We all have different genetic dispositions, and through the science of epigenetics, we are learning how these genes can be switched on and off through environmental triggers. Many times, we don't consciously know why we feel the way we do; that is an emotional pattern at work. It's like the emotion has worn a groove in the brain, so it settles into that specific track without much prompting.

Each of us has emotions, good and not so good, and these emotions can drastically affect the quality of our lives.

We all love the good emotions – love, joy, peace, compassion, humility, anticipation, gratitude, awe, empathy, happiness, wonder, etc. – but oh, those negative ones – disgust, anger, frustration, hate, fear, shame, guilt, distrust, grief, envy, rage, worry – those are the ones that tie us up in knots.

Dr. Joseph Mercola, D.O., writes, "When you feel an emotion, what you're really sensing is the vibration [frequency] of a particular energy. Each emotion has its own vibratory signature, and when intense emotions are felt, they can become trapped in your body. Trapped emotional energy will typically result in physical dysfunction."[19] In other words, feeling bad emotionally can lead to feeling bad physically.

> *Proverbs 14:13 TPT*
> *Superficial laughter can hide a heavy heart, but when the laughter ends, the pain resurfaces.*

This scripture is a good reminder that our coping mechanisms only mask emotional pain but never heal it. I want to introduce you to a technique

that will get to the root of unwanted emotions using essential oils and allow you to release them permanently.

Aroma Freedom Technique

Aroma Freedom Technique (AFT) was developed by Dr. Benjamin Perkus, Ph.D.,[20] a clinical psychologist who discovered that, because scent acts as a signal that automatically triggers responses in the brain, the scent of essential oils can be used intentionally to cause emotional changes.

Dr. Perkus says that AFT is effective at "releasing negative thoughts, feelings, and memories. It has to do with the brain's natural process of memory reconsolidation. AFT alters the perception of danger or stress that had been stored in the original memory and actually promotes a re-wiring of the memory itself, naturally and easily."

Smell can trigger memories. We've all experienced this. Whenever I smell coffee and bacon together, I'm instantly transported in my mind back to my Mimi's kitchen. It's this feature of instant and irresistible triggering of memories and their associated feelings that makes the AFT process so effective.

I've been using AFT to successfully deprogram negative emotions. It's simple, quick, and effective. You can do it in your own home all by yourself or you can get someone to guide you. If you're interested in learning more about this process, Dr. Perkus' book is available at https://AromaFreedom.com.

Forgiveness

In her book, *The Armor of Victory*, Janet M. Magiera states,

> A fellow minister told me of a vision she received which I believe is very powerful. This minister saw "wounds of the heart" that had been buried in the cemetery and had tombstones erected to memorialize them. The wounds were buried, but unlike a dead body, they continued to fester and boil under the earth. Not only did the wound need to be unburied and have forgiveness applied

CHAPTER 29 – BENEFITS OF ESSENTIAL OILS

> to it, but the tomb stone needed to be pushed over and broken into tiny pieces so that there was no longer a memorial to the wound.
>
> Jesus came to heal the brokenhearted with forgiveness and to further set the captives free. He summarized his whole mission at the beginning of his ministry by quoting Isaiah 61:1 and Isaiah 58:6.
>
> *Luke 4:18 APNT*
> *The Spirit of the Lord [is] on me and because of this, he has anointed me to preach to the poor and has sent me to heal the broken-hearted and to preach forgiveness to the captives and sight to the blind and to strengthen the broken with forgiveness.*
>
> In order for a person to be healed of a physical wound or cut, the cut first needs to be cleansed. If the cut is deep, it needs to be sewn up or cauterized. Then ointment or salve can be applied to the wound and it can be bandaged. Once a cut is healed, there may be a scar, but there is no further pain. The same process applies to dressing wounds in our soul.[21]

Have we erected any memorials to our wounds? A good indicator that forgiveness needs to be applied is if there's pain in a memory. Just as with the healing of a physical wound, healing a mental/emotional wound may require repeated applications of forgiveness.

One day, I was having some prayer time with Father and consciously forgiving people as He brought them to my mind (I had asked Him to do this). Then, he brought to mind one situation, and my response was nothing. I felt nothing about it. It was like watching something that had happened to someone else. So, I asked Father why He had brought it up. He showed me that He wanted me to know what real forgiveness felt like. I could remember what happened, but it had no emotional impact on me at all. No pain, no regret. It's just ... over. That's forgiveness.

When we fail to forgive, send away, the offenses caused by others, we retain them. They affect our emotions, our health, our peace, and our

CHAPTER 29 – BENEFITS OF ESSENTIAL OILS

confidence. We cannot experience healing while holding onto an offense that is making us sick. Dealing with the trespasses of others is a key to being able to forgive [send away] our own trespasses.

I believe that using essential oils while applying forgiveness to our wounds will help us diffuse negative emotions associated with the memory by quickly accessing the limbic system.

Zyto Balance Biomarker Report

I wanted to support my body with essential oils, but how could I know which oils my body needed? I was tired of guessing. I wanted to know how to use my oils more effectively. I was taking a shotgun approach to my wellness based on my symptoms. But I knew that's not the best way to use essential oils.

Essential oils are designed to support, maintain, and protect our health on the physical, mental, emotional, and yes – even spiritual level. They're designed to support, enhance, and strengthen our body systems.

So, I needed a way to ask my body what it needs. I found a scanning system that provides a comprehensive personalized wellness report that goes into specific detail of what physical and emotional stress the body is currently experiencing and an explanation of why specific essential oils can help.

The Zyto Balance Biomarker Report gives a 40-page report that goes over body systems and emotions in detail, as well as a report that details which vertebrae in the spine are attached to any underlying bodily stressors. It's a great reference if you receive chiropractic care.

From the report, I'm able to identify the specific Young Living supplements and essential oils my body is craving, as well as identify areas in which my body needs additional support.

If you're ready to get real results with essential oils, please contact me at Carol@3Jn2Wellness.com and I'll put you in touch with the person who does the Zyto scans for me.

CHAPTER 29 – BENEFITS OF ESSENTIAL OILS

Important Considerations When Purchasing Essential Oils

I've mentioned the dangers of the adulterated essential oils currently being sold everywhere. Avoiding these fake oils is essential if you want to receive therapeutic benefits.

Be sure to follow all label warnings and instructions. You can't find therapeutic grade essential oils in stores or on websites like Amazon. You must go to the producer or their representative.

Always dilute essential oils with a vegetable oil – such as V-6, fractionated coconut oil or pure virgin olive oil before applying it to the skin. If redness or irritation occurs when using essential oils topically, apply more vegetable oil to the affected area. Water will not help.

Essential oils can be used aromatically (by smelling or diffusing), topically on the skin, or internally (in food or supplements).

If it's cheap (low cost), it's probably cheap (adulterated). Know your supplier.

Quality is key, not quantity. Quality essential oils are very potent, far more potent than dried herbs.

Because they are very powerful, start slowly and listen to God's guidance for you.

Can Essential Oils be Used on Children?

Many essential oils are appropriate for use with children and should always be diluted with a carrier oil prior to use. Some Young Living products are pre-diluted with a carrier oil as indicated on the label and are intended for direct application to children. Children generally respond well to essential oils.

Can Essential Oils be Used During Pregnancy or While Nursing?

Prior to using essential oils, seek the advice and recommendation of a competent, trained health care advisor who is experienced in essential oil usage. Generally speaking, pregnant/nursing women should avoid overuse/excessive use of clary sage (*Salvia sclarea*), sage (*Salvia officinalis*), tansy (*Tanacetum vulgare*), hyssop (*Hyssopus officinalis*), fennel (*Foeniculum vulgare*), and wintergreen (*Gaultheria procumbens*), as well as the blends and supplements that contain these oils.

Conclusion

Essential oils aren't a magic solution to all one's problems; they're a doorway to a whole new way of being. Essential oils don't cure disease. Learning to use essential oils is about lifestyle, a paradigm shift, about strengthening the body. When we do this, the body will take care of itself because God designed the body to heal itself.

Everyone is different and no two essential oils are the same; therefore, no two people respond to essential oils in the exact same way. By simply supporting and strengthening the body with a healthy lifestyle and proper nutrition, everyone can have his or her own individual experience without trying to narrow it down to a specific oil for a specific problem.

**There is treasure to be desired and oil in the dwelling of the wise.
Proverbs 21:20 KJV**

I own and recommend the following reference books:

Reference Guide for Essential Oils, by Connie and Alan Higley. Available at AbundantHealth4You.com. An abbreviated version is also available.

Full-Color 7th Edition Essential Oils Pocket Reference, from Life Science Publishing. Available at DiscoverLSP.com.

Healing Oils of the Bible, by David Stewart Ph.D. Widely available online and in bookstores.

CHAPTER 29 – BENEFITS OF ESSENTIAL OILS

Abundant Health 4 You has an app called *Reference Guide for Essential Oils* that I use regularly. Check your app store.

If you have any questions about essential oils, feel free to contact me at Carol@3Jn2Wellness.com.

CHAPTER 30

THE BE IN HEALTH MEAL PLAN

This sample 7-day healthy eating plan will give you an idea of the types of foods I eat each day. The wonderful thing about this is that I can choose whatever food I happen to like from each category. Some days I prefer turkey to chicken or coconut yogurt to coconut kefir. I use the foods I like that fit within these guidelines.

Foods I Eat

A list of what I ate (and still eat) to regain (and maintain) my health is in chapter 24.

Foods I Avoid

A list of the top foods I avoid is in chapter 19.

Water

I drink at least eight 8-oz. glasses of purified (never tap) water every day. Water is my first, and in many cases only, beverage. My drinking water is room temperature; it's much easier on the gut than ice cold water. There are many quality water purifiers on the market to fit every budget. Don't skimp here.

Cooking Double

I try to cook a double portion of food so I have leftovers. This works out well because my husband takes the leftovers with him to work the next day. I freeze anything I'm not going to use within 2 days.

Meals

Refer to the recipes in chapter 50.

Breakfast

- Super Restoring Smoothie + supplements (I add many of my supplements to my smoothie – especially essential oils.)

CHAPTER 30 – THE BE IN HEALTH MEAL PLAN

- I mix up the types of fruit and veggies I add to my smoothie so I'm not having the same thing every day.
- I include several types of berries in my smoothie, as berries are very beneficial to the body and are easy on the digestive system.
- On days I prefer hot food for breakfast, I make a hot smoothie or a sweet potato and beet hash or a Farmer's Wife Breakfast with lamb sausage.

Lunch

My favorite lunch is a sweet potato with ghee, Himalayan pink salt, Ceylon cinnamon, and pecans. I enjoy this with a mug of bone broth.

Dinner

Dinner is usually very simple: a protein and vegetables. For example, I'll scramble some eggs and add asparagus, avocado, and sauerkraut. My husband's favorite meal is taco salad. I enjoy a Waldorf chicken salad. All these recipes are in chapter 50.

Snacks

Because I practice intermittent fasting (chapter 36), I usually don't get hungry between meals. But if I do snack, I have either applesauce (see my recipe in chapter 50) or a nut mix that I make from raw, unsalted walnuts, pistachios, and macadamia nuts.

Salad Dressing

Salad dressing is a problem for those avoiding unhealthy oils, sugars, additives, and flavorings. There's not much available commercially that I would buy. So, I make my own.

My recipe for Taco Salad Dressing is in chapter 50. If I want a non-creamy dressing, I simply mix balsamic vinegar with EVOO (extra virgin olive oil). If I feel like getting fancy, I add fresh garlic and other herbs. I like to keep things simple.

CHAPTER 30 – THE BE IN HEALTH MEAL PLAN

For Vegans/Vegetarians

The Be in Health healthy eating plan is based on Old Testament dietary principles, which include meat. If you're a vegan/vegetarian, it's possible to follow this plan, but it's more limited.

The main concern for vegetarians is getting enough calories from healthy fat and protein each day. Many vegan/vegetarian diets are rich in grains, legumes, wheat, and soy, which I eliminate since they tend to cause digestive upset. Legumes and grains are heavy with toxins such as lectins and alpha-amylase inhibitors, and often cause acid reflux, gas, and bloating. In many studies, these have been shown to contribute to or cause leaky gut syndrome.

If you're a vegetarian who wants to follow this eating plan, try including more good saturated fats, such as coconut oil, avocado, and olives. That's the best fuel for our bodies overall, even more than protein. Starchy vegetables like carrots, beets, acorn squash, butternut squash, pumpkin, and peas are great complex carbohydrate options. Protein can come from eggs, quinoa, lentils, spirulina, bee pollen, nuts/seeds, and/or protein powders from rice, hemp, or pea. Although lentils and peas are legumes, they tend to be better tolerated than many other beans, but test for your own particular gut issues since everyone is different.

Above all, I always listen to my body and am open to trying new things and making adjustments. I developed the Be in Health lifestyle because something was not working in my body (my gut). I'm open to trying new foods or eating schedules since they may be part of the solution and may lead to optimal health restoration.

Snack/Dessert Ideas

- Chia Seed Coconut Milk Pudding*
- Slow Cooker Cinnamon Applesauce*
- Veggies like carrots, celery
- A handful of raw unsalted nuts/seeds (walnuts + pistachios + macadamia nuts is a great combo)

CHAPTER 30 – THE BE IN HEALTH MEAL PLAN

- Water (sometimes I'm just thirsty)

Be in Health Sample 7-Day Menu

Day	Breakfast	Lunch	Dinner with Bone Broth
1	Super Restoring Smoothie*	Grilled Salmon with Vegetables of Choice	Waldorf Chicken Salad*
2	Farmer's Wife with Lamb Sausage*	Avocado Stuffed Meatballs*with Sweet Potatoes	Leftover Grilled Salmon over Leafy Greens
3	Baked Apple Smoothie*	Garlicky Spaghetti Squash with Chicken, Mushrooms, and Kale*	Cauliflower Soup* with salad
4	Sweet Potato/Beet Hash*	Cilantro Salmon Burger* with vegetables	Leftover Meatballs over Leafy Greens
5	Super Restoring Smoothie*	Leftover Spaghetti Squash	Pumpkin-Ginger Soup*
6	Farmer's Wife with Lamb Sausage*	Egg Scramble with Asparagus, Avocado, and Sauerkraut*	Green Tea Chicken Soup*
7	Super Restoring Smoothie*	Lemon Basil Chicken* with Vegetables of Choice	Taco Salad*

* - Included in recipes in chapter 50.

CHAPTER 31

MY SHOPPING LIST

Food Shopping Guidelines

- God made cattle and sheep/lambs to feed on grasses. Therefore, I buy only 100% grass-fed and finished beef and lamb. If the label says 'Grass-fed,' but not '100% Grass-fed,' there's a good chance that the animals are initially grass-fed, but then the last few months they are grain-fed. These grains are most likely GMO and gluten-filled. I am what the thing I eat, ate. There are many local ranchers and co-ops where I can buy 100% grass-fed and finished beef and lamb. Check online.
- I buy pasture raised chicken and turkey. This means they are allowed to roam freely and eat naturally.
- I buy organic produce as much as possible, paying attention to The Clean 15 List and The Dirty Dozen List.[1] This saves money on shopping because I know which foods should always be purchased organic and which I can get non-organic. The budget doesn't always allow for 100% organic or sustainable food.
- I don't buy already prepared, processed foods. I cook from scratch at home. I control the ingredients in what I make.
- I always soak my fruits and veggies after purchase even if they're organic. I don't know who (or what) has touched the food or if it was dropped on the floor. I use either white vinegar diluted in water or a premade produce soak.

I buy according to the above rules in this order:

- 100% grass-fed and finished meat, before I buy
- A2, raw dairy products, before I buy
- Organic fruits and vegetables, before I buy
- Gluten-free products

CHAPTER 31 – MY SHOPPING LIST

Be in Health Shopping List

Vegetables

- ☐ Artichoke
- ☐ Arugula
- ☐ Asparagus
- ☐ Avocados
- ☐ Beets/Beet Greens
- ☐ Bok Choy
- ☐ Broccoli
- ☐ Broccoli Rabe
- ☐ Brussels Sprouts
- ☐ Cabbage
- ☐ Carrots
- ☐ Cauliflower
- ☐ Celery
- ☐ Collards
- ☐ Cucumber
- ☐ Garlic
- ☐ Green Beans
- ☐ All dark, leafy greens
- ☐ Jerusalem Artichoke
- ☐ Kale
- ☐ Mushrooms
- ☐ Olives
- ☐ Onions
- ☐ Parsnips
- ☐ Pumpkin
- ☐ Radish
- ☐ Romaine Lettuce
- ☐ Rutabaga
- ☐ Sea Vegetables
- ☐ Spinach
- ☐ Sprouts
- ☐ Squash
- ☐ Turnip Greens
- ☐ Watercress
- ☐ Wheatgrass juice

Fish – Wild-Caught Only, No Farm-Raised

- ☐ Anchovies
- ☐ Bass Cod
- ☐ Grouper
- ☐ Haddock
- ☐ Halibut
- ☐ Herring
- ☐ Mackerel
- ☐ Mahi Mahi
- ☐ Red Snapper
- ☐ Salmon
- ☐ Sardines
- ☐ Seabass
- ☐ Trout
- ☐ Tuna
- ☐ Walleye

NO SHELLFISH

Starches

- ☐ Cassava
- ☐ Plantains
- ☐ Sweet potatoes
- ☐ Yams

CHAPTER 31 – MY SHOPPING LIST

Seeds/Nuts – Sprouted (or sprout/soak your own)

- ☐ Chia
- ☐ Flax
- ☐ Hemp
- ☐ Almonds
- ☐ Pecans
- ☐ Walnuts
- ☐ Pumpkin
- ☐ Sesame
- ☐ Sunflower
- ☐ Macadamia nuts
- ☐ Pistachios
- ☐ Seed/nut butters

Low Fructose Fruits (in moderation)

- ☐ Apples (only Granny Smith)
- ☐ Blackberries
- ☐ Blueberries
- ☐ Cantaloupe
- ☐ Clementines
- ☐ Casaba Melon
- ☐ Grapefruit
- ☐ Guava
- ☐ Lemons
- ☐ Limes
- ☐ Honeydew Melon
- ☐ Nectarines
- ☐ Oranges
- ☐ Papaya
- ☐ Peaches
- ☐ Plums
- ☐ Tangerines
- ☐ Raspberries
- ☐ Strawberries

Meat – Organic, 100% Grass Fed

- ☐ Beef
- ☐ Bison
- ☐ Pasture raised chicken
- ☐ Ducks
- ☐ Eggs
- ☐ Lamb
- ☐ Pasture raised turkey
- ☐ Quail
- ☐ Venison & other wild game

NO PORK

Dairy – Raw or Low Temp Processed

- ☐ A2 Cow's cheese/milk
- ☐ Amasi (from A2 cows)
- ☐ Goat's milk products
- ☐ Sheep's milk products

Sweeteners (In Moderation)

- ☐ Local, raw (unpasteurized) honey
- ☐ Stevia
- ☐ Maple syrup (Grade A: Dark Color & Robust Flavor)

CHAPTER 31 – MY SHOPPING LIST

Spices and Herbs

- ☐ Basil
- ☐ Cilantro
- ☐ Coriander seeds
- ☐ Cinnamon
- ☐ Cloves
- ☐ Cumin
- ☐ Dill
- ☐ Fennel
- ☐ Garlic
- ☐ Ginger
- ☐ Mint
- ☐ Mustard seed
- ☐ Nutmeg
- ☐ Oregano
- ☐ Parsley
- ☐ Peppermint
- ☐ Rosemary
- ☐ Sage
- ☐ Tarragon
- ☐ Thyme
- ☐ Turmeric

Fats/Oils – Organic Unrefined

- ☐ Avocado oil
- ☐ Almond oil
- ☐ Butter (pasture raised, A2)
- ☐ Coconut oil
- ☐ Ghee
- ☐ Macadamia oil
- ☐ Extra virgin olive oil
- ☐ Sesame oil

NO canola oil, corn oil, or vegetable oils

Condiments

- ☐ Apple cider vinegar
- ☐ Balsamic vinegar
- ☐ Coconut vinegar
- ☐ Coconut Aminos
- ☐ Cacao nibs/powder (contains gluten)
- ☐ Extracts (vanilla/almond)
- ☐ Guacamole
- ☐ Himalayan pink salt
- ☐ Mustard (stone ground)

Beverages

- ☐ Coconut kefir
- ☐ Coconut milk
- ☐ Herbal teas
- ☐ Raw vegetable juices
- ☐ Sparkling water
- ☐ Spring or filtered water

Supplements

- ☐ Digestive enzymes
- ☐ Probiotics
- ☐ Fish Oil
- ☐ L-glutamine

PART 8

LIVING THE LIFESTYLE

**Who forgiveth all thine iniquities; who healeth all thy diseases.
Psalm 103:3**

CHAPTER 32

THE AMAZING HEALTH BENEFITS OF BONE BROTH

What is bone broth? Simply, it's broth (clear soup) made from bones. Any type of bones can be used, but I usually use chicken. I will use a whole fryer, but many people add extra feet, knuckles, and other joints to get more gelatin (a rich source of dietary collagen, which is a key protein). Other people prefer to use beef, lamb, turkey, or fish bones.

I've been asked if there's a substitute for bone broth for vegans and vegetarians, and while there's no vegan substitute for gelatin, you can make a mineral-rich plant-based broth.[1]

Restore the Gut to Health with Bone Broth

The main reason I started consuming bone broth is because of leaky gut syndrome, which I was diagnosed with over 15 years ago via a camera I swallowed that gave doctors a tour of my digestive system. (Yes, that really happened.) Leaky gut syndrome occurs when tight junctions in the gut (small intestine), which control what passes through the lining of the small intestine, don't work properly, letting substances leak into the bloodstream.

What is usually leaked into the bloodstream are proteins, specifically gluten (from certain grains) and casein (from dairy products). The body doesn't know what to do with these 'foreign' proteins, so it tucks them into various organs/tissues/glands. This can lead to an autoimmune disorder, in which the immune system identifies the foreign proteins, but then attacks the entire organ/tissue/gland where the foreign proteins are stored. The immune system essentially confuses the foreign proteins with the proteins that make up you.

Bone broth also contains collagen and gelatin, which help to 'seal up' the gut and prevent the leaks by supporting the mucous lining of the gut. Gelatin decreases inflammation,[2] allowing your intestinal cells to heal.

CHAPTER 32 – THE AMAZING HEALTH BENEFITS OF BONE BROTH

Bone Broth Supports Immune Health

Bone broth has been called a superfood due to its high concentration of minerals. Bone marrow can help strengthen the immune system (no surprise to chicken soup aficionados). A Harvard study[3] showed that some people with autoimmune disorders experienced relief of symptoms when drinking bone broth, with some achieving complete remission.

Have you ever noticed how well chicken soup works[4] when you don't feel well? It's because broth made with chicken bones contains nutrients that support immune function while decreasing inflammation and oxidative stress. Bone broth contains amino acids like L-glutamine, glycine, arginine, and cysteine. Remember that amino acids are the building blocks of protein.

Taking Glucosamine and Chondroitin? Try Bone Broth Instead

Many people take supplements to get glucosamine sulfate and chondroitin sulfate into their systems to support joint health. Both of these nutrients are in bone broth, and the chondroitin sulfate in bone broth has been shown to help prevent osteoarthritis. The National Institutes of Health [5] states that glucosamine sulfate is as effective in treating OA as over-the-counter painkillers, as well as being able to slow the progression of OA. (Rheumatoid arthritis is an autoimmune disorder, so bone broth can help for the reasons discussed above.) Instead of taking pills, why not drink bone broth instead?

Look Younger, Sleep Better, Feel Better

Collagen helps form elastin and other compounds within the skin that are responsible for maintaining the skin's youthful tone, texture, and appearance. Many people spend a lot of money to plump up the lines on their faces with collagen, but bone broth is naturally rich in collagen. Why spend the money and endure the needles?

CHAPTER 32 – THE AMAZING HEALTH BENEFITS OF BONE BROTH

The glycine in bone broth[6] has also been shown in several studies to help people sleep better and improve memory.

Get a Jump on Detoxing with Bone Broth

Bone broth is considered by many to be a powerful detoxifier. It helps the digestive system expel waste while it supports the liver's ability to remove toxins. It also helps maintain tissue integrity and improves the body's use of antioxidants.

Some of the ways bone broth boosts detoxification are by supplying sulfur and glutathione.[7] (The Preventative Research Center of the CDC [8] has found that glutathione helps with the elimination of fat-soluble compounds, especially heavy metals like mercury and lead.)

Bone broth contains potassium and glycine, which support both cellular and liver detoxification.[9] It also contains minerals in forms that the body can easily absorb: calcium, magnesium, phosphorus, silicon, sulfur, and others. It contains chondroitin sulfates and glucosamine, the same compounds sold as pricey supplements to reduce inflammation, arthritis, and joint pain.[10,11]

These are some of the wonderful benefits of bone broth. See my recipe in chapter 50.

CHAPTER 32 – THE AMAZING HEALTH BENEFITS OF BONE BROTH

CHAPTER 33

HOW TO OVERCOME A SUGAR ADDICTION

Are you the type of person who, once you start eating something sugary, can't stop? Me, too (or at least, I used to be). I used to consider ice cream and chocolate cake to be major food groups. Yikes! I had a MASSIVE addiction to sugar.

It's easy to see how that could happen. Sugar is everywhere. They put it in almost every processed food imaginable: cereals, ketchup, pasta sauce, salad dressings, barbeque sauce, smoothies, crackers, etc. Need some help? Here are some ways to overcome a sugar addiction.

Positive Mental Attitude

Recognizing the need to cut processed sugar out of your life is your first step. "But, Carol, sugar tastes so good. Why should I stop eating it?" I'm so glad you asked. Did you know that the average American consumes 20 teaspoons of added sugar every day (that doesn't count naturally-occurring sugar, such as in fruit)? That's three times more than Dr. Joseph Mercola, D.O. recommends.[1]

Sugar is what is fueling our current epidemics of obesity and type 2 diabetes.[2] Not to mention that it's cancer's favorite food. Dr. Yella Hewings-Martin, Ph.D., says, "Evidence pointing [to sugar causing cancer] was discovered in a study funded by the sugar industry nearly 50 years ago — but the work was never published."[3] Even if you don't currently have these diseases, sugar is a gateway that opens the door to them.

Your health, present and future, is the number one reason to cut out sugar. Once you've made that decision, you will need some ammunition to help you deal with sugar cravings and withdrawal symptoms. It sounds like you're getting off a drug. Guess what? You are.

According to Dr. William Cole, D.C., sugar (no matter the source) stimulates the brain's pleasure center, the nucleus accumbens, with

CHAPTER 33 – HOW TO OVERCOME A SUGAR ADDICTION

dopamine, the same way that sex and doing drugs does.[4] "The problem with all this sugar stimulation is that prolonged dopamine signal creates a tolerance," Dr. Cole says. "Over time, this creates deeper neuronal pathways, [so] we need more sugar to give us the same euphoric fix."

Sugar will be lurking everywhere, around every corner, trying to lure you back into its web. Knowing that you're getting healthier can help you overcome the urges, but you're going to need some big guns.

Exercise

Exercise is the best 'cure' for sugar cravings. It falls into the category of taking care of yourself. When you're eliminating something from your life, it's wise to add in things that nourish you. You must exercise self-love and self-care in addition to exercising your body. Be full emotionally so you don't come to this process drained.

Bodily exercise can reduce insulin levels,[5] which will decrease your desire for sugary foods. "Moderate exercise, like walking, makes you breathe a little harder and your heart beat a little faster. Your muscles use more glucose, the sugar in your bloodstream. Over time, this can lower your blood sugar levels," according to WebMD.[6]

Eat Sour Foods

Eating something sour, like cultured vegetables or kefir, helps reduce cravings for something sweet.[7] Try some coconut yogurt, coconut kefir, sauerkraut, a pickle, add some lemon or lime to your water. An additional benefit of eating sour foods is that they're probiotic-rich.

Eat Fat/Starchy Foods

Dr. Cole suggests fat bombs[8] (see recipe in chapter 50) as a way of curbing cravings. He also says that starchy tubers like sweet potatoes are a great way to get your carbs in whole food form.[9]

Make Sure You're Getting Enough Minerals

Krystelle Fournier, a Board Certified Holistic Health Counselor, recommends eating foods that are high in magnesium (dark leafy greens,

CHAPTER 33 - HOW TO OVERCOME A SUGAR ADDICTION

nuts and seeds, avocado), chromium (broccoli, sweet potatoes, pasture raised eggs), and zinc (pumpkins seeds, Brazil nuts, pasture raised eggs) to reduce sugar cravings.

Here are some things to avoid when quitting sugar:[10]

Don't Overdo It on Fruit

You may think that the sugar in fruit is good so it's okay to have as much as you want. But, it's still sugar, and it still has an effect on your blood sugar levels. The fructose in fruit doesn't spike the blood sugar levels like processed table sugar or high fructose corn syrup (HFCS) does, but too much fruit in a short amount of time isn't the answer. Try sour foods instead (see above).

Don't Replace Sugar with Artificial Sweeteners

Artificial sweeteners like Splenda® (sucralose), Sweet'N Low® (saccharin), Equal® and NutraSweet® (aspartame, now being called Amino Sweet®), acesulfame K, and neotame are NOT a good replacement for sugar. Each comes with their own negative health implications. If you absolutely must sweeten something, use stevia, maple syrup, raw (unpasteurized), local honey (up to 1 Tbsp. per day) or coconut sugar (sparingly). My choice is stevia. I prefer NOW Better Stevia because it has no added ingredients. It also has the USDA organic seal and the Non-GMO Project Verified butterfly.

There are many, many names for sugar that are unfamiliar to most people but are used by manufacturers. Get the low-down in Appendix 2.

Soothe the Detox

Detox symptoms from sugar withdrawal can include fatigue, headaches, digestive issues, moodiness, and flu-like symptoms. Don't give in to the sugar monster just to alleviate them. The body is detoxing and that's a good thing. See chapter 44 for ways to handle detox symptoms. (**Always check with your doctor if symptoms are too much.**)

Healthy fats are your friend. They will supply energy. Bone broth can help with digestive issues. Supplements like NAC (N-Acetyl Cysteine),

CHAPTER 33 – HOW TO OVERCOME A SUGAR ADDICTION

dandelion root, milk thistle, and cilantro (add to food) will help soothe the detox symptoms. Turmeric and magnesium can help with headaches. Foods that are rich in electrolytes like avocados and leafy greens can help with muscle aches.[11] Be sure to keep hydrated and eat real, whole food.

Once you've gotten through the initial withdrawal symptoms (about 3 days), your taste buds will start to return to normal and sugar will start to taste bad. Real food will start to taste good. Congratulations! You're on your way to a healthier future. You can overcome a sugar addiction.

CHAPTER 34

HOW TO QUIT COFFEE

I had my last cup of coffee on December 31, 1994. That's because, on January 1, 1995, I started a doctor-supervised 10-day fast. Going cold turkey like I did is like jumping into a pool filled with ice cubes. It's a shock to the system but at least it's over quickly. I don't recommend cold turkey for everyone; for some people, weaning is a better way to go. I'm going to discuss both ways to quit coffee.

Why Should I Quit Drinking Coffee?

It seems that no one agrees if coffee is good or bad for health. There are too many contradictory studies. While healthy people may benefit from coffee, those with leaky gut syndrome, chronic inflammation, and/or autoimmune disorders may find that coffee does more harm than good.[1]

According to Dr. Mark Hyman, M.D., these are reasons to quit coffee:[2]

- Caffeine increases stress hormones, which elicit cortisol and increase insulin. Insulin increases inflammation, which is already a problem for those with an autoimmune disorder. Cortisol can lead to belly fat.[3]

- Coffee addiction is an addiction to a drug, caffeine.

- Caffeine addiction decreases insulin sensitivity, making it difficult for cells to respond appropriately to blood sugar.

- The acidity of coffee is associated with digestive discomfort, indigestion, heartburn, GERD (acid reflux), and dysbiosis (imbalances in the gut flora).

- There are many associations with coffee like cream and sugar. I quit coffee for good after my fast when my doctor told me I could go back to coffee but not the cream and sugar I put in it. I thought, "What's the point?" I viewed coffee as a delivery method for cream and sugar. I'll bet I'm not alone in that.

CHAPTER 34 – HOW TO QUIT COFFEE

- Coffee interferes with serotonin production, which is necessary for restful sleep, which is critical for those with an autoimmune disorder.

- Coffee causes an imbalance in electrolytes, which can cause irregular/fast heartbeat, fatigue, lethargy, nausea, vomiting, diarrhea and/or constipation.

- Constituents in coffee can interfere with normal drug metabolism and detoxification in the liver, making it difficult to regulate the normal detoxification process in the liver.

Switching to organic coffee doesn't eliminate the caffeine. Switching to decaf still doesn't get rid of all the caffeine (the USDA allows coffee with 3% caffeine to be called decaffeinated), plus it adds toxins depending on the decaffeination process used.[4]

These are just some of the reasons to quit coffee. But how?

Cold Turkey Method

Going 'cold turkey' means "the abrupt and complete cessation of taking a drug to which one is addicted." This is how I quit both coffee (in 1995) and cigarettes (in 1985); I'm an 'all or nothing' kind of person. Quitting coffee cold turkey meant drinking my usual amount of coffee one day, and the next day and from then on, nothing. Just stop. It's the fastest way to detox from caffeine.

Why is it called 'cold turkey'? One symptom of opioid withdrawal is goose flesh (small bumps on the surface of the skin usually resulting from being cold; also called goosebumps). When someone discontinued opioids abruptly (cold turkey), they would exhibit these visible symptoms and it was noticed their skin looked like a cold turkey.[5]

The biggest symptom I had quitting coffee cold turkey was a massive headache that lasted for days. What made it worse was having to go to work and be productive. Mood swings and fatigue were other not-so-pleasant symptoms.

CHAPTER 34 – HOW TO QUIT COFFEE

The best way to quit cold turkey is to do it over a long weekend or even a week-long vacation. Let the people around you know what you're doing so they can be supportive.

Be especially kind to yourself during this time. Drink as much purified water as you possibly can to flush the toxins out. You will have to weigh the pros and cons of taking pain relievers. Sleep as much as you can and eat easily digestible foods, like bone broth or soup.

The key to going cold turkey is to avoid all caffeine including in chocolate (which has sugar, another reason not to eat it), or medications, other beverages (like tea, soda, and energy drinks), or food with added caffeine. Just the smallest amount will bring detox to a halt.

If all this sounds too overwhelming, there's another, easier way to quit.

Weaning Method

The weaning method means gradually cutting back the amount of caffeine consumed until you're no longer consuming it. It takes longer to accomplish but the withdrawal symptoms are less severe than with the cold turkey method.

You can do the weaning method by yourself or you can use one of the weaning aids available commercially. If you do use an aid, be sure to read the labels so you know what you're ingesting (and, yes, if it's a skin patch you're still ingesting it; anything that goes on the skin ends up in the blood just like anything we eat).

If you're doing it by yourself, you will need to track your caffeine intake. You can use the Food – Mood – Poop Journal (chapter 49) for this. Aim for cutting back by 10-30 mg of caffeine per day.

The website http://CaffeineInformer.com has these suggestions:[6]

- Coffee should be reduced by 1/4 of a cup every two to three days. (This is easier if you make coffee at home.)
- Energy drinks can be reduced by about 1/4 of a can every two to three days.

CHAPTER 34 – HOW TO QUIT COFFEE

- Soda can be reduced by cutting back by 1/2 of a can every two to three days or by 1/4 of a bottle if drinking a 16 Fl.oz. size.
- Tea can be reduced by cutting back 1/2 cup every two to three days. Most decaffeinated teas have some caffeine in them.[7]

Benefits of Quitting Coffee

- Better sleep and more energy. Many people drink coffee for energy, but the truth is that "caffeine from coffee is not an energy-generating substance, metabolically speaking," according to Dr. Tina M. St. John, M.D. "In other words, your body cannot metabolize caffeine to power your cells... The stimulatory effects of caffeine on the brain, however, give the perception of increased energy because you feel more mentally alert."[8] Once you stop drinking coffee, your metabolism will level off so you won't get those caffeine highs and lows.
- Feeling calmer. Wesley Delbridge, R.D., a spokesperson for the Academy of Nutrition and Dietetics, says, "Caffeine is a stimulant, meaning it hits your nervous system's gas pedal. Caffeine triggers a release of adrenaline, needlessly putting you into 'fight or flight' mode. Plus, since caffeine is a vasoconstrictor, narrowing your blood vessels, it raises your blood pressure."[9]
- Digestion will improve. Coffee poops[10] are a real and ever-present threat to coffee lovers everywhere. That's because, Delbridge says, "Apart from the fact that caffeine speeds things up in your digestive system, coffee is very acidic, which can also increase your risk of the runs." Eliminating caffeine from your diet will do a lot to prevent emergency trips to the bathroom.[11]
- You'll save money that can be spent on better quality, real, whole foods. According to the Caffeine Informer,[12] you can save between $237 and $1,332 per year depending on what types of caffeine you consume and how much.

These are just some of the reasons to improve health by quitting coffee.

CHAPTER 35

WHY (THE RIGHT KIND OF) FAT IS HEALTHY

For more years than I care to admit, I bought into the lie that eating fat will make you fat. It made sense to me only because I didn't understand how the body works and how it assimilates fats and other nutrients. I'm not going to give you a biology lesson here, I'm just going to show you why (the right kind of) fat is healthy.

For many years it was thought that consuming less fat would increase health and reduce weight, but the opposite has happened. According to the Centers for Disease Control and Prevention, no state in the country has less than 20% obesity today.[1]

Why was eating fat assumed to be bad? After World War II, research came out that seemed to link saturated fats to coronary heart disease. Soon, the American Heart Association recommended that people reduce their fat intake. In 1976, the U.S. Senate held a series of committee meetings on Diet Related to Killer Diseases.[2] Subsequent USDA food guidelines recommended eating less saturated fat and more carbohydrates. The war on fats had begun.

It is now known that the right kind of fat is healthy.[3]

Saturated Fats

There's no evidence that saturated fat is associated with increased risk of cardiovascular disease or coronary heart disease, as was previously thought.[4] Before this became well known, many people stopped eating saturated fats and replaced them with hydrogenated and partially hydrogenated oils (also called trans fats), which have now been shown to increase heart disease, obesity, and Type 2 diabetes, which are at near-epidemic proportions in the U.S.[5]

In the past, colorectal cancer was said to be associated with diets high in saturated fats. However, there is no correlation. The Women's Health Initiative Dietary Modification Trial studied postmenopausal women for more than eight years and found that a low-fat diet did not reduce the risk of colorectal cancer.[6]

Dr. Joseph Mercola, D.O., says the benefits of eating saturated fats include improved cardiovascular risk factors, stronger bones, improved liver health, healthy lungs, healthy brain, proper nerve signaling, and a strong immune system.[7] Additionally, energy from medium-chain fatty acids helps to burn other fats.

I avoid vegetable oils, including corn, peanut, soybean, and canola oil, and replace them with healthy oils, including coconut oil (a medium-chain fatty acid that is easily digested), ghee (or clarified butter, which is butter with the proteins removed), sesame oil, grass-fed A2 butter, and extra virgin olive oil.

The American Heart Association Strikes Again

Despite having been previously proved wrong about the relationship between healthy dietary fats and cardiovascular disease, in June 2017 the AHA declared, "We advise against the use of coconut oil." [8]

Hilda Bastian, who works at the National Institutes of Health making clinical effectiveness research accessible to the public as the lead for the PubMed Health team, believes the AHA got it wrong on coconut oil for these reasons:[9]

- Inadequate research and method of choosing studies
- Not being equally critical of all studies
- Incorrect representation of the results of the coconut oil review
- Making strong conclusions based on weak evidence

The AHA made their declaration about coconut oil despite their conclusion that

> Finally, we note that **a trial has never been conducted** to test the effect on CHD (Coronary Heart Disease) outcomes of a low-fat diet that increases intake of healthful nutrient-dense carbohydrates and fiber-rich foods such as whole grains,

CHAPTER 35 — WHY (THE RIGHT KIND OF) FAT IS HEALTHY

vegetables, fruits, and legumes that are now recommended in dietary guidelines.

That's right; the health guidelines the government has been promoting for the last 20-30 years have never been tested!

So, why is the AHA demonizing coconut oil? Let's follow the money trail. Dr. Tania Dempsey, M.D., an expert in chronic disease, autoimmune disorders, and mast cell activation syndrome, writes that

> *Pharmaceutical companies Pfizer, Glaxo-Smith Kline, AstraZeneca, Amgen and many more are listed as providing research grants for the authors. It just so happens that these companies manufacture cholesterol-lowering medications, like statins and the new drug Repatha. Why would they want to know whether coconut oil is good or bad for patients? Or whether eating carbohydrates is better than eating saturated fat? Well, for one, they will be well-positioned to market their drugs to the people who keep changing their diet based on the latest "research."*

> *And it just so happens that the Canola Oil Council and the California Walnut Commission also helped fund the research—which apparently showed that canola oil and other mono and polyunsaturated fats lowered LDL. Never mind that canola oil is genetically modified and high in erucic acid, a very long-chain fatty acid that can disrupt our cell membranes and has been found to cause heart disease in animals.*[10]

Eggs and Cholesterol

There's no relationship between egg consumption and coronary heart disease.[11] Further, egg consumption is unrelated to blood cholesterol levels.[12] A study published in the *American Journal of Clinical Nutrition* found that egg consumption does not influence the risk of cardiovascular disease in men,[13] while another study shows that dietary cholesterol is not related to coronary heart disease incidences or mortality.[14]

CHAPTER 35 – WHY (THE RIGHT KIND OF) FAT IS HEALTHY

Some eggs are better than others. The way the chickens are raised and what they eat are contributing factors. I buy eggs labeled 'pasture raised' (which is **not** the same as pasteurized) or locally farmed eggs whenever possible. This means the chickens are allowed to roam freely and eat naturally. 'Cage-free' doesn't mean the chickens are allowed to roam; it simply means they aren't in cages. They're still cooped up (literally).

The color of the egg depends on the breed of chicken. It's not a reflection of the nutritional value of the egg.[15]

Eggs are a remarkable food, packed with high-quality protein, healthy fats, vitamins A, B5, and B12, folate, phosphorus, and selenium.

The Best Healthy Fats

Avocados

Did you know that avocado is a fruit? Botanically, it's a large berry. Avocados are rich in monounsaturated fats, which raise levels of good cholesterol while lowering levels of bad cholesterol and triglycerides.[16] They also provide the benefits of vitamin E: preventing free radical damage, boosting immunity, and acting as an anti-aging nutrient for the skin.[17]

Additionally, avocados are a healthy protein; in fact, they have more protein than any other fruit. For pregnant women, avocado is also one of the great folate foods; this vitamin can help reduce the risk of birth defects. Avocados contain more potassium than bananas and the fat in them can help you absorb more nutrients from other plant foods.

I eat avocados every day.

Coconut Oil

Coconut oil is an amazing food. It's rich in medium-chain fatty acids,[18] which are easy for the body to digest. They're not easily stored by the body as fat and provide almost instant energy.

These medium-chain fatty acids improve brain and memory function. Plus, the high amount of natural saturated fats in coconut oil means it

CHAPTER 35 – WHY (THE RIGHT KIND OF) FAT IS HEALTHY

promotes heart health and increases good cholesterol. The antioxidants found in coconut oil make it an effective anti-inflammatory food.

Adding coconut oil to my diet was easy; I simply use coconut oil in place of the vegetable oils I had been using. Because it has a high smoke point, it's much better to use in cooking than olive oil or butter. I also use it to add flavor to food after cooking instead of butter. I like putting it on vegetables and cooked salmon.

Some people don't like the taste of coconut oil and think it alters the taste of the food it's cooked with. If you find this is the case, you can try experimenting with different brands, or simply use another type of oil, like sesame, olive, or avocado.

Butter and Ghee

Butter became a victim of the war on fats, but lately, it's been experiencing a comeback as a healthy fat.[19] The omega-6 and omega-3 fatty acids found in butter help the brain function properly and improve skin health. (These two fatty acids are considered essential, meaning the body needs them but can't produce them on its own; they must be derived from food sources.) Butter is rich in fat-soluble vitamins (A, B12, D, E, K2) and trace minerals (including selenium and iodine).

Unlike the trans fats in processed foods, dairy trans fats are healthy. Butter is the richest dietary source of dairy trans fats.[20]

Ghee, or clarified butter, is an ideal choice for those, like me, who cannot digest the A-1 casein protein in most dairy products, including butter. Ghee is butter with the protein removed, leaving only the fat. It has butter's naturally decadent flavor and a high smoke point, making it ideal for cooking at high temperatures. Ghee's benefits include being loaded with the fat-soluble vitamins A, D, and E.[21]

Ghee is a fantastic alternative to butter because it doesn't promote lactose sensitivity or intolerance. I prefer it to butter, even A2 butter (from southern France or Italy).

CHAPTER 35 – WHY (THE RIGHT KIND OF) FAT IS HEALTHY

A Note About Margarine

Hippolyte Mège-Mouriès created margarine in France in 1869 when responding to a challenge by Emperor Napoleon III to create a butter substitute from beef tallow for the armed forces and lower classes.[22]

Butter is a mechanically processed food made from milk, comprised mostly of saturated (healthy) fat. Modern margarine is made from vegetable oils that are chemically processed to stay solid at room temperature. The chemical process is known as hydrogenation, which forms unhealthy trans fats. Some margarine is processed using interesterification instead of hydrogenation. Interesterification doesn't form trans fats, but its health effects are unknown at this time.[23]

Healthline says, "In addition to hydrogenated or interesterified vegetable oils, modern margarine may contain several food additives, including emulsifiers and colorants. Put simply, modern margarine is a highly processed food product made from vegetable oils, while butter is basically concentrated dairy fat." [24]

Extra Virgin Olive Oil

I include olive oil in my diet because of its many benefits. Extra virgin olive oil (EVOO) is great for heart health. A 2013 study found that when people supplemented a Mediterranean diet with EVOO, it reduced the incidence of heart attack or dying of heart disease, probably due to its high levels of monounsaturated fats.[25] EVOO has high amounts of antioxidants, meaning it protects cells from free radical damage. It also helps improve memory/cognitive function and works as an anti-inflammatory. Since so much disease results from chronic inflammation, this is important.

Unfortunately, buying EVOO isn't as easy as just grabbing the first bottle off the shelf. I buy only extra virgin olive oil. This means no chemicals are involved when the oil is refined. Unfortunately, many common brands are diluted.[26] A 2011 study by UC Davis[27] found that many top-selling brands failed the standards for extra virgin olive oil; many lawsuits against olive oil companies have been filed.[28]

CHAPTER 35 – WHY (THE RIGHT KIND OF) FAT IS HEALTHY

Some tips for recognizing real EVOO are to be wary of any brand that costs less than $10 a liter; look for a seal from the International Olive Oil Council; check the harvesting date on the label; if it's labeled as 'light,' 'pure,' or a 'blend,' it isn't virgin quality; and finally, opt for dark bottles, as they protect the oil from oxidation. I only use Bariani brand EVOO.

EVOO isn't good for cooking at high temperatures because of its low smoke point, but it's great for low-temperature cooking, making salad dressings, and drizzling over cooked foods.

Improved Health Markers

For decades, my cholesterol levels were borderline high. I resisted taking statin drugs. Turns out, all I needed to do was change the way I eat. Over the last couple of years, my doctor tells me my cholesterol levels are now "outstanding" (her word) and my triglycerides are good. In fact, I'm now the healthiest I've ever been in my life. The praise goes to God; I credit eating foods He made instead of fake 'food' that man makes.

CHAPTER 35 – WHY (THE RIGHT KIND OF) FAT IS HEALTHY

CHAPTER 36

THE SURPRISING BENEFITS OF INTERMITTENT FASTING

I found a way of eating that allows me to eat until I'm satisfied, gives me more energy, helps me lose weight, and may even help me live longer. What am I talking about? Read on to learn about the surprising benefits of intermittent fasting.

I've been practicing intermittent fasting since July 2015. I started because I wanted to lose weight and restore my health. I knew that the body prioritizes digestion[1] over other functions because it's necessary for survival; so if I limited the time my body spent digesting food, there would be more time for my body to work on healing itself, as God designed it to do.

What is Intermittent Fasting?

Intermittent fasting isn't about *what* you eat, it's about *when* you eat. I eat all my daily meals within a 6 to 8-hour time frame. The rest of the time, I'm fasting. (24 hours per day minus 8 hours eating time frame = 16 hours of fasting per day.) Currently, I eat breakfast around 11 am, lunch at 3 pm, and dinner at 7 pm. Allowing only 4 hours between meals eliminates the desire to snack, which cuts down on caloric intake and expense.

Some people may prefer to start and end their meals earlier in the day, for example, breakfast at 8 am, lunch at noon, and dinner at 4 pm.

Others fast for 24-hours every few days, or once a week, or one week per month. When I do a 24-hour fast, this schedule seems to work best: on day one, I eat breakfast and lunch, then skip dinner. On day two, I skip breakfast and lunch, then eat dinner. I go 24 hours without eating, yet I eat on both day one and day two. This way I don't feel deprived.

CHAPTER 36 – SURPRISING BENEFITS OF INTERMITTENT FASTING

I've found that the 16-hour daily fast works better for me on a regular basis than the other types. People who want to try intermittent fasting can experiment to find what works best for them.

Intermittent fasting isn't for everyone. Those who are hypoglycemic, have diabetes, are pregnant/nursing, have a history of eating disorders, get poor sleep, or are chronically stressed, should not practice intermittent fasting. Always ask your doctor before you make diet changes.

Here are some of the benefits of intermittent fasting.

Weight Loss

Simply put, when someone eats every few hours, whether small meals throughout the day or constant snacking or 'grazing,' the body remains in a 'fed' state. This means the body is constantly being called upon to digest the food that is constantly being eaten.

The fed state begins when eating starts in the morning and ends approximately 3-5 hours after eating stops at the end of the day. Insulin levels drop when the body isn't busy with digestion, thus making it easier for the body to burn fat.

If one eats a 'midnight snack' at 11 pm and breakfast at 6 am, the body has only 2-4 hours of digestive rest. This simply isn't enough time for the body to repair all the damage it sustains through daily toxin exposure.

Many people find that they can lose weight easily without changing the types of food eaten simply by practicing intermittent fasting. I do, however, eat real, whole foods, which increased my weight loss when combined with intermittent fasting.

Health Restoration

Health benefits of intermittent fasting include:

- Reduced risk of chronic disease, from diabetes to heart disease and cancer [2]

CHAPTER 36 – SURPRISING BENEFITS OF INTERMITTENT FASTING

- Decreased inflammation and free radical damage [3]
- Helps keep weight off by reducing overeating [4]
- Increased levels of HGH (human growth hormone) [5]
- Increased insulin and leptin sensitivity may reverse diabetes [6]
- Decreased blood pressure and resting heart rate [7]

Spiritual/Mental Clarity

Many people fast to cleanse, detox, and/or purify their bodies. Some extol the spiritual virtues of fasting. Fasting is less about what I give up and more about what I gain. Since my body does not belong to me (1 Corinthians 6:19), fasting takes the focus off me and allows me to focus on God.

Fasting has been found to significantly reduce symptoms of anxiety for 80% of patients that have chronic pain.[8] It can play a preventive and therapeutic role in mood disorders like anxiety and depression.[9]

Dr. Dale Bredesen, M.D., director of neurodegenerative disease research at the UCLA School of Medicine, and author of *The End of Alzheimer's: The First Program to Prevent and Reverse Cognitive Decline* developed a protocol to prevent and reverse cognitive decline, which includes an eating plan called ReCODE.[10] The plan calls for fasting 12 hours per day and not eating for 3 hours before going to bed.

Dr. Brady Salcido, D.C., brain optimization expert, outlines these benefits of intermittent fasting for the brain:[11]

- Reduces inflammation
- Creates more brain cells
- Boosts BDNF, an important protein known as 'Miracle-Gro® for the brain.' BDNF helps to produce new brain cells, protect brain cells, stimulate new connections and synapses while also boosting memory, improving mood, and learning.[12]
- Burns fat for fuel instead of sugar

CHAPTER 36 – SURPRISING BENEFITS OF INTERMITTENT FASTING

- Boosts HGH (human growth hormone)
- Supercharges your energy

Making the Change

How do I deal with not eating until late in the morning or noon? It did take me several days to get used to it. I found that if I structured my morning time and included my workouts at that time, the time until I ate my first meal went by quickly without much agony. Now, it's just habit/routine for me.

> *Diets are easy in the contemplation, difficult in the execution. Intermittent fasting is just the opposite — it's difficult in the contemplation but easy in the execution. Intermittent fasting is hard in the contemplation, of that there is no doubt. "You go without food for 24 hours?" people would ask, incredulous when we explained what we were doing. "I could never do that." But once started, it's a snap. No worries about what and where to eat for one or two out of the three meals per day. It's a great liberation. Your food expenditures plummet. And you're not particularly hungry. ... Although it's tough to overcome the idea of going without food, once you begin the regimen, nothing could be easier. – Dr. Michael R. Eades, M.D.*[13]

**"The best of all medicines is resting and fasting."
Benjamin Franklin**

CHAPTER 37

THE 10 BEST ANTI-INFLAMMATION FOODS

Inflammation is the immune system's healthy response to injury or foreign invaders like bacteria and viruses, and to proteins that escape the gut leading to autoimmune disorders. In a person with a properly functioning immune system, the inflammation goes away once the situation is resolved. It becomes a problem when the inflammation doesn't go away, signaling that the immune system isn't working properly. Because chronic inflammation can be caused by diet, here are the 10 best anti-inflammation foods.

Inflammation is the root cause[1] of many diseases. It's the common link between such debilitating conditions as Alzheimer's, heart disease, cancer, and arthritis. While there can be other causes of chronic inflammation, such as low-grade bacterial, viral, and fungal infections, food allergies or food sensitivities, stress, and environmental toxicity, diet and lifestyle play a huge role that cannot be underestimated.

Because food plays such a significant role in overall health, incorporating as many of these anti-inflammatory foods into one's diet can only have a beneficial effect.

- **Healthy Fats**, such as Extra Virgin Olive Oil (EVOO), organic unrefined coconut oil, avocados, and organic pasture raised butter (preferably from A2 cows) or ghee. In a study in India, the high levels of antioxidants present in virgin coconut oil reduced inflammation and healed arthritis more effectively than leading medications.[2] See chapter 35 for more information.

- **Fatty/Oily Fish** (wild-caught), such as salmon, mackerel, tuna, and sardines, are rich in omega-3 polyunsaturated fatty acids, which have been shown to reduce inflammation and potentially lower the risk of heart disease, cancer, and arthritis.[3]

- **Nuts and seeds** properly prepared (soaked/sprouted).[4] Flax, hemp, chia, sunflower, and pumpkin seeds, as well as walnuts,

CHAPTER 37 – THE 10 BEST ANTI-INFLAMMATION FOODS

almonds, and pecans, are great choices. They're "chock full of the polyunsaturated and monounsaturated fats but contain very little unhealthy saturated fat. As a result, nuts have major anti-inflammatory effects." [5]

- **Dark Leafy Green Vegetables** are rich in antioxidants that restore cellular health, as well as anti-inflammatory flavonoids.[6] I eat only organic or follow the Clean 15 and Dirty Dozen lists.[7] I put a lot of dark leafy greens (kale, chard, spinach, beet greens, etc.) in my smoothies.

- **Beets.** According to the National Institutes of Health, "Beetroot is also being considered as a promising therapeutic treatment in a range of clinical pathologies associated with oxidative stress and inflammation." [8]

- **Mushrooms** (organic). Shitake and Maitake are great and button mushrooms are, as well. The polysaccharides, terpenoids, and phenolic compounds in mushrooms contribute to their anti-inflammatory properties.[9] I like to sauté them with garlic, ginger, and turmeric for a delicious side dish.

- **Blueberries.** The best fruit to eat (only organic). They contain the anti-inflammatory flavonoid quercetin.

- **Garlic, ginger, and turmeric.** These are three of the best anti-inflammation spices. See chapter 47 for more detailed information.

- **Green tea.** Matcha green tea is excellent, as well as white and oolong teas. Dr. Andrew Weil, M.D., says, "Tea is rich in catechins, antioxidant compounds that reduce inflammation." [10]

- **Bone broth.** See chapter 32.

Always ask your doctor before you make diet changes.

CHAPTER 38

FOOD PREPARATION TIPS

Following the Be in Health Lifestyle means preparing foods from scratch, just as our grandparents and great-grandparents did. Having a plan is key.

- Prepare a menu and shopping list every week.
- Pick a day or two and cook things ahead of time. Lots of items freeze well.
- Pre-prepare what you can.
- Use the farm ideology of something always needs to be growing (or cooking, prepping, etc.) while you're sleeping (or away from the house).
- Use a slow cooker and always cook twice as much as you need.
- Start with mastering one meal (breakfast or evening meal) then move on to get a different meal figured out.
- Most of all, make meals simple. Meals don't have to be huge affairs. Eat simply and eat well. It really doesn't take that much longer. I found that once I started doing it, it's a breeze. Cooking from scratch and being mindful of food showed me much time I previously devoted to meaningless tasks. Now, I spend even more time with my husband because we prepare meals together.

This is a lifestyle change, a new paradigm, not a temporary undertaking. Going back to the old ways will simply recreate the old problems. I asked myself the question, "Do I love myself (spouse, kids, God) enough to do this for myself/them?"

CHAPTER 38 – FOOD PREPARATION TIPS

CHAPTER 39

COOKING WITH ESSENTIAL OILS

Have you ever wanted to cook with essential oils but didn't know where to begin? You looked at the label and it didn't say it was okay to ingest or worse, it warned against ingestion? Or perhaps you've tried cooking with essential oils, but it didn't turn out as expected? Here's a brief intro on how to cook with essential oils.

Are Essential Oils Ingestible?

Whether an essential oil is ingestible depends on the brand of oil used and the classification the oil has. I only use oils that are certified by the FDA as GRAS (Generally Regarded as Safe), FA (Food Additive), or FL (Flavoring Agent).[1]

> **If the label says, "Not for internal use," do NOT use that oil because it has been adulterated with chemicals that make it unsafe for ingestion.**

Ingestion of essential oils also depends on which school of thought you subscribe to. There are three main perspectives[2] about essential oils:

- The German school of thought uses essential oils mainly by way of inhalation. They tend to avoid ingestion and topical use.

- The British believe in using essential oils mainly for inhalation and topical application, such as massage. They dilute all essential oils for topical application.

- The French believe in inhaling, applying topically, and taking internally using only therapeutic grade essential oils. They also believe in using oils as therapy, not just in aromatherapy (see chapter 29).

I follow the French school of thought that believes in using essential oils for complete well-being. This is a safe method if you use a common-sense approach and read safety precautions.

Tips for Cooking with Essential Oils

- Use food grade essential oils. I only use Young Living Essential Oils that have been tested and labeled safe in my foods. Young Living has made this easy with their Vitality™ dietary essential oils. So, I know that ingesting any of the Vitality™ line of essential oils is safe.

- Essential oils are highly concentrated. It only takes a little essential oil when cooking. In some cases, I put a drop on a toothpick and swirl it in... a little will go a long way.

- Young Living essential oils are very potent, far more potent than dried herbs and spices. In fact, one drop of Young Living Peppermint Vitality™ Essential Oil is equal to 28 cups of peppermint tea. It's very highly concentrated.

- When drinking water or smoothies with essential oils, I use only glass or stainless-steel containers. I never use plastic or Styrofoam™. The essential oils will eat away the petrochemicals of the cup because therapeutic grade oils scrub away chemicals.

Substituting with Essential Oils

The simplest way to start using essential oils in cooking is to substitute them for dried herbs and spices in recipes. When a recipe calls for less than a teaspoon of herbs, I dip a toothpick in the essential oil and then swirl it in the recipe to blend. (I don't put the toothpick back in the oil after stirring the food.) I always use this method for cinnamon bark oil, clove oil, ginger oil, and nutmeg oil. These are much stronger than the dried spices.

CHAPTER 39 – COOKING WITH ESSENTIAL OILS

- If I want to replace the juice or zest of one lemon, orange, tangerine, or grapefruit, I use 1 drop of the essential oil per serving. In other words, if the recipe will serve 10 people, 10 drops is fine. I always use glass, ceramic, or stainless-steel bowls when mixing with essential oils, so toxins don't get drawn out from plastic into the food.

- I'm careful when dropping an oil into other ingredients; some oils come out quickly, some very slowly. So, I'm careful to be ready to tip the bottle up quickly or move it away from the bowl so I don't end up with too many drops.

- When cooking, I add essential oils at the very end before serving. When baking, I add them in the order shown in the recipe.

- Therapeutic grade essential oils are safe when used as directed. I always read the complete label before using.

- One tablespoon or more of basil, oregano, rosemary, thyme, fennel, dill, black pepper, or celery seed can be replaced with 1/2 – 1 drop of its companion oil.

I also enjoy adding essential oils to my drinking water.

I like to experiment with dietary grade essential oils in my cooking and baking. It's surprisingly easy and delicious.

Note: Pregnant women should consult their health care professional before using essential oils containing constituents with hormone-like activity such as Fennel, Clary Sage, Sage, Idaho Tansy, and Juniper. Epileptics and those with high blood pressure should consult their health care professional before using some essential oils. Avoid Hyssop, Fennel, and Idaho Tansy oils.

CHAPTER 39 – COOKING WITH ESSENTIAL OILS

CHAPTER 40

HACKS THAT HELP ME SLEEP

Not getting at least 7-9 hours of uninterrupted sleep per night (at night) can be just as bad as eating poorly and not exercising. *Medical News Today* says that women working the night shift have a 19% higher risk of cancer.[1]

Those who sleep less than 7 hours per night increase their chances of getting sick,[2] especially those struggling with sleep disruption from autoimmune disorders/leaky gut syndrome. Here are some hacks that help me sleep:

- I diffuse essential oils all night. My favorites are Cedarwood, Stress Away™ blend, Clary Sage, Lavender, Peace & Calming® blend, Valerian, Frankincense, Vetiver (a thick oil, so inhale directly instead of clogging up the diffuser), and Tranquil (a roll-on blend for the bottoms of the feet).

- I keep the sleeping room dark. I use light-blocking curtains and cover the light of all electronics that emit a light with duct tape. It's really dark in my bedroom.

- I don't keep a clock in my bedroom. If I wake during the night to use the bathroom, I don't check the time. This eliminates the anxiety that comes from knowing I only have X number of hours until I have to get up.

- I turn off all blue-light devices (mobile phone, tablet, computer, TV) one hour before going to bed. The light from these devices is 'short-wavelength-enriched,' meaning it has a higher concentration of blue light than natural light; blue light affects levels of the sleep-inducing hormone melatonin more than any other wavelength. Some people use these apps to improve sleep:

    o **lux**[3] reduces blue light (blight) on a device after the sun goes down.

CHAPTER 40 – HACKS THAT HELP ME SLEEP

- - **Sleep Cycle** [4] analyzes sleep patterns and wakes you during your lightest sleep phase.
  - **Koala Web Browser** [5] filters out blue light.
- I try to go to bed at the same time every night and get up at the same time every morning. Doing this helps balance circadian rhythms so I will be more alert during the day and sleep better at night.
- I supplement with magnesium within 1 hour of going to bed. I use Natural Vitality's Natural Calm.
- I release negative thoughts before getting into bed. Racing thoughts will keep you awake. I write my thoughts down, plan out the next day's tasks, and pray and forgive others and myself when necessary so I can sleep peacefully.

Psalm 127:2 KJV
It is vain for you to rise up early, to sit up late, to eat the bread of sorrows: for so he giveth his beloved sleep.

Psalm 4:8 KJV
I will both lay me down in peace, and sleep: for thou, LORD, only makest me dwell in safety.

Proverbs 3:24 KJV
When thou liest down, thou shalt not be afraid: yea, thou shalt lie down, and thy sleep shall be sweet.

CHAPTER 41

REDUCING TOXIN EXPOSURE

The principle of 'put off, put on' (Ephesians 4, Colossians 3) tells us that before we put on the new man, we must first put off the old man. Likewise, I needed to reduce the toxins my body was exposed to if I expected the good foods, probiotics, essential oils, and supplements I had started using to have their full, positive effect on me.

It seems like toxins are everywhere. They're in our environment, they're in our thoughts, and sometimes they are the people around us. And who wants to be around toxins? Merriam-Webster.com defines toxin as "a poisonous substance and especially one that is produced by a living thing." Read on for examples of how I reduced toxins in my life.

Reducing Toxins in My Environment

Our environments are filled with toxins; it's hard to escape them. Every day we hear about toxins in our air, water, and food.

But many haven't considered the toxins in their own homes. Many of the materials used to build our homes release toxic substances into the home environment. This is known as outgassing and it can continue for years after the home is built. New materials added in renovations, like carpet, hardwood or engineered flooring, paint, and kitchen cabinets continue to out-gas. This means we are breathing toxins in our sleep.

Our homes are our sanctuaries, so it was important to me to limit my toxin exposure at home. I hadn't considered that many of the household and beauty products used in my home daily were toxic. Sure, we know that bleach and ammonia are toxic, but what about shaving cream and hand lotion? Laundry soap and that expensive face cream? Toothpaste and sunscreen? What are people using to clean their houses and themselves and their children? Are we sure it's safe?

CHAPTER 41 – REDUCING TOXIN EXPOSURE

Replacing Toxic Thoughts

Toxic thoughts are so common that many don't even recognize them. Every thought that we allow to take root in our minds and our hearts affects us. Sometimes we don't see the effect until it's too late.

Dr. Carol Morgan, Ph.D., lists these toxic thoughts to eliminate:[1]

- Thinking that you're a victim
- Thinking that you can change other people
- Thoughts that constantly resist the unchangeable
- Thinking that "the grass is always greener on the other side"
- Having expectations of other people
- Thinking that having a significant other will complete you
- Feeling that you always need to prove that you're right
- Worrying about what other people think of you
- Thinking there's only ONE right and ONE wrong
- Worrying about the future because you feel unprepared
- Thinking that money equals happiness
- Believing that the past determines your future

Once you've identified the toxic thought, how do you get rid of it? First, you have to realize that you're not responsible for every thought that drops into your mind. You are, however, responsible for every thought that you allow to stay there and take root.

The Bible calls these toxic thoughts that have taken root in our minds "strongholds" (2 Corinthians 10:4). The Greek word for "stronghold" is only used here and means "anything on which one relies."

CHAPTER 41 - REDUCING TOXIN EXPOSURE

2 Corinthians 10:4-5 APNT
For the equipment of our service is not of the flesh, but of the power of God and by it, we overcome rebellious strongholds.

And we pull down reasonings and all pride that elevates [itself] against the knowledge of God and we lead captive all thoughts to the obedience of Christ.

We are to cast down these toxic thoughts and lead them away to Christ. This requires action on our part: we must recognize the thought for what it is (toxic) and cast it down. We must not allow it to stay. However, when you remove a thought, you must replace it with another one or it will come back. Our minds can't be empty; there can't be a vacuum.

We must put off the negative before we can put on the positive. We must send away the toxic thought and replace it with a thought that is in alignment with Christ.

Removing Toxic People from Your Life

'Toxic people' is a fairly new concept. Not that toxic people being around is new, it's just new that we as a society recognize them as such. Toxic people are negative people who drain the joy out of the people around them. We all know (or knew) someone like that. We all secretly wish that person wasn't in our life, but often, we suffer in silence.

It's very important to remove from your life anyone who is using you or hurting you. The first step is to recognize what is happening and then make a decision to change it. Establish boundaries with these people. Tell them what the consequences will be if they violate those boundaries. You will have to learn to say, "No." I'm not saying it will be easy, but it will be freeing when you do it. Get support if you need it.

Surround yourself with people who will lift you up and encourage you, who will support your dreams and goals. You deserve to be happy.

Removing toxic people from your life will benefit you greatly, allowing you to live the life you deserve to live.

CHAPTER 41 – REDUCING TOXIN EXPOSURE

The Facts About Chemicals

I want to share a few statistics and facts with you about chemicals in the home that negatively affect health. Did you know that Americans now spend between 80-90% of their time inside [2] and that the average American home contains over 63 hazardous products? [3]

In addition to the 7,000,000 accidental poisonings each year in America from chemicals in the home, [4] chemically-manufactured household cleaners are the number one contributor to indoor air pollution,[5] where the concentrations of some pollutants are often 2 to 5 times higher than typical outdoor concentrations,[6] even when factoring in pollution caused by vehicles and factories. These figures come from the EPA.

Liquid dish soap is the leading cause of poisonings[7] in the home for children under the age of 6 (over 2.1 million accidental poisonings per year). Most brands contain formaldehyde and ammonia.

A 15-year study[8] revealed that stay at home moms and women who work at home have a 54% higher risk of developing certain health problems than women who work away from the home. The only thing linked to this increased risk is increased exposure to household cleaners.

Did you know that the average newborn baby has 287 chemicals[9] found in their umbilical cord blood, 180 of which cause cancer in humans or animals? 217 are toxic to the brain and nervous system.

It gets worse when you consider the toxic chemicals in our personal care products. From antiperspirants to perfumes, from toothpaste to skin care products, Americans have been unwittingly poisoning themselves and their families with hundreds of chemical compounds that the body is unequipped to deal with.

Experts agree that anyone serious about experiencing improved health today and in the long-run must begin to replace products made with toxic chemicals[10] with personal care and household products that are safer for the health of the body.

CHAPTER 41 - REDUCING TOXIN EXPOSURE

Bayer Buys Monsanto

In 2018, the U.S. Justice Dept. approved a $66 billion deal for Bayer AG (a German pharmaceutical company and offshoot of IG Farben) to buy Monsanto (an American agrochemical company responsible for glyphosate (Roundup®) and Agent Orange). The new company will be the world's biggest seed and agricultural-chemicals company in the world.[11]

According to Mute Schimpf, a spokeswoman for Friends of the Earth Europe, "The merger will create the biggest platform of its kind — and give Bayer-Monsanto a 'first mover' advantage similar to Facebook, in the way that it affects competitors. The new platform allows Bayer-Monsanto to control how, where, when, and by whom food is produced. As Facebook's algorithms decide which newsfeeds we see, so 'Baysanto' will decide which pesticides are used, and which seeds are planted."[12]

In June 2018, Bayer announced that "Bayer will remain the company name. Monsanto will no longer be a company name. The acquired products [like Roundup®] will retain their brand names and become part of the Bayer portfolio."[13] So, the Monsanto name is no more but toxic products like Roundup® live on.

Glyphosate/Roundup®

You may have heard about glyphosate, the active ingredient in Monsanto/Bayer's Roundup® weed killer products. It's the most widely used pesticide worldwide. Since 1974, 3.5 billion pounds of Roundup® has been used in just the U.S.[14]

A group of 94 scientists recently published a study that strongly suggests that glyphosate is a carcinogen,[15] meaning it causes cancer. Glyphosate is in our water and in our food. It's been found in umbilical cord blood[16] and breast milk.[17] We don't yet know the complete ramifications of Roundup® use.

In August 2018, Monsanto was ordered to pay $289 million in damages when a jury ruled that the active ingredient in Monsanto's Roundup®, glyphosate, caused a man's cancer.[18]

255

CHAPTER 41 – REDUCING TOXIN EXPOSURE

The Guardian reports that weed killer products are more toxic than their active ingredient:

> *U.S. government researchers have uncovered evidence that some popular weedkilling products, like Monsanto's widely-used Roundup®, are potentially more toxic to human cells than their active ingredient is by itself. ...*
>
> *The tests are part of the US National Toxicology Program's (NTP) first-ever examination of herbicide formulations made with the active ingredient glyphosate, but that also include other chemicals. While regulators have previously required extensive testing of glyphosate in isolation, government scientists have not fully examined the toxicity of the more complex products sold to consumers, farmers, and others.*[19]

So, glyphosate is very bad, but when you combine it with other things, it's even worse. Do you have this product in your garage? Is it sprayed on grass that your kids, your grandkids, or your pets play on?

Problems with Standard Household Cleaners

One common name-brand all-purpose spray with bleach warns to "avoid prolonged or repeated skin contact" and "prolonged breathing of vapor." But this product is designed to be used in areas that can often have poor ventilation (bathrooms and kitchens), and who wants to break out a gas mask and industrial-strength rubber gloves every time you wipe down your counters or sink?

Let's look at one common name-brand bathtub cleaner that has been used in millions of American households for decades. It gives off chlorine fumes for up to two weeks after use and leaves behind a gritty residue. The label on this product says it can cause "coughing or irritation of nose and throat" and contact with the skin may cause "superficial temporary irritation." In individuals with lung issues this product may lead to "reduced lung function." One of the ingredients in this product is a known carcinogen in animals. How many kids are bathed in tubs cleaned

CHAPTER 41 - REDUCING TOXIN EXPOSURE

with this product? Do you scrub the tub before you settle in for a long soak?

Last, but definitely not least, let's look at the warnings on common brands of toilet bowl cleaners. You can't have any skin contact with this product or even inhale it without it causing some sort of problem. For any contact with your skin, the label says to "IMMEDIATELY flush with plenty of water for at least 15-20 minutes." If accidentally ingested, you must call the Poison Control Center and face "mucosal damage." If this product has any accidental contact with the eyes, you must flush your eyes for 15-20 minutes with water and then call the Poison Control Center. If this product is accidentally mixed with any other cleaning product, "hazardous gases may be released."

Are these products you want in your home?

We've all been sold a line that there's no alternative — the only way to have a clean toilet bowl is to work with a poisonous substance that gives off toxic fumes well after you're done using it. This is complete nonsense.

Thieves® Line

I use and recommend Thieves® Household Cleaner. For general use, I take an empty 32 oz. spray bottle, add 1 oz. of Thieves® Household Cleaner, fill the bottle with water and I'm ready to go. The 14 oz. bottle of concentrated Thieves® Household Cleaner will make 14 bottles of cleaner when diluted, each one lasting for months. Because it doesn't have harsh chemicals, it's safer for the environment and less expensive in the long run.

14 Easy, Fun, and Inexpensive Solutions

1. To use in the bathtub where grime can accumulate, first sprinkle about ½ c. of baking soda in the tub, then spray with the Thieves® Household Cleaner and start scrubbing.

2. To clean the toilet bowl, dump in about ¼ c. of baking soda along with a couple of drops of Thieves® Essential Oil. Scrub the toilet bowl, then let it sit for a minute or two before flushing. You can also pour a small

CHAPTER 41 – REDUCING TOXIN EXPOSURE

amount of Thieves® Household Cleaner right into the toilet bowl, then scrub.

3. For glass cleaner, use the Thieves® Household Cleaner in a spray bottle or add 1/10 oz. Thieves® Household Cleaner to 32 oz. of water and add a splash of white vinegar.

4. For a mold and mildew remover, use a couple of drops of Thieves® Essential Oil directly on the site if the area is small. For larger areas, such as driveways or sidewalks, fill a bucket with a tsp. of Thieves® Household Cleaner in warm water, apply to the area, and clean.

5. For a natural and non-toxic dishwashing liquid, add 1/3 oz. of Thieves® Household Cleaner and 4 drops of Thieves® Essential Oil or 5-6 drops of Lemon Essential Oil to 32 oz. of water. I use Thieves® Dish Soap.

6. One cap full of Thieves® Household Cleaner will clean one load of laundry. I use Thieves® Laundry Soap. To get out stubborn spots, I pretreat with Thieves® Laundry Soap.

7. For a natural and non-toxic fabric softener, add 1-2 drops of Thieves® Essential Oil to a woolen dryer ball and place in the dryer with the laundry to be dried. Or take a jar and add 3 cups white vinegar, 1/4 cup rubbing alcohol (or vodka), and 20 drops of Thieves® Essential Oil (you can also use other essential oils such as Purification® blend or Lavender or Lemon). Shake before use and add ½-¾ cup to the fabric softener dispenser in the washing machine.

Did you know that of the 3-10 gallons of toxic household cleaning products[20] in an average home, the chemicals in dryer sheets and fabric softeners are among the most toxic? [21] They contain the known carcinogens benzyl acetate, chloroform, and dichlorobenzene, as well as several chemicals on the EPA's Hazardous Waste List.[22]

8. To freshen the air, diffuse your favorite essential oils instead of plug-ins, candles, or sprays. These products can cause DNA mutations, tumors, and asthma.[23]

CHAPTER 41 - REDUCING TOXIN EXPOSURE

9. For a non-toxic carpet freshener, Thieves® Essential Oil can be sprinkled on straight for heavy duty deodorizing. For medium to light freshening, mix a few drops of Thieves® Essential Oil with baking soda. Sprinkle on carpet, let sit several hours, then vacuum up. (Make sure to do a color test first.)

10. For a fruit and vegetable wash, fill your sink with cool water and add 2 drops of Thieves® Essential Oil along with 1 Tbsp. of apple cider vinegar. Wash your produce in this solution, then rinse with pure water. Insects, parasites, and some pesticide residues will wash right away. I use Thieves® Fruit and Veggie Wash.

11. For a spot or stain remover on carpets or clothing, use Thieves® Essential Oil straight on the stain after testing the fabric or carpet in an inconspicuous location to make sure it retains its proper color. You may also try the All-Purpose Thieves® Household Cleaner described above or the Thieves® Spray.

12. For a non-toxic paint remover, sprinkle Thieves® Essential Oil straight on the affected area to help paint come off more easily.

13. For a toxin-free dishwasher detergent, put 4 to 6 drops of Thieves® Dish Soap in the detergent compartment. Add vinegar and/or Lemon Essential Oil or Thieves® Household Cleaner to the rinse aid area. You can also use Thieves® Automatic Dishwasher Powder.

14. What about stinky smells in the bathroom? Do you use air fresheners, candles, or plug-ins? Some reports say they're more toxic than cigarettes. They contain high levels of phthalates, which are known to be especially harmful to children.[24] These chemicals were even present in sprays which were claimed to be 'All-Natural' and 'unscented.' Instead, use Purification® Essential Oil Blend. Keep a bottle by the toilet and add a drop to the toilet water when you flush.

Soap

Have you heard the news that antibacterial soaps and hand sanitizers may not be all they were cracked up to be?[25] It's true. Antibacterial products can be harmful to the immune system in the long-run. That's

CHAPTER 41 – REDUCING TOXIN EXPOSURE

why I use Thieves® Foaming Hand Soap and Hand Purifier instead of those chemical-laden products.

Thieves® Spray is great to use on countertops and other surfaces such as doorknobs. Take Thieves® Spray with you and spray on your hands while traveling or spray on grocery cart handles while shopping, or use the Thieves® Hand Purifier designed specifically for hands.

Oral Care

Have you ever noticed that your tube of toothpaste has a warning on it that if you swallow this product, you should call the Poison Control Center?

Drug Facts		Drug Facts (continued)
Active Ingredient	**Purpose**	pea sized amount in children under 6. Supervise children's brushing until good habits are established. Children under **2 yrs.: ask a dentist.**
Sodium monofluorophosphate 0.76%	Anti-cavity toothpaste	
Use: Helps prevent against cavities		**Inactive Ingredients:** Sorbitol, Silica, Water, Sodium Lauryl Sulfate, Flavor, PEG-32, Mica, Sodium Methyl Cellulose, Saccharin, Trisodium Phosphate, FD&C Blue No. 1, Calcium Glycerophosphate
Warnings: Keep out of reach of children under 6 years of age. If you accidentally swallow more than used for brushing, get medical help or contact a Poison Control Center immediately.		

The first thing to note on the toothpaste label above is that it's called a drug ("Drug Facts"). Toxic toothpaste ingredients include sorbitol (a GMO sugar substitute), sodium lauryl sulfate (used to create the foam during brushing; can cause skin irritation,[26] among other things), saccharin (made from coal tar), and sodium fluoride (listed as sodium monofluorophosphate).

Fluoride

A recent study published in *The Journal of Epidemiology and Community Health*[27] discovered that individuals who consumed fluoride-rich water had a 30 percent higher risk of hypothyroidism than those who consumed water that had natural levels of fluoride. The findings also suggest that serious side effects from excessive fluoride in drinking water include weight gain, tiredness, depression, and painful muscles.[28]

CHAPTER 41 - REDUCING TOXIN EXPOSURE

Fluoride has been implicated in lowered IQ, hindered thyroid function, impaired gastrointestinal function, and more.[29] In fact, in 2018, the Supreme Court of New Zealand ruled by majority vote that water fluoridation is compulsory mass medication, in breach of human rights.[30]

Besides fluoride, other toxic chemicals and additives are routine ingredients in toothpaste and mouthwashes, making them some of the most toxic substances in our homes. The irony is we're putting it in our mouths where we don't even have to swallow it for it to poison us slowly. Many of these toxins can be absorbed into the bloodstream right through the lining of the cheeks.

I personally use the non-toxic Thieves® AromaBright Toothpaste. With Thieves® Mouthwash, I don't have to worry about calling the Poison Control Center if I accidentally ingest it.

Making Your Own Products

There are many sources for making your own personal care products, such as http://DrAxe.com and http://WellnessMama.com. The books *The Chemical Free Home*, *The Chemical Free Home 2*, and *The Chemical Free Home 3* by Melissa M. Poepping have many recipes you can use instead of toxic substances. You can order her books at http://AbundantHealth4You.com.

Top Toxins to Avoid

The Environmental Working Group[31] has up-to-date information on toxins found in household and personal care products. Below are ingredients the EWG rates as 'high hazard' and where they're found.

- **1,4-Dioxane**. Found in 'natural' and 'organic' brand shampoos, body washes, and lotions; bubble bath, sunless tanning products, moisturizers, baby soap, anti-aging products, hair relaxers.
- **Parabens (ethyl, methyl, propyl, and butyl)**. Found in deodorants/antiperspirants, shampoos/conditioners, spray tans/lotions/sunscreens, makeup/other cosmetics, pharmaceutical drugs, food additives.

CHAPTER 41 – REDUCING TOXIN EXPOSURE

- **Phthalates (diethylhexyl phthalate, dibutyl phthalate).** Found in plastics like PVC, toys, food packaging, shower curtains, vinyl flooring/wall coverings, household cleaners, cosmetics, personal care products such as nail polish, hair spray, lipstick, nail polish remover, perfumes, hoses, raincoats, lubricants, adhesives, detergents, food such as meat and milk packaged with plastic tubing at dairy farms, tap water, medical equipment such as IV tubing and bags, nasogastric tubes, umbilical artery catheters, tubing used in cardiopulmonary bypass procedures, blood bags and infusion tubing, ventilator tubing, enteral nutrition feeding bags, tubing used during hemodialysis.

- **Toluene.** Found in synthetic fragrances, printing, leather tanning processes, volatile petrochemical solvents/paint thinners, paint, nail polish, hair dye, lacquers, adhesives, rubber.

- **Triclosan.** Found in toothpaste, deodorant, antibacterial soap, body washes, cosmetics, waterless hand sanitizer, furniture, kitchenware, clothing, toys, many industrial uses.

Toxins in Personal Care/Beauty Products

The personal care/beauty industry is "highly unregulated," says Vanessa Cunningham, nutrition and wellness expert. "There is no pre-product approval before a product hits the market and enters your home. A minuscule approval process exists, but only for color additives and ingredients classified as over-the-counter drugs." [32]

These are the products found in common personal care/beauty products like shampoo, soap, and makeup that I avoid:

- Parabens
- Synthetic colors
- Fragrance
- Phthalates
- Triclosan

- Sodium lauryl sulfate (SLS) / Sodium laureth sulfate (SLES)
- Formaldehyde
- Toluene
- Propylene glycol
- Sunscreen chemicals

Note that this list contains 3 of the 5 top toxins to avoid. Appendix 3 has a comprehensive list of ingredients I avoid.

Tattoos/Permanent Makeup

Tattoos have become very popular lately, with the Pew Research Center reporting that 40% of millennials have at least one tattoo.[33] Let's talk about the health implications of tattoos.

Note that permanent makeup is a form of tattooing, so the same precautions apply.

According to the Mayo Clinic,[34] the negative health effects of tattoos are not insignificant. Here are some of the risks:

- Allergic reactions to the colored dyes used in tattooing can last for years. (Refer to chapter 6 for more information on synthetic dyes.) Consider whether you want the chemicals used in making these synthetic dyes to be in your body permanently.

- Infections. Symptoms include fever, shivering, swelling of the tattooed area, pus coming out of the tattooed area, red lesions around the tattooed area.

- Other possible skin problems include inflammation called granuloma[35] and keloids (raised areas caused by an overgrowth of scar tissue).

- If the equipment used to create your tattoo is contaminated with infected blood, you can contract various bloodborne diseases — including methicillin-resistant *Staphylococcus aureus* (MRSA), hepatitis B and hepatitis C.

CHAPTER 41 – REDUCING TOXIN EXPOSURE

For those with inflammation or autoimmune disorders, tattoos can aggravate symptoms or cause new ones to manifest.

Making the Change

Our nation, really the whole western world, has never been sicker than we are now. Lifestyle matters. If we continue to layer more and more toxins on our already-weakened bodies, we will just get sicker. But if we break free of the chains of the chemical-laden world that we live in, our bodies will start to get healthier and will work better.

I recently had a very telling experience. Years after I had removed toxic cleaners and personal care items from my life, I happened to go into a chain drugstore one day to get some cotton balls. I couldn't stop coughing the whole time I was in there. Just that brief airborne exposure to all the chemicals in the household cleaners and personal care/beauty products in that store hit me like a ton of bricks and made me realize how much my body had been cleansed from those poisons. And my body certainly didn't like being exposed again.

The choice is ours. We can continue to do what we've always done and continue to get the same results. Or we can make the change. Slowly incorporate healthier products into the home and replace old items. (Some people like me want to throw out all the bad stuff immediately. That's an option, too.)

Here's a simple way to do it; it's called the rule of three. Each month I replaced three of my toxic products with items that can replace those products. Many of Young Living's Thieves® products can replace multiple toxic products. Sooner than I realized, I had a chemical-free home and I was feeling so much better.

If you need information on how to switch out your toxic personal care and house cleaning products for toxin-free products, please email me at Carol@3Jn2Wellness.com.

CHAPTER 42

THE BODY WAS MADE TO MOVE

Moving one's body is crucial to feeling better. Moving helps the lymphatic system do its job, which is to transport lymph, a fluid containing infection-fighting white blood cells, throughout the body, and to help rid the body of toxins, waste, and other unwanted materials.

God did not design us to sit all day. We were made to move. The NET version of 1 Timothy 4:8 says, "physical exercise has some value." Science is just now starting to tell us about the detrimental effects of sitting all day.[1]

Some benefits of moving your body regularly:

- Prevents your muscles from stiffening [2]
- Boosts happiness levels [3]
- Naturally reduces the risk of heart disease [4]
- Helps you sleep better [5]
- Gives you an energy boost [6]
- Increases strength and flexibility [7]
- Improves memory [8]
- Increases self-confidence [9]
- Makes you less susceptible to disease [10]
- Helps you perform better at work [11]
- Helps you live longer [12]

These exercises are very gentle, yet effective.

- Walking – inside or outside, walk every day for at least 20 minutes. I also use this time for:

CHAPTER 42 – THE BODY WAS MADE TO MOVE

- - Oil pulling. [13] I like to add clove, lemon, orange, and peppermint essential oils to the coconut oil. Oil pulling is easy. Put a small amount of coconut oil/essential oils in your mouth and swish it around and back and forth through your teeth for 10-20 minutes. Spit in the trash when done, then brush your teeth.
  - Prayer/business meeting with God. I may be the COO (chief operating officer) of my business/ministry/life, but God is my CEO and Chief Advisor.
- Pilates – I love Winsor Pilates and have been doing it since 2005. It has strengthened my core so that my back no longer bothers me.
- DDP Yoga – Diamond Dallas Page combines yoga with strength training for an amazingly simple but effective workout.

"Food is the most widely abused anti-anxiety drug in America, and exercise is the most potent yet underutilized antidepressant."
Bill Phillips

CHAPTER 43

HOW TO EAT HEALTHY WHEN EATING OUT

Dining out can be fun. The camaraderie of friends and family: laughter, intimacy; new experiences in new places; familiar foods; exotic, unfamiliar foods. What's not to love? Americans love to eat out, but now that I'm eating healthy, am I doomed to be excluded forever from these culinary adventures? Not since I learned how to eat healthy when eating out.

Mindset

When I'm planning to eat out, it's important to know why. I *always* ask myself, "What is the purpose of this occasion?"

Am I eating out because I want to spend time with friends and family? I'll suggest some restaurants that I know I can eat at. I research a list ahead of time, so I'll always have suggestions available.

Am I eating out to try something new? God has given us such an abundance of healthy foods and many cultures use healthy foods in their cooking. Again, I research ahead of time, so I'm not thrown off by an unfamiliar menu.

Am I eating out because I'm tired of eating healthy and I'm secretly (or not-so-secretly) trying to sabotage myself? If so, it's time to put on the brakes and find out why I'm trying to sabotage myself. I need to find out what is happening that is causing me to sabotage myself, so I don't eat out until I find out why I'm doing this. Chapter 54 is about self-sabotage and how to overcome it.

Sometimes, eating out is a celebration, like a birthday, anniversary, or date night. In this case, I can suggest an alternative activity. If I do find myself faced with 'celebratory foods' like cake and alcohol, I must decide if a 'cheat' is worth it. I did (or rather, overdid) it once, and I've decided that the resulting symptoms weren't worth it.

CHAPTER 43 – HOW TO EAT HEALTHY WHEN EATING OUT

If I know why I'm eating out and I have a plan, it's easy to stick to my healthy eating agenda.

I Ask for What I Want

Many restaurants nowadays provide a great deal of nutritional information to their customers. If it's not on the menu, all I need to do is ask. Do I need a low-sodium meal? Gluten-free? Dairy free? Sugar-free? Vegan? Organic and GMO-free? There are many options available and some restaurants even cater to specific eating plans. (Doing a web search for the city and the type of restaurant I want is easy; e.g., "Tucson organic restaurants.") But what happens when I find myself in a generic restaurant and I don't want to blow all the hard work I've put into becoming healthier?

I've found that I can simply ask for what I want. For instance, I don't eat grains, dairy, or sugar. So, depending on the type of restaurant I'm at, I've asked for and received these not-on-the-menu meals:

- A salad with a grilled chicken breast, balsamic vinegar on the side.
- Grilled chicken breast, salmon, or steak with grilled vegetables.
- A beef patty with avocado slices and sweet potato fries.
- A Cobb salad without cheese, bacon, or other processed meats.
- Scrambled eggs or an omelet with vegetables.

Those are seven options that I can ask for at just about any restaurant. Even most fast food restaurants can give me a salad, a grilled chicken breast, or a plain hamburger patty. It just takes thinking outside the box.

Snacks When I'm Away from Home

What do I do if I'm going to be away from home for a long period of time without the possibility of eating a healthy meal? Fortunately, I don't have to starve to death because there are many options.

CHAPTER 43 – HOW TO EAT HEALTHY WHEN EATING OUT

Personally, I follow an intermittent fasting schedule (see chapter 36), eating three meals per day about four hours apart. Because of this, I'm always full and I don't need to snack. But sometimes I'm away from home at what would normally be a mealtime for me. What do I do?

The first thing I've realized is that I won't die if I skip a meal. There are some medical conditions, like hypoglycemia and diabetes, where you absolutely should eat more often. **Please follow your doctor's instructions for this.** Since I don't have any medical reasons, it's okay for me to skip a meal every now and then.

Here are some ideas for take-along snacks. Some require an ice pack in a tote bag, some can live in my purse indefinitely. Again, like with eating out, snacks require advance planning. Eventually, it became second nature to me.

- Hard-boiled eggs
- Carrots, celery, jicama sticks
- Nuts and seeds
- Homemade kale chips
- Berries
- Citrus fruits
- Granny Smith (sour) apples

I avoid traditional snacks like dried fruits, which have high concentrations of sugar, and protein bars. There are some good protein bars on the market, but research of the ingredients is needed to make sure it's not an unhealthy food in a healthy-food disguise. I also don't use pre-prepared smoothies, which may have dairy and sugar in them. I don't eat edamame because it's an under-ripe soybean; soybeans are known endocrine disruptors.[1] See chapter 12 on soy.

When I eat healthfully, my cells are satiated, and I don't need to overeat. That's why eating healthy means I can eat until I'm satisfied and not have to go hungry. I can eat out, stick to my eating plan, and enjoy myself. It

CHAPTER 43 – HOW TO EAT HEALTHY WHEN EATING OUT

just takes a little forethought and planning, and you, too, can learn how to eat healthy when eating out.

PART 9

PRACTICAL APPLICATION

The best-kept secret of medicine is that the body will heal itself IF we provide the right conditions **and** stop doing the things that caused the sickness in the first place.

CHAPTER 44

WHAT IS A HERXHEIMER REACTION?

I was feeling good about myself. I had started my new Be in Health lifestyle of real, whole foods. My body was slowly adapting to my new way of life when, suddenly, I woke up sick one morning. I had a headache and flu-like symptoms. (Another time, I developed an itchy rash over most of my body.) I wondered why I felt this way. After all, I made this change in my eating habits so I could feel better. What was happening? I came to find out I was experiencing a Herxheimer reaction.

A Herxheimer reaction, technically known as a Jarisch-Herxheimer Reaction, or Herx for short, is a short-term detoxification reaction in the body. It can last anywhere from a few days to a few weeks, maybe a few months, depending on how severe one's toxin load is. But don't worry, it's not permanent; it's the body's way of sloughing off toxins. Simply put, it meant I would feel worse before I felt better.

What is Happening to Me?

A Herxheimer reaction occurs when the body is detoxifying and the released toxins either exacerbate the original symptoms or create their own symptoms. The important thing to note is that worsening symptoms don't indicate that what you're doing has failed; in fact, usually, just the opposite is true.[1]

Adolf Jarisch and Karl Herxheimer, both dermatologists, working separately, noted that as their patients underwent treatment for skin lesions, the lesions first became worse before improving. They both also found that **those who had the most extreme reactions ending up healing faster, with better results**.

When experiencing a Jarisch-Herxheimer Reaction, it's important to remember that the positive health changes you've made (whether a supplement or the Be in Health lifestyle) is NOT the cause of the reaction. Rather, the reaction is part of the detoxification process. When one stops eating artificial, processed, chemical-laden food and starts eating real,

CHAPTER 44 – WHAT IS A HERXHEIMER REACTION?

whole food, the body starts to release endotoxins (toxins that are present inside a bacterial cell that are released when the cell disintegrates) it has stored up from the bad, fake food. These endotoxins find various ways to escape the body, whether through the elimination process (urination and bowel movements) or the skin (fever, rashes, blisters, pimples, etc.). As endotoxins stored in the muscles are released, the muscles start to ache, mimicking flu symptoms.

How Do I Deal with This?

It was hard to convince myself that something that made me feel so bad was necessary, but these toxins needed to leave my body in some way. I remembered how many years I ate toxic food and took prescription medicines. The release of those toxins did not last as long as it took to store them.

Mindset is very important when experiencing a Herx reaction. I needed to be especially kind to myself during this period. I didn't berate myself or put unrealistic expectations on myself. I slowed down and let my body heal. I told my body how much I love and appreciate it. I enlisted the support of my loved ones.

Here are some specific things I did to lessen the symptoms.

- **Water.** I drank plenty of purified water. This is crucial to help the body flush out the endotoxins. I set a timer on my phone for every half hour to remind myself to drink water.

- **Detox baths.** I took hot detox baths every night before bed. I combined 1 cup Epsom salts and 1 cup baking soda with various essential oils, such as frankincense, rosemary, helichrysum, lavender, peppermint, or any of my favorites. I soaked for at least 20 minutes with soothing music in the background.

- **Lots of rest.** I slept as much as my body needed. Serious healing takes place during sleep.

- **Sauna**. If you have access to a far infrared sauna, begin with no more than 15 minutes at a time. Dry brush your body beforehand and shower immediately afterward.

- **Nutrients**. The body needs extra nutrients like vitamins A, C, E, and NAC (N-Acetyl Cysteine) during the detox process. The herb milk thistle is particularly helpful during detoxification.

- **Bowels**. When my body started to reabsorb the toxins that were being released, I became constipated. Dr. Jill Carnahan, M.D., has the following suggestions to get the bowels moving:[2]

  - Ingest 500-1000 mg magnesium citrate daily or until you have normal, soft bowel movements at least once daily. You may also add 5-10 grams of ascorbic acid daily to bowel tolerance.
  - Start every morning with a tall glass of warm water.
  - Drink a few tablespoons of extra virgin olive oil several times daily on an empty stomach.
  - Stir 2 tablespoons of ground flax or chia seed into water and let sit for 10 minutes. Stir again and drink on an empty stomach.

WARNING: If you experience any *serious* symptoms such as cardiac irregularity, breathing difficulties including chest, lung, or throat constriction, or significant swelling, **please seek immediate medical attention.**

Ongoing Detoxification

Detoxification is something that should be happening for the rest of our lives because, no matter how clean we eat and how many toxins we avoid, we will always be subject to stress and toxins in our daily living. We can't live in a bubble. This isn't a reason to avoid the Be in Health lifestyle, rather it's a reason why the Be in Health lifestyle is so critical for our overall well-being. Continuing to live this lifestyle can help lessen the daily detox symptoms.

CHAPTER 44 – WHAT IS A HERXHEIMER REACTION?

According to Dr. Brian R. Clement, Ph.D., N.M.D., L.N.C., in *Hippocrates Life Force: Superior Health and Longevity*,[3] "A complete and total detoxification of the body can take up to seven years, the same period of time it takes for us to replace all the cells in our body. More than half of the accumulated wastes in our body will be released the first seven days of a detox program, but complete healing and restoration of the body can be broken down into [the following] stages."

Number of Years After Detox	Results
Up to 1.5 years	Major digestive cleansing with removal of fat deposits and calcifications
1.5 to 2 years	Deep tissue and joint cleansing
2 to 5 years	Bone structure, cartilage, and further joint cleansing
5.5 to 6 years	Organ repositioning and renewal
6 to 7 years	Brain tissue and neurological cleansing

Dr. Clement continues, "As layer after layer of contaminants are stripped away, the release of toxins will periodically affect how you feel. But as time passes, your overall health and feelings of wellness will markedly improve. Due to the body's cellular intelligence, every part is affected by the whole. When one part of us is renewed, our entire body benefits from greater harmony and integration."

Whatever happens, please don't start eating bad, fake food again. While this may temporarily ease Herx symptoms, it will just set you up for failure. There's a reason (or multiple reasons) why you started the Be in Health lifestyle. Don't sabotage yourself just for temporary relief.

CHAPTER 45

IS HEALTHY FOOD REALLY TOO EXPENSIVE?

The number one reason I hear from people about why they don't eat healthy food is that it's too expensive. Everyone defines 'too expensive' differently, depending on their budget. What I've discovered is that it all depends on what types of food someone is talking about, whether they're willing to prepare homemade food, and what they're comparing. So, let's dive in and find out if healthy food is really too expensive.

Types of Food

Let's start with a definition of healthy food. When I speak of healthy food, I'm referring to food in the form it's found in nature, without preservatives or added flavorings, colors, or other chemicals, food that doesn't come in boxes or cans. In other words, real food. The Standard American Diet (SAD) consists of mostly pre-prepared and pre-packaged foods. Healthy food and SAD food are two very different things.

Many people have the mistaken impression that eating healthy food means substituting one package of processed food for another. Just because a label says 'Gluten-Free' or 'Non-GMO' doesn't necessarily mean it's a healthy food. Processed food is processed food, regardless of the label. If a food is processed, that means it has been taken from its original form as found in nature and turned into something else. A simple example is applesauce. Applesauce is a food processed from apples (real food). Another example is cheese, which is a processed food. The real food is raw milk.

Why is Most Processed Food Unhealthy?

Unless you're doing the processing, like making your own applesauce or soup, you don't know how the food you buy was processed and with what. Most processed foods have large amounts of unhealthy, cheap fats that are often hydrogenated, which means they become trans fats.[1]

CHAPTER 45 – IS HEALTHY FOOD REALLY TOO EXPENSIVE?

According to the Mayo Clinic,[2] "Trans fat is considered by many doctors to be the worst type of fat you can eat. Unlike other dietary fats, trans fat — also called trans-fatty acids — both raises your LDL ("bad") cholesterol and lowers your HDL ("good") cholesterol. A diet laden with trans fat increases your risk of heart disease, the leading killer of men and women."

Vegetable oils are extremely unhealthy, and most people eat way too much of them.

Another problem with processed foods is the process itself. As I talked about in chapter 10, when the modern steel roller mill was invented, it changed the nutritional quality of wheat flour forever. This is why I don't eat food that's been processed by anyone other than myself or someone I know and trust.

When processed food is taken out of the equation, all that's left is real food. Now the comparison is between the cost of real food that isn't organic and probably GMO and real food that is organic and non-GMO.

Organic Food vs. Non-Organic Food

Many people who are considering the switch to eating healthy food think that every single item they purchase must be organic, non-GMO, and of the very best quality. If this is within your budget, then, yes, do that. But it's not an either/or situation. Just because you can't buy everything organic and non-GMO doesn't mean you should buy nothing organic and non-GMO.

Did you know that not all produce is heavily contaminated with pesticides? EWG.org[3] has a list of what they call the Dirty Dozen and the Clean Fifteen; it's updated yearly. The Dirty Dozen is a list of 12 foods that should always be purchased organic because of high pesticide content. The Clean Fifteen is a list of 15 foods that have low pesticide contamination so getting them organic isn't necessary. See, you just saved money because now you know which produce you should buy organic and which it doesn't matter.

CHAPTER 45 – IS HEALTHY FOOD REALLY TOO EXPENSIVE?

The least healthful foods we consume are dairy products and meat (you are what the thing you eat, ate). This is because of how the animals are fed. Most are fed GMO grains, which means the products that come from these animals are GMO. Most of the animals are also given hormones and antibiotics, which end up in the meat and dairy products we consume. If you can afford nothing else, get 100% grass-fed and finished, organic, pasture raised dairy products and meat. This alone will make a huge difference in one's health. Personally, I don't consume dairy products because I'm allergic to them. (Many, many people are allergic to the A1 casein protein in most dairy products; see chapter 11.)

Are You Willing?

Food preparation is another big area that makes people think they can't eat healthfully. We are a society consumed with busyness. We rush from here to there and grab a quick bite on the go. All that rushing around and what do we get for it? We get sick and tired.

When I first made the switch to healthy eating, I didn't know how I was going to do it. I wasn't used to preparing homemade meals. Every. Single. Day. Where would I find the time?

You know what? I did find the time because it was important to me. And I found that the important things in my life like my marriage, my business, and my ministry, didn't suffer. Now, I spend even more time with my husband because we prepare meals together. I realized that I had been wasting a lot of time. I've also come to realize that many people simply don't want to change, no matter how they might benefit from it.

I realized that I didn't need to prepare a super-fancy meal every day. Simple is good. How about some scrambled eggs for dinner? I'll sauté up some veggies, add some avocado (a healthy fat) and sauerkraut (a probiotic-rich food) on the side, and I have an amazing dinner (or lunch or breakfast). My favorite lunch is a sweet potato smothered with ghee, some Ceylon cinnamon, and pecans.

It all comes down to, what's more important to you? Is health more important to you than some (possible) inconvenience?

CHAPTER 45 – IS HEALTHY FOOD REALLY TOO EXPENSIVE?

What Are You Comparing?

Is healthy food really too expensive? Not compared to eating out. Eating out used to be a big part of our budget. In the past few years, my husband and I have gone out to dinner, on average, twice a year. Why? Because the food we make at home tastes much better than what we can get at a restaurant. Not to mention, it's healthier, and yes, less expensive than eating out.

Many people are willing to eat junk and take a pill to help alleviate the symptoms caused by the crappy food. I'm not willing to do that anymore. My health is more important than convenience. Is healthy food all that expensive compared to the cost of being sick, the cost of doctor and hospital visits, the cost of drugs that may make you even sicker?

So, is healthy food really too expensive? Not if you want to be healthy. Not if you compare it to the alternative. Are you willing to change? Or, are you using the supposed cost as an excuse not to change?

CHAPTER 46

KITCHEN MAKEOVER

Instead of That, Eat This

- Instead of sugar, I use stevia or raw (unpasteurized), local honey (up to 1 Tbsp. per day). I make sure the stevia I buy doesn't have chemical additives.
- Instead of processed meat, I eat fresh 100% grass-fed and finished beef and lamb, and pasture raised poultry.
- Instead of farm-raised fish, I eat wild-caught fish.
- Instead of tilapia, I eat wild-caught salmon.
- Instead of regular cow/goat/sheep dairy, I eat cultured 'dairy' products like coconut milk kefir.
- Instead of gluten-filled flour products, I eat coconut flour and almond flour products I make myself (no store-bought processed foods).
- Instead of hydrogenated oils like canola oil, I eat coconut oil, avocado oil, and olive oil.
- Instead of butter, I eat coconut oil or ghee.
- Instead of white potatoes (including French fries), I eat sweet potatoes (sweet potatoes fries are delicious).
- Instead of soy products (like soy sauce, tofu, or soy protein), I eat soy-free Coconut Aminos.
- Instead of iodized table salt, I use Himalayan pink salt.
- Instead of eating raw food, I eat cooked food.
- Instead of coffee or soda, I drink purified water and herbal teas.

CHAPTER 46 – KITCHEN MAKEOVER

- In other words, I eat fresh, real, whole food instead of dead, processed, GMO food.

If you're avoiding eggs, here are some substitutions you can use in recipes.

Ground Flax Seed	Chia Seed	Ripe Bananas	Applesauce
1 Tbsp. ground flax seeds	1 Tbsp. chia seeds	½ mashed banana	¼ c. unsweetened applesauce
PLUS	PLUS		
3 Tbsp. water	1/3 c. water		
EQUALS	EQUALS	EQUALS	EQUALS
1 Egg	1 Egg	1 Egg	1 Egg
(Blend until mixture is thick, creamy, & egg-like)	(Mix & let sit for 15 minutes)		

Kitchen Gadgets

The following kitchen gadgets/appliances/utensils will come in handy for food preparation:

- Heavy duty blender, like a Vitamix®, for smoothies and chopping. If I could have only one appliance, this would be it.
- Food processor for chopping veggies
- Spiralizer for making veggie 'noodles'
- Heavy duty stock pot with strainer insert for making bone broth
- Mason jars for freezing bone broth
- Cookware: stainless steel or cast iron for all stovetop cooking
- Crockpot for applesauce, soups, stews

CHAPTER 46 – KITCHEN MAKEOVER

- Dehydrator for drying fruits, veggies, sprouted/soaked nuts & seeds, making beef or salmon jerky
- Immersion blender for pureeing soups in the pot, mixing batters
- Glass mixing bowls, baking dishes, storage containers, mason jars to avoid using plastic

You don't have to get everything at once. Figure out your immediate needs and go from there. A good source for glass mixing bowls and jars is yard sales/estate sales.

Where to Shop

Changing what you eat often means changing where you shop. I'm blessed to live in an area with Sprouts Farmers Market, Natural Grocers, and Whole Foods Market®. There may be other natural food markets in the area you live in.

Other good sources of wholesome foods include ethnic markets (Asian, Mexican, Mediterranean) and local farmers markets and food co-ops. Check there to find local, raw (unpasteurized) honey in your area.

You can get pantry items online through Amazon.com, Vitacost.com, and ThriveMarket.com.

There are services that deliver fresh, organic food to your doorstep. Check online to find something in your area.

CHAPTER 46 – KITCHEN MAKEOVER

CHAPTER 47

6 SPICES TO IMPROVE AND MAINTAIN HEALTH

Mankind has used herbs and spices as medicine since the very beginning. Herbs come from the leafy green part of the plant. Spices are parts of the plant other than the leaves, such as the root, stem, bulb, bark, or seeds.

> *Genesis 1:11 NIV*
> *Then God said, "Let the land produce vegetation: seed-bearing plants and trees on the land that bear fruit with seed in it, according to their various kinds." And it was so.*
>
> *Ezekiel 47:12 KJV*
> *And by the river upon the bank thereof, on this side and on that side, shall grow all trees for meat [food], whose leaf shall not fade, neither shall the fruit thereof be consumed: it shall bring forth new fruit according to his months, because their waters they issued out of the sanctuary: and the fruit thereof shall be for meat [food], and the leaf thereof for medicine.*
>
> *Revelation 22:2*
> *In the midst of the street of it, and on either side of the river, was there the tree of life, which bare twelve manner of fruits, and yielded her fruit every month: and the leaves of the tree were for the healing of the nations.*

Here are six spices highly regarded for their health-restoring properties.

Turmeric Root

Turmeric, a member of the ginger family and the main spice in curry, has become all the rage among spices lately, and with good reason. Here are some of the things turmeric and curcumin, its chief constituent, can help with:

CHAPTER 47 – SPICES TO IMPROVE AND MAINTAIN HEALTH

According to the Linus Pauling Institute at Oregon State University,[1] curcumin "modulates numerous molecular targets and exerts antioxidant,[2] anti-inflammatory,[3] anticancer, and neuroprotective activities."

According to a clinical trial conducted by the Johns Hopkins University School of Medicine, curcumin can help shrink precancerous lesions[4] known as colon polyps when taken with a small amount of quercetin, a powerful antioxidant found in onions, apples, and cabbage. The average number of polyps dropped more than 60% and those that remained shrank by more than 50%. In a 2006 study, researchers at UCLA also found that curcumin helps clear the brain of the plaques that are characteristic of Alzheimer's disease.[5]

Curcumin and other chemicals in turmeric may decrease swelling (inflammation).[6] Because of this, turmeric may be beneficial for treating conditions that involve inflammation like autoimmune disorders.

Because turmeric/curcumin isn't readily absorbed[7] into the human body, adding a spice that contains piperine (like black pepper) will make it more bioavailable to human cells. I use 1 teaspoon of powdered turmeric in my smoothie every morning and add 1-2 drops of Vitality™ Black Pepper Essential Oil[8] to increase absorption.

Garlic

Garlic is used to help prevent heart disease,[9] including atherosclerosis or hardening of the arteries (plaque buildup in the arteries that can block the flow of blood and may lead to heart attack or stroke), high cholesterol, high blood pressure, and to boost the immune system. Garlic may also help protect against cancer.[10]

Experiments have shown that garlic — or specific chemical compounds found in garlic — is highly effective at killing countless micro-organisms[11] responsible for some of the most common and rarest infections, including tuberculosis, pneumonia, thrush, and herpes. Because of its antiviral properties, garlic can be used to treat eye infections and as a natural ear infection remedy.[12]

Other raw garlic benefits[13] include its ability to reduce the risk of cancer, control hypertension, boost cardiovascular health, and fight hair loss.[14]

Some ways to get more garlic into your diet include making a garlic oil infusion: crush garlic cloves and add them to a carrier oil (like olive oil). Let the mixture sit for about five hours, then strain the pieces of garlic out and keep the oil in a jar with a lid.

Astragalus Root

Astragalus root, another powerful antiviral spice, has been used in traditional Chinese medicine for centuries. Its main use is to boost the body's immune system.[15] Scientific studies have shown that astragalus has antiviral properties[16] and stimulates the immune system, suggesting that it may help prevent the common cold or flu.

A 2004 study evaluated the effects of astragalus on herpes simplex virus type 1 [17] and found that the spice has "obvious inhibiting efficacy." Another study published in the *Chinese Medical Sciences Journal* concluded that astragalus can inhibit the growth of coxsackie B virus[18] in mice. Astragalus has antibacterial and anti-inflammatory properties, and it's used on the skin for wound care. It's also one of the seven adaptogen (helps the body adapt to stress) spices to lower cortisol.[19]

Ginger Root

Ginger can prevent stomach upset[20] from many sources, including pregnancy, motion sickness, and chemotherapy.[21] "This is one of Mom's remedies that really work," says Dr. Suzanna M. Zick, N.D., M.P.H., a research investigator at the University of Michigan.

A powerful antioxidant,[22] ginger works by blocking the effects of serotonin, a chemical produced by both the brain and stomach when you're nauseated, and by stopping the production of free radicals, another cause of upset in your stomach. In one study of cruise ship passengers traveling on rough seas, 500 mg of ginger every 4 hours was as effective as Dramamine®,[23] the commonly used OTC motion-sickness medication. In another study, where subjects took 940 mg, it was even more effective than the drug.

CHAPTER 47 – SPICES TO IMPROVE AND MAINTAIN HEALTH

Ginger might also decrease blood pressure,[24] arthritis pain,[25] and cancer risk.[26] Ginger helps regulate blood flow, which may lower blood pressure, says Zick, and its anti-inflammatory properties might help ease arthritis.

I put a chunk of fresh, raw ginger in my daily smoothie.

Ashwagandha Root

Ashwagandha is also referred to as Indian ginseng. Often used in Ayurvedic medicine, ashwagandha regulates the immune system[27] and eases anxiety.[28] Ashwagandha has been used in eastern medicine for over 2,500 years and has immuno-modulating effects that boost the immune system and aid the body in lowering cortisol levels.[29]

There have been over 200 studies on ashwagandha's ability to improve thyroid function [30] and treat adrenal fatigue. [31] According to OrganicFacts.net, ashwagandha "has a wide range of health benefits, including its ability to fight against cancer and diabetes, as well as reduce inflammation, arthritis, asthma, hypertension, stress, and rheumatism. Furthermore, it boosts your supply of antioxidants and regulates the immune system. It also has antibacterial and anticonvulsant properties." [32]

Ashwagandha is an adaptogenic spice,[33] meaning it greatly enhances the body's ability to deal with stress. Ashwagandha should be taken with care.[34] It should not be taken if you're pregnant or wish to become pregnant.

Cinnamon Bark

Besides tasting delicious, cinnamon has many beneficial properties. In a recent study of type 2 diabetics,[35] those taking 1, 3, or 6 gm of cinnamon per day saw a reduction in serum glucose, triglycerides, LDL cholesterol, and total cholesterol, which also reduces the risk of heart disease.

Cinnamon contains large amounts of highly potent polyphenol antioxidants,[36] even more than garlic and oregano. These antioxidants have anti-inflammatory effects [37] which may help lower the risk of disease.

CHAPTER 47 – SPICES TO IMPROVE AND MAINTAIN HEALTH

Cinnamon has been shown to lead to various improvements for Alzheimer's disease [38] and Parkinson's disease [39] in animal studies. Cinnamaldehyde, the main active component of cinnamon, may help fight various kinds of infection. [40]

I use Ceylon cinnamon (known as the 'true' cinnamon). Most cinnamon sold in the U.S. is actually a combination of cinnamon and cassia, which is a cousin of cinnamon. Cassia contains coumarin, "a toxin that could damage your liver if eaten regularly. Coumarin is also a potential carcinogen. Cassia cinnamon has very high levels of coumarin. Ceylon has none or very little coumarin. To avoid this toxin, go with Ceylon cinnamon." [41]

Another type of cinnamon called Saigon or Vietnamese cinnamon is more closely related to cassia than to true Ceylon cinnamon. Expect to pay more for Ceylon cinnamon.

CHAPTER 47 – SPICES TO IMPROVE AND MAINTAIN HEALTH

CHAPTER 48

APPS TO HELP US GET AND STAY HEALTHY

You've found a great recipe and now you need to shop for the ingredients. Unfortunately, labels don't tell the whole story of what is in a product. Knowing that healthy foods (and healthy personal care and cleaning products) are available doesn't mean you will know them when you're confronted with an array of choices at the store. So, here are 6 apps to help you get and stay healthy. The first five are free to download. Find them all in your app store.

EWG's Healthy Living

The Healthy Living app comes from EWG.org (Environmental Working Group), an organization dedicated to helping people live healthier lives in a healthier environment. This app lets you scan a product's barcode, read a review, and make a healthy choice. You can scan both personal care and food items in a database of around 200,000 items or browse through the database. You will be given reviews based on allergy concerns, cancer concerns, and developmental concerns, as well as a score from 1 (good) to 10 (worst).

Think Dirty.

The Think Dirty. app is for personal care and cleaning products. Scan the barcode and get a rating from 0 (neutral) to 10 (dirty) based on carcinogenicity, developmental and reproductive toxicity, and allergies and immunotoxicity. It will give you the reason for the rating based on each ingredient (in other words, each ingredient is also rated 0-10). You will receive recommendations for items rated 0-2 (neutral) in the same category as the item you scanned. If your item isn't in the database, you can submit it for review and get the result in a day or two. You can also shop on Amazon for the product you choose directly from the app. This is my favorite app in this category (personal care and cleaning products).

CHAPTER 48 – APPS TO HELP US GET AND STAY HEALTHY

Non-GMO Project Shopping Guide

The Non-GMO Project is a non-profit organization that offers North America's only third-party verification and labeling for non-GMO (genetically modified organism) foods and products. GMO foods, also called GE (genetically engineered) or BE (bio-engineered) are created in a lab by altering the genetic makeup of a plant or an animal. The vast majority of corn, soy, canola, and sugar beets grown in the U.S. are now genetically engineered, and they're often used as ingredients in processed foods.[1] The food industry is also pushing to further expand the use of genetic engineering. This app allows you to scan products to find out if they're genetically modified or not. You can also search by product category, brand, and product name.

EWG's Food Scores

Another great app from EWG, Food Scores rates products based on nutrition, ingredient concerns, and processing, combining these three areas into an overall score from 1 (best) to 10 (worst). To come up with a score, nutrition is weighed most heavily, followed by ingredient concerns, then processing. Considerations include the likely presence of key contaminants (pesticides, hormones, and antibiotics) and possible health implications of food additives. It took the engineers at EWG three years to build this app and it includes over 80,000 foods, 5,000 ingredients, and 1,500 brands.

Healthyout

Eating out is one of the biggest challenges facing those dedicated to healthy eating. HealthyOut from Rise Labs, Inc. helps you find the better options on a menu and makes meal modification suggestions, so you won't fill up on the bad stuff. It lets you search your local area for restaurants offering healthy items. You can choose from meals that fall within a specific calorie range or ones that adhere to your dietary plan (vegetarian, Paleo, gluten-sensitive, South Beach, Zone, etc.). The app currently covers over 500 cities nationwide.

CHAPTER 48 – APPS TO HELP US GET AND STAY HEALTHY

Real Plans

Whether you're stuck in a rut for inspiration or just can't get organized to cook, Real Plans is a game-changer. It's a meal planner with superpowers. It creates a custom plan to suit your family's size, busy schedule, and ever-changing needs. Real Plans gives you access to over 1,500 carefully curated recipes to suit every taste and occasion. Pick your meals or import your own recipes. It then generates a shopping list for you. Real Plans costs $14/month, or $33/quarter, or $72/annually.

CHAPTER 48 – APPS TO HELP US GET AND STAY HEALTHY

CHAPTER 49

FOOD - MOOD - POOP JOURNAL

My Food – Mood – Poop Journal			
Date:			
	Food/Drink Consumed (list time of day)	How I Feel (Mood, Stomach/Digestion, Energy Level, Sleep Quality, Skin, Aches/Pains, etc.)	Poop*
After Waking			
Breakfast			
Snack			
Lunch			
Snack			
Dinner			
Snack			
Water			

CHAPTER 49 – FOOD – MOOD – POOP JOURNAL

*Use the Bristol Stool Chart below to give it a number and describe the color.

You may be a busy person on the go who doesn't have time to write down everything you eat, drink, feel, and poop. Enter Cara, a personal food and symptom diary that lets you track what you eat and how you feel. The app makes it easy to enter foods, track symptoms, digestion, and elimination details to get a daily score. Used consistently, Cara users can share trends with medical professionals and may learn to avoid the symptom triggers altogether. Though the food database is somewhat limited, users can easily add their own foods to the database.

Cara is available in the Apple app store (Android coming soon). Best of all, it's free.

There are other apps available to help you keep your FMP journal updated. They include:

- Bowelle – free
- PoopLog – free

BRISTOL STOOL CHART

	Type 1	Separate hard lumps	Very constipated
	Type 2	Lumpy and sausage like	Slightly constipated
	Type 3	A sausage shape with cracks in the surface	Normal
	Type 4	Like a smooth, soft sausage or snake	Normal
	Type 5	Soft blobs with clear-cut edges	Lacking fibre
	Type 6	Mushy consistency with ragged edges	Inflammation
	Type 7	Liquid consistency with no solid pieces	Inflammation

CHAPTER 50

GUT-RESTORING RECIPES

Applesauce

Total Time: 4 hours. Serves: 6-8

- 10 large green apples, peeled, cored, and chopped
- ½ cup water
- 1 tsp. Ceylon cinnamon
- Stevia

Directions:

- In a slow cooker, combine all ingredients, sweetening with stevia to taste. Cook on low for 4 hours.
- Mix applesauce well and mash any clumps of apples to reach desired consistency.

Avocado-Stuffed Meatballs

- Coconut oil (for greasing pan)
- 1 pound 100% grass-fed and finished ground beef
- 1 egg (for those who don't eat eggs, combine 1 Tbsp. ground flax seed with 3 Tbsp. water, mix, and let sit for 5 minutes until it has an egg-like consistency)
- 3 Tbsp. fresh chopped parsley
- 4 cloves minced garlic
- 1 Tbsp. organic Dijon mustard
- 1 tsp. Himalayan pink salt
- 1/2 diced avocado

CHAPTER 50 – GUT RESTORING RECIPES

Directions:

- Preheat oven to 400° F. Lightly grease sheet pan with coconut oil.
- In large bowl, combine all remaining ingredients except avocado. Mix well and use wet hands to form 8 to 12 meatballs.
- To stuff meatballs, make a hole in center, insert avocado cube, and close up the hole, making sure avocado is fully surrounded by meat.
- Place meatballs on prepared sheet pan and bake until cooked through, about 12 minutes.

Recipe from Dr. Josh Axe, D.N.M., D.C., C.N.S.

Baked Apple Smoothie

- 1 Granny Smith apple
- ¼ cup coconut milk
- 1 Tbsp. flax meal
- 2 Tbsp. vanilla protein or collagen powder
- ½ tsp. Ceylon cinnamon
- ½ tsp. vanilla extract
- Pinch ginger
- Stevia or raw (unpasteurized), local honey

Directions:

- Bake apple in oven at 350° F for 30 minutes.
- In a high-powered blender, combine all ingredients, sweetening with stevia or honey to taste. Puree on high until smooth.

Recipe from Dr. Josh Axe, D.N.M., D.C., C.N.S.

CHAPTER 50 - GUT-RESTORING RECIPES

Carol's Homemade Holy Guacamole

- 2 ripe avocados cubed
- 2 Tbsp. red onion finely chopped
- 2 Tbsp. fresh cilantro chopped
- 1/4 tsp. Himalayan pink salt
- 1 tsp. lemon juice
- 1 drop Young Living Lime Vitality™ Essential Oil
- 1 drop Young Living Jade Lemon Vitality™ Essential Oil

Mix all ingredients and serve.

Cauliflower Soup

- 1 Tbsp. coconut oil
- 2 medium yellow onions diced
- 1 bay leaf
- 1 1/4 tsp. ground cumin
- 1 tsp. Himalayan pink salt
- 1 tsp. ground turmeric
- 1 drop Young Living Black Pepper Vitality™ Essential Oil (to increase the bioavailability of turmeric)
- 1/2 tsp. ground coriander
- 1/8 tsp. ground cardamom
- 4 garlic cloves minced
- 4 1/2 cups bone broth
- 1 large head of cauliflower roughly chopped to the same size
- 1 cup canned coconut milk
- 1 Tbsp. apple cider vinegar

CHAPTER 50 – GUT RESTORING RECIPES

Directions:

- In a large soup pot, heat the oil over medium-low. Add the onions and all the spices except for the garlic. Sauté, stirring occasionally until the onions become translucent, about 10 minutes. Then, add the garlic and sauté another few minutes.
- Add the broth and cauliflower and bring to a boil over high heat. Reduce to a simmer and allow to cook for about 15 minutes, until the cauliflower is tender.
- Remove from heat and transfer carefully to a Vitamix® blender. Blend on high (allowing steam to vent) for a few minutes, until silky and smooth.
- Transfer back to the soup pot and stir in the coconut milk and vinegar. Bring back to heat over low, ensuring it doesn't boil.

Chia Seed Coconut Milk Pudding

Make this in advance because it needs time for the chia seeds to soak up the liquid. Let it do its work in the refrigerator overnight.

- 1/4 cup chia seeds
- 1 cup full fat coconut milk
- 1 cup frozen organic blueberries
- Pinch cardamom
- Stevia to taste

Directions:

- Blend everything by hand and put into a glass bowl, seal, and refrigerate overnight.

Makes a great snack. Add a little bit of fresh fruit on top or a few sprouted/soaked nuts.

CHAPTER 50 - GUT-RESTORING RECIPES

Chicken Bone Broth

- 2 whole raw pasture raised chickens
- 1 package gizzards or chicken feet (optional)
- 3 – 4 onions (Cut in half or quarters to fit in pot. I leave the skins on but take off any stickers.)
- 8 + large carrots cut in 1/2 to 1/3 (skin on)
- 6+ large celery stalks cut into 1/2 or 1/3
- 3-4 (or more) cloves garlic (I keep the paper on them and smash them once with my knife and throw them in the pot.)
- 2-3 drops Young Living Vitality™ Black Pepper essential oil (to increase the bioavailability of turmeric)
- 1 tsp. turmeric
- 1 large bunch of fresh lemon thyme. (Use your judgment. I just throw it in. I don't chop or remove from stems.)
- 1 large bunch of fresh rosemary (same as the thyme)
- 1 Tbsp. Himalayan pink salt
- 2 Tbsp. apple cider vinegar (don't leave this out; it leaches the calcium out of the bones and into the broth)
- 2-3 Tbsp. coconut oil
- 2-inch chunk fresh ginger sliced (no need to peel first)
- 3-4 bay leaves
- Fresh Parsley

Directions:

- Put it all in the pot and fill with water till covered. Turn on high. Bring to a boil. Boil 1 minute then turn the heat down to simmer and put the lid on.

CHAPTER 50 – GUT RESTORING RECIPES

- In about 1.5 – 2 hours pull out the chicken and take the meat off to use later. Put the bones/skin back in the pot. Put the lid back on and continue to simmer for the remainder of the 24 hours. About an hour before it's done, stir in a bunch of fresh parsley.
- Take off heat and let cool then strain through cheesecloth/strainers.
- Store in quart size glass mason jars. Leave about 1-2 inches at the top for expansion. Bone broth is best consumed within 4 days, so put any you won't eat within 4 days in the freezer.

Watch a video of me making bone broth at https://3Jn2Wellness.com/Bone-Broth/

Cilantro Salmon Burgers

- 2 cans (6–7 ounces each) wild-caught Alaskan salmon, drained
- 2 Tbsp. scallions finely chopped
- 3 cloves garlic minced
- 2 tsp. chopped cilantro
- 3 pasture raised eggs (for those who don't eat eggs, combine 1 Tbsp. ground flax seed with 3 Tbsp. water, mix, and let sit for 5 minutes until it has an egg-like consistency; multiply this by 3 to replace the 3 eggs in this recipe)
- 2 drops Young Living Lime Vitality™ Essential Oil
- 1 Tbsp. organic Dijon mustard
- 1 tsp. Himalayan pink salt
- ¼ cup coconut flour
- Coconut oil

Directions:

- In a bowl, combine salmon, scallions, garlic, and cilantro and mix well.

- In another bowl, whisk together eggs, lime essential oil, mustard, and salt. Add to bowl with salmon and mix until well combined. Add coconut flour and mix again.
- In a skillet with coconut oil over medium-high heat, drop mixture in 3 or 4 portions to form burgers. Cook, turning once until browned and heated through, about 8 minutes.

Recipe from Dr. Josh Axe, D.N.M., D.C., C.N.S.

Coconut Milk Kefir

- Heat 2-3 cans of coconut milk. Be sure to buy BPA-free cans – I use Native Forest Organic or 365 Organic.
- For a thicker kefir, use less of the liquid from the cans or add some collagen protein.
- Heat it to about 160° F either in a blender with that option or on the stovetop.
- Cool to a temperature that allows you to comfortably stick your finger in and it's warm to the touch.
- Pour into a large mason jar, mix in the Kefir Starter packet or 1/3 cup from the last batch, and stir rapidly with a wire whisk.
- Cover with a breathable cloth such as cheesecloth or a towel and secure with a rubber band. It needs to be kept between 70° F - 100° F to ferment. If your home tends to be cool, you can leave it in an oven and turn it on warm occasionally.
- After 24 hours, stir and test to taste until the tartness is present at the level you like. Note that coconut milk kefir will not be as tart as cow's or goat's milk kefir.
- Cover with the jar lid and place in the fridge after stirring rapidly with a wire whisk. It will thicken quite a bit after refrigeration, but not as much as goat or cow's milk kefir.
- Save about 1/3 of a cup from each batch to culture the next one.

CHAPTER 50 – GUT RESTORING RECIPES

I get my Kefir Starter from Body Ecology.[1] It's very economical because each box will provide about 42 batches of kefir. You use 1/3 cup from each batch to culture the next one. Each kefir starter packet makes a total of 7 batches. I add ¼ to ½ cup of Coconut Milk Kefir to my Super Restoring Smoothie every day.

Egg Scramble with Asparagus, Avocado, and Sauerkraut

Serves 1–2. Time: 10 minutes

- 1 bunch asparagus chopped
- 2 tsp. coconut oil
- 4 eggs
- 2 Tbsp. water
- ½ tsp. Himalayan pink salt
- ½ avocado, peeled and sliced
- ¼ cup sauerkraut

Directions:

- Heat a skillet to medium heat and add the coconut oil. Once the oil is hot, add the chopped asparagus and sauté for 2–3 minutes or until asparagus is slightly softened.
- Whisk together the eggs, water, and salt, and add the mixture to the asparagus.
- Let the eggs cook for 1 minute and then use a spatula to scramble the mixture.
- Scoop the egg scramble onto a plate and top with sauerkraut and avocado.

Farmer's Wife with Lamb Sausage

Make sausage:

- 1 Tbsp. ghee

- 1 lb. 100% grass fed and finished ground lamb
- 1 tsp. Himalayan pink salt
- 2 tsp. ground fennel seed
- 2 Tbsp. apple cider vinegar
- 2 Tbsp. Coconut Aminos (available in Sprouts, Whole Foods, and other natural food locations)

Directions:

- Mix all ingredients (except for the ghee), kneading well. Taste and adjust flavors as you like.
- Shape your sausage to your desired form – round or long.
- Heat up a skillet with ghee in it.
- Add sausages and fry them for approximately 7 minutes on one side and 4 minutes on the other.

Make salad:

- ½ avocado
- Handful of organic green mix (e.g. arugula, mizuna, baby kale, etc.)
- 1 cup sauerkraut
- Olive oil
- Balsamic vinegar

Drizzle olive oil and balsamic vinegar (or other healthy dressing) over the greens. Arrange the items on your plate with sausage and enjoy.

Recipe from Magdalena Wszelaki

Fat Bombs

- ½ cup melted organic coconut oil
- ½ cup organic cacao powder

- ½ cup almond butter

Directions:

- Melt the coconut oil.
- Whisk in the cacao powder and almond butter until homogeneous and smooth.
- Roll into balls.
- Refrigerate or freeze until hard, then store in refrigerator until ready to consume.

You can experiment by adding in more flavorful ingredients—stevia, honey, vanilla bean powder/vanilla extract, Peppermint Vitality™ Essential Oil,[2] etc.

Recipe from Brian Comstock [3]

Garlicky Spaghetti Squash with Chicken, Mushrooms, and Kale

- 1 spaghetti squash
- 2 Tbsp. coconut oil
- 8 garlic cloves minced
- 3 cups mushrooms chopped
- 2 chicken breasts sliced into strips (I used the chicken I have frozen after making bone broth)
- 4 cups kale
- 1 tsp. Himalayan pink salt
- 1 Tbsp. parsley

Directions:

- Preheat oven to 425° F. Poke spaghetti squash with fork numerous times and place on a pan in oven to bake for 45- 90

- After it's cooked, remove from oven. Once it has cooled, cut it in half length-wise. Remove the guts with a spoon, then use a fork to comb against the 'spaghetti' strands to separate them and remove from skin. Set aside.
- In a skillet with coconut oil over medium heat, add garlic and mushrooms. Sauté for 5 minutes until browned.
- Add the chicken and cook for 1 minute. Add the kale and continue to cook until chicken is cooked through.
- Add the Himalayan pink salt, and parsley. Stir well and cook for another minute.
- Add the chicken mixture to the bowl of spaghetti squash strands and toss together.

Recipe from Dr. Josh Axe, D.N.M., D.C., C.N.S.

Green Tea Chicken Soup

- 2 quarts chicken bone broth
- 6-7 bags green tea
- 2 Tbsp. coconut oil
- 1 red onion chopped
- 4 garlic cloves finely chopped
- 2 carrots peeled and chopped
- 1 cup chopped celery (about 2 stalks)
- 1 tsp. fresh thyme chopped
- 1 bay leaf
- 2 chicken breasts chopped into medium sized pieces
- 2 tsp. Himalayan pink salt

CHAPTER 50 – GUT RESTORING RECIPES

Directions:

- Bring broth to a boil, then turn off the heat and add tea bags. Allow tea to steep for 10 minutes, uncovered, then remove tea bags.
- Place chicken into pot and bring to a boil again, then turn down to a low simmer for 20 minutes to cook the chicken.
- Add the remaining ingredients and cook for another 20 minutes till chicken is cooked through.
- Serve hot or store refrigerated in glass containers for 4-5 days.

Recipe from Dr. Josh Axe, D.N.M., D.C., C.N.S.

Kale Chips

- 1 bunch kale chopped
- 1 Tbsp. lemon juice
- 2 Tbsp. coconut oil
- ¼ tsp. Himalayan pink salt

Directions

- Preheat oven to 350° F.
- Chop kale into ½-inch pieces.
- Place all ingredients in a large bowl and massage the oil, lemon juice, and salt into the kale using your hands to get into all the crannies of the kale.
- Place on parchment-lined baking sheets and bake for 12 minutes.

Recipe from Dr. Josh Axe, D.N.M., D.C., C.N.S.

Lemon Basil Chicken

- 3 Tbsp. coconut oil
- 4 skinless boneless chicken breast halves

- 3 Tbsp. fresh lemon juice
- 4 garlic cloves chopped
- 1 tsp. (packed) grated lemon peel
- 1 cup chicken bone broth
- 1/2 cup chopped fresh basil or 1 Tbsp. dried basil

Directions:

- Heat coconut oil in a heavy, large skillet over medium-high heat. Sprinkle chicken with salt. Add chicken to skillet and sauté until brown and cooked through, about 5 minutes per side. Transfer chicken to platter; tent with foil.
- Add lemon juice, garlic, and lemon peel to same skillet. Stir over medium-high heat until fragrant, about 30 seconds. Add bone broth, boil until reduced to sauce consistency, about 8 minutes, stirring constantly. Mix basil into sauce. Season to taste with salt.
- Spoon sauce over chicken and serve.

Mayonnaise

- 3 egg yolks
- 1/2 tsp. Himalayan pink salt
- 2 Tbsp. lemon juice
- 1 Tbsp. water
- 1 1/2 cups avocado/olive/coconut oil.

Directions

- Drop the egg yolks into the basin of your food processor, then sprinkle them with salt. Spoon in the lemon juice and water.
- Close the food processor and pulse it once or twice to combine, and then turn it on so that the blade continues moving smoothly. Working a half cup at a time, pour the oil of your choice into the feeder tube of the food processor, allowing it to drip into the egg

CHAPTER 50 – GUT RESTORING RECIPES

- yolks in a very thin, smooth stream until the mayonnaise thickens and all the oil is incorporated into the egg yolks, about 2 or 3 minutes.
- Scrape the mayonnaise into a jar with a tight-fitting lid and store in the fridge no longer than a week.

Pumpkin-Ginger Soup (Recipe from Dr. Josh Axe)

Total Time: 45 minutes. Serves: 8

- 1 Tbsp. coconut oil
- 1 medium onion sliced
- 1 bulb fennel, stalks removed, cored, and sliced
- 2 green apples peeled and chopped
- 2 cups cubed pumpkin
- 1 knob fresh ginger peeled and minced
- 1 tsp. Himalayan pink salt
- 4 cups chicken bone broth
- ½ cup coconut milk kefir

Directions:

- In a stockpot over medium heat, cook onions in coconut oil, stirring occasionally, until translucent. Add ginger and garlic and cook, stirring, until fragrant.
- Stir in pumpkin and add broth to reach desired consistency.
- Bring to a boil, reduce heat, and simmer 10 minutes or longer (the longer the simmering time, the more flavorful the soup). If desired, transfer to blender (or use immersion blender) and, working in batches if necessary, puree until smooth.
- Return soup to pot, stir in kefir, and season to taste with salt. Warm through.

Super Restoring Smoothie

This great smoothie will help restore health with all these wonderful ingredients. I'll give you broad categories, so you can decide which specific ingredients are right for you.

1. Liquid Base

This is the liquid in your smoothie. I use ¼ to ½ cup coconut milk kefir. According to Dr. Josh Axe, D.N.M., D.C., C.N.S., kefir will boost immunity, build bone strength, potentially fight cancer, support digestion, combat IBS, improve allergies, heal skin, and improve symptoms of lactose intolerance.[4]

Kefir is also rich in probiotics, which, according to Dr. Mary Jane Brown, Ph.D., R.D. (UK), help balance friendly bacteria in the digestive system, can prevent and heal diarrhea, can keep the heart healthy, may reduce the severity of certain allergies and eczema, can help reduce symptoms of IBS, ulcerative colitis, and Crohn's disease, may help boost the immune system, and may help weight loss and loss of belly fat.[5]

Additionally, I add an ounce or so of Aloe Vera Juice. Aloe Vera is healthful for the digestive system, supportive of the immune system, and detoxifies the body. I also add some purified water if the smoothie gets too thick.

2. Protein?

Many people like to add a protein powder to their smoothies thinking they need the protein. However, most Americans get far too much protein. "Current protein intake is above the recommended dietary allowance for protein," says Jamie I. Baum, an assistant professor of nutrition in the food science department at the University of Arkansas. The excess gets turned into body fat because your system can't use it. "Without exercise [...] extra protein isn't going to do much for you as far as physical fitness and physique are concerned," Baum says. "[In fact], too much protein when trying to get in shape can lead to excess weight gain."[6]

CHAPTER 50 – GUT RESTORING RECIPES

Protein powder is a mechanically and chemically processed food. I've never met anyone who makes their own. Additionally, many people are sensitive to whey protein (a dairy product), so they opt for a vegan protein powder that usually contains legumes (peas) and/or grains (rice), both of which can cause/irritate leaky gut syndrome, or one that contains soy (see chapter 12). That said, everyone must decide for themselves if they want to add a protein powder.

Heather McClees, certified nutritionist and dietetic specialist, suggests the following to add protein to smoothies.[7]

- Spinach
- Hemp Seeds
- Kale
- Pumpkin Seeds
- Almond Butter
- Chia Seeds

3. <u>Fiber</u>

Fiber is so important for the gut. It creates bulk which aids in moving stool and harmful carcinogens through the digestive tract. Without enough fiber in the diet, irregularity, constipation, and sluggishness can result. Insufficient fiber can also increase the risk of colon cancer, as well as other serious health issues. According to the *Journal of the American Medical Association* (JAMA), we should be eating anywhere from 20 to 35 grams of fiber per day.[8]

I use several types of seeds for fiber, all soaked/sprouted and ground. About 2 tablespoons total is all that's needed, so I mix and match from chia seeds, flax seeds, pumpkin seeds, sunflower seeds, and sesame seeds.

You can buy seeds already sprouted/soaked and ground, but it's easy to do yourself. I soak my seeds overnight in purified water, then rinse them off. I blot them with paper towels then spread them out on a cookie sheet

CHAPTER 50 - GUT-RESTORING RECIPES

and put them in the oven at the lowest temperature (my oven goes down to 170° F.) It usually takes between 1 and 2 hours before the seeds are dry. (If you have a food dehydrator, you can use that to dry the seeds.) I add the seeds whole with all the other ingredients because my Vitamix® blender is powerful enough to grind them this way. Pre-grind if you find it necessary. Store remaining seeds in glass containers.

4. <u>Herbs/Spices</u>

Here's a place you can go wild. I add 1/2 to 1 teaspoon of ground organic Ceylon cinnamon and the same amount of ground organic turmeric, plus a 1-inch slice of fresh peeled organic ginger. What herbs and spices do you like? Fennel? Basil? Mint? Add them to your smoothie. Fresh or powdered is fine. Or substitute with essential oils. I always add DiGize Vitality™ Essential Oil blend to support digestion, Copaiba Vitality™ Essential Oil to support overall health, and EndoFlex Vitality™ Essential Oil blend to support the endocrine (hormonal) system. Longevity Vitality™ Essential Oil blend is perfect for those looking to make the most of their silver years, supporting a healthy immune system and overall wellness.

5. <u>Greens</u>

Another place to go wild. Do you like kale? Spinach? Beet greens? Chard? Add 'em! I also like to add fresh parsley. Not only is it rich in many vital vitamins, including vitamins C, B-12, K, and A, parsley keeps your immune system strong, tones your bones, and heals the nervous system, too. It helps flush out excess fluid from the body, thus supporting kidney function.

You can add a super green powder if you'd like. I add fresh cilantro, which has good amounts of antioxidants, essential oils, vitamins, and dietary fiber, which may help reduce LDL or 'bad' cholesterol levels in the blood. It's also helpful for heavy metal detoxification.

Many people think that greens are too bitter and don't put them in their smoothies because of that. I agree that many greens are too bitter to eat alone, but I truly can't taste them in the smoothie. For me, it's the best way to get the vital health benefits of greens.[9]

CHAPTER 50 – GUT RESTORING RECIPES

Here's a way to keep your fresh herbs fresher longer. After you wash and dry them, place them stem down in a mason jar and fill with a couple of inches of purified water. Then put a baggie over the top and secure with a rubber band. They will keep in the refrigerator fresh like this for a week or so.

For larger greens like kale, chard, and spinach, once I've washed and dried the leaves and stems, I freeze them. It's easy to break off frozen pieces to add to my smoothie. I always include the stems in my smoothie.

6. Berries

I add a handful each of frozen organic strawberries and blueberries to my smoothie. Some people like to add raspberries, but I don't like the little seeds. It's all about personal choice.

Blueberries are packed with antioxidants, called anthocyanins, that may help keep memory sharp as you age, and raspberries contain ellagic acid, a compound with anticancer properties. Strawberries are a true superfood. They're an excellent source of vitamin C, are chock full of antioxidants, and they contain powerful heart health boosters. All berries are great sources of fiber, a nutrient important for a healthy digestive system.

7. Additional Ingredients for Your Specific Health-Restoring Needs

I also add organic cacao powder, a superfood containing a rich supply of antioxidants, magnesium, polyphenols, and dietary fiber. Omit if you're sensitive to gluten.

For those who like their smoothie sweeter, you can add stevia or local, raw (unpasteurized) honey. (Don't use more than 1 tablespoon of honey PER DAY. Although it's far healthier than table sugar, it's still sugar.)

So, there you have it. I add a couple of ice cubes and some purified water, then put it in the Vitamix® and enjoy.

Sweet Potato/Beet Hash

Total Time: 45 minutes. Serves: 2-4

- 1 cup peeled and cubed sweet potatoes
- 1 large beet peeled and cubed
- 1 Tbsp. coconut oil melted
- Himalayan pink salt to taste
- 1 cup cooked diced turkey
- 1 onion diced

Directions:

- Preheat oven to 400° F.
- On a baking sheet, toss sweet potatoes and beets with coconut oil and season with salt. Spread in a single layer and roast until golden brown and fork-tender, 25–30 minutes.
- In a skillet over medium heat, cook onion and season with salt, stirring occasionally until onions caramelize. Add the cooked diced turkey and stir in roasted vegetables. Cook for another 5 minutes. Serve.

Taco Salad

This is a very mild taco salad, so add more spices if you like it hotter.

- 1 pound 100% grass-fed and finished ground beef or cooked, shredded pasture raised chicken
- ½ tsp. taco seasoning (see below)
- Makings for salad (lettuce, onions, etc.)
- 1 recipe Carol's Homemade Holy Guacamole
- Taco Salad Dressing (see below)

CHAPTER 50 – GUT RESTORING RECIPES

Directions:

- Brown the ground beef. If you prefer, use cooked, shredded chicken instead of beef (it's a great way to use the cooked chicken left over from making bone broth).
- Add ½ tsp. taco seasoning and mix.
- Spoon mixture over salad makings.
- Spoon Taco Salad Dressing over salad.
- Top with Carol's Homemade Holy Guacamole.

Taco Seasoning (nightshade free recipe follows)

- 1 tsp. paprika
- 1 tsp. cumin
- 1/2 tsp. oregano
- 1/2 tsp. chili powder
- 1/4 tsp. cayenne pepper

This will make a good supply of seasoning that will keep in the pantry.

Taco Salad Dressing

- 1 cup homemade mayonnaise (recipe in chapter 50)
- ½ tsp. Taco Seasoning (above)
- Water to thin

Add ingredients to bowl, whisk to combine. Serve over salad.

Nightshade Free Taco Seasoning[10]

- 1 1/2 tsp. organic onion powder
- 1 tsp. organic cilantro (can substitute parsley, if desired)
- 1/2 tsp. Himalayan pink salt
- 1/2 tsp. organic oregano

- 1/4 tsp. organic turmeric

Waldorf Chicken Salad

- 5 Granny Smith apples chopped (skin on)
- 2 stalks celery chopped
- ½ to 1 cup walnuts chopped
- ½ c organic, unsweetened dried cranberries, reconstituted with stevia (I buy the cranberries on Amazon.com since most store-bought dried cranberries have sugar and unhealthy oils.)
- 1 cup shredded cooked chicken (leftover from making bone broth)
- Mayonnaise to moisten (recipe in chapter 50)

Mix all ingredients and serve.

CHAPTER 50 – GUT RESTORING RECIPES

PART 10

THE BE IN HEALTH MINDSET

"I think anything is possible if you have the mindset and the will and desire to do it and put the time in."
Roger Clemens

CHAPTER 51

STOP TRYING TO BE PERFECT

Many times, when we start a lifestyle of health, we become very rigid. Perfectionism creeps in. Are you a perfectionist? Always trying to do the right thing, always wanting to please others? I'm here to tell you that you can stop trying to be perfect.

Where Does Perfectionism Come From?

Being a perfectionist is so rewarding. Not only do you get to work yourself to exhaustion, you get to lord it over others who don't do things as perfectly as you do.

And the biggest reward? You just know that God is looking at you and smiling, so pleased with all your effort.

Right? No? That's not how it works?

Then why do we still do it? Why do we feel compelled to be perfect?

It all goes back to Cain and Abel.

> *Genesis 4:3-7 NIV*
> *In the course of time Cain brought some of the fruits of the soil as an offering to the LORD. And Abel also brought an offering—fat portions from some of the firstborn of his flock.*
>
> *The LORD looked with favor on Abel and his offering, but on Cain and his offering he did not look with favor. So Cain was very angry, and his face was downcast.*
>
> *Then the LORD said to Cain, "Why are you angry? Why is your face downcast? If you do what is right, will you not be accepted? But if you do not do what is right, sin is crouching at your door; it desires to have you, but you must rule over it."*

Cain got all down in the mouth and pouty when God didn't accept his offering. Making it even worse for Cain, God accepted Abel's sacrifice.

CHAPTER 51 – STOP TRYING TO BE PERFECT

From Cain's viewpoint, he had worked so hard to raise those crops that he brought to God. For a perfectionist, this is the ultimate disappointment: not having your work and your effort recognized.

What was the difference between Cain's offering and Abel's? Hebrews 11 tells us.

> Hebrews 11:4 NIV
> By faith Abel brought God a better offering than Cain did. By faith he was commended as righteous, when God spoke well of his offerings. And by faith Abel still speaks, even though he is dead.

The difference was faith. Abel believed what God had told them about sacrifices, that blood must be shed (Leviticus 17:11, Hebrews 9:22), and he offered an appropriate sacrifice. Cain decided to offer his own efforts instead.

What Perfectionism Does to Us

Perfectionism drives us to make decisions based on fear of failure, fear of making mistakes, or on other people's opinions about us. We want to be flawless in everything so no one thinks badly of us. The problem is, the one who ends up thinking badly of you is you. Ironically, the compulsion of perfectionism causes us to feel imperfect.

The reality is that perfectionism is fear. We are afraid of rejection, criticism, failure. So, we do everything in our power to avoid them. And when we can't measure up to this new level of perfection that we've set for ourselves, we shift the focus and the blame onto others. "Look at what Johnny's doing."

At the heart of perfectionism is the desire for love and acceptance.

Self-Righteousness

Righteousness is to be fully accepted by God. Perfectionism is self-righteousness. What happens is, you set up – many times, unknowingly – a system of right and wrong for yourself and those around you. People

CHAPTER 51 – STOP TRYING TO BE PERFECT

who don't live up to your expectations disappoint you and you pass judgment on them.

In Romans 10, Paul describes this concerning the Israelites.

> *Romans 10:3-4 KJV*
> *For they being ignorant of God's righteousness, and going about to establish their own righteousness, have not submitted themselves unto the righteousness of God.*
>
> *For Christ is the end of the law for righteousness to every one that believeth.*

We no longer need to keep the law to earn our righteousness; Christ did that for us. But many times, we act as if we don't know this and we set up our own systems of (self) righteousness.

Those who are self-righteous view themselves as better than others. Since everyone else messes up, how could they possibly be trying as hard as I am? This is also known as Phariseeism.

> *Luke 11:37-44 KJV*
> *And as he spake, a certain Pharisee besought him* [Jesus] *to dine with him: and he went in, and sat down to meat.*
>
> *And when the Pharisee saw it, he marvelled that he had not first washed before dinner.*
>
> *And the Lord said unto him, Now do ye Pharisees make clean the outside of the cup and the platter; but your inward part is full of ravening* [extortion, robbery] *and wickedness.*
>
> *Ye fools, did not he that made that which is without make that which is within also?*
>
> *But rather give alms of such things as ye have; and, behold, all things are clean unto you.*
>
> *But woe unto you, Pharisees! for ye tithe mint and rue and all manner of herbs, and pass over judgment and the love of God: these ought ye to have done, and not to leave the other undone.*

CHAPTER 51 – STOP TRYING TO BE PERFECT

> *Woe unto you, Pharisees! for ye love the uppermost seats in the synagogues, and greetings in the markets.*
>
> *Woe unto you, scribes and Pharisees, hypocrites! for ye are as graves which appear not, and the men that walk over them are not aware of them.*

Phariseeism, self-righteousness, perfectionism, are all about outward appearances.

Here is what Jesus said about it.

> *Matthew 7:1-5 KJV*
> *Judge not, that ye be not judged.*
>
> *For with what judgment ye judge, ye shall be judged: and with what measure ye mete, it shall be measured to you again.*
>
> *And why beholdest thou the mote that is in thy brother's eye, but considerest not the beam that is in thine own eye?*
>
> *Or how wilt thou say to thy brother, Let me pull out the mote out of thine eye; and, behold, a beam is in thine own eye?*
>
> *Thou hypocrite, first cast out the beam out of thine own eye; and then shalt thou see clearly to cast out the mote out of thy brother's eye.*

Jesus said that the same measure we use against others in judgment will come back to us in judgment. Not from God, but from man. If you're experiencing judgment from others, consider what judgment you're giving to others. Perfectionism is hypocrisy.

Here is God's view:

> *Isaiah 64:6 KJV*
> *But we are all as an unclean thing, and all our righteousnesses are as filthy rags; and we all do fade as a leaf; and our iniquities, like the wind, have taken us away.*

CHAPTER 51 – STOP TRYING TO BE PERFECT

> *Isaiah 52:1 KJV*
> *Awake, awake; put on thy strength, O Zion; put on thy beautiful garments, O Jerusalem, the holy city: for henceforth there shall no more come into thee the uncircumcised and the unclean.*

Who wants to dress in the filthy rags of self-righteousness when you can dress like royalty?

Doomed to Fail

The problem with self-righteousness is that man can never be righteous by his own works, so, perfectionism is doomed to fail.

> *Job 22:1-3 KJV*
> *Then Eliphaz the Temanite answered and said [to Job],*
>
> *Can a man be profitable unto God, as he that is wise may be profitable unto himself?*
>
> *Is it any pleasure to the Almighty, that thou art [self] righteous? or is it gain to him, that thou makest thy ways perfect?*

The NIV of verses 2 and 3 says,

> *Job 22:3-3 NIV*
> *Can a man be of benefit to God? Can even a wise person benefit him?*
>
> *What pleasure would it give the Almighty if you were righteous? What would he gain if your ways were blameless?*

Our trying to be righteous by our own works means nothing to God. It doesn't give Him any pleasure. That's a dagger to the heart of the self-righteous. You mean God doesn't care about all the work I do to make myself approved in His sight? "But, I try so hard. I just want God to love me and accept me."

> *Jeremiah 17:10 NIV*
> *"I the LORD search the heart and examine the mind, to reward each person according to their conduct, according to what their*

CHAPTER 51 – STOP TRYING TO BE PERFECT

deeds deserve."

Oh, good, He'll see how hard I work and accept me.

> *Romans 3:10-12 KJV*
> *As it is written, There is none righteous, no, not one:*
>
> *There is none that understandeth, there is none that seeketh after God.*
>
> *They are all gone out of the way, they are together become unprofitable; there is none that doeth good, no, not one.*

It's very disheartening for a perfectionist to hear these words.

So, if all our efforts to become righteous, accepted, in God's sight, fail, what can we do?

The Righteousness of God

First, remember that righteousness is credited to your account, so to speak, by faith.

> *Romans 4:1-3 KJV*
> *What shall we say then that Abraham our father, as pertaining to the flesh, hath found?*
>
> *For if Abraham were justified* [made righteous] *by works, he hath whereof to glory; but not before God.*
>
> *For what saith the scripture? Abraham believed God, and it was counted unto him for righteousness.*

Glorying in yourself because of your works fits with the model of perfectionism. Perfectionists love to praise themselves for their hard work.

But God says that righteousness comes from believing God. Let's keep reading.

> *Romans 4:4-22 KJV*
> *Now to him that worketh is the reward not reckoned of grace, but*

CHAPTER 51 – STOP TRYING TO BE PERFECT

of debt.

But to him that worketh not, but believeth on him that justifieth the ungodly, his faith is counted for righteousness.

Even as David also describeth the blessedness of the man, unto whom God imputeth righteousness without works,

Saying, Blessed are they whose iniquities are forgiven, and whose sins are covered.

Blessed is the man to whom the Lord will not impute sin.

Cometh this blessedness then upon the circumcision only, or upon the uncircumcision also? for we say that faith was reckoned to Abraham for righteousness.

How was it then reckoned? when he was in circumcision [works of the flesh], or in uncircumcision? Not in circumcision, but in uncircumcision.

And he received the sign of circumcision, a seal of the righteousness of the faith which he had yet being uncircumcised: that he might be the father of all them that believe, though they be not circumcised; that righteousness might be imputed unto them also:

And the father of circumcision to them who are not of the circumcision only, but who also walk in the steps of that faith of our father Abraham, which he had being yet uncircumcised.

For the promise, that he should be the heir of the world, was not to Abraham, or to his seed, through the law [works], but through the righteousness of faith.

For if they which are of the law be heirs, faith is made void, and the promise made of none effect:

Because the law worketh wrath: for where no law is, there is no transgression.

CHAPTER 51 – STOP TRYING TO BE PERFECT

> *Therefore it is of faith, that it might be by grace; to the end the promise might be sure to all the seed; not to that only which is of the law, but to that also which is of the faith of Abraham; who is the father of us all,*
>
> *(As it is written, I have made thee a father of many nations,) before him whom he believed, even God, who quickeneth the dead, and calleth those things which be not as though they were.*
>
> *Who [Abraham] against hope believed in hope, that he might become the father of many nations, according to that which was spoken, So shall thy seed be.*
>
> *And being not weak in faith, he [Abraham] considered ~~not~~ his own body now dead, when he was about an hundred years old, ~~neither yet~~ [and] the deadness of Sara's womb:*

Abraham did consider the ages of both himself (99) and Sarah (90); he did acknowledge that they were too old to have children. Nevertheless,

> *He [Abraham] staggered not at the promise of God through unbelief; but was strong in faith, giving glory to God;*
>
> *And being fully persuaded that, what he [God] had promised, he [God] was able also to perform.*
>
> *And therefore it was imputed to him [Abraham] for righteousness.*

What is it that we are to believe? Keep reading.

> *Romans 4:23-25 KJV*
> *Now it was not written for his sake alone, that it was imputed to him;*
>
> *But for us also, to whom it shall be imputed, if we believe on him that raised up Jesus our Lord from the dead;*
>
> *Who was delivered for our offences, and was raised again for our justification [our being made righteous].*

CHAPTER 51 – STOP TRYING TO BE PERFECT

Our Response to God's Righteousness

Righteousness comes by faith, by believing on him whom God sent (Jesus Christ, the Messiah). Do you still want some works to do?

> *John 6:28-29 KJV*
> *Then said they unto him, What shall we do, that we might work the works of God?*
>
> *Jesus answered and said unto them, This is the work of God, that ye believe on him [Jesus Christ] whom he hath sent.*
>
> *Ephesians 2:10 KJV*
> *For we are his [God's] workmanship, created in Christ Jesus unto good works, which God hath before ordained that we should walk in them.*

There's your work: believe on Jesus Christ and his finished work. We have to do this Every. Single. Day. Still have some time left that day? Then, do the good works God has planned for you.

Will doing these good works make you righteous? No.

> *Acts 15:10 KJV*
> *Now therefore why tempt ye God, to put a yoke upon the neck of the disciples, which neither our fathers nor we were able to bear?*

Trying to keep the law of good works puts a yoke on us. It weighs us down. It also tempts God because it disregards the finished work of Jesus Christ.

Only faith in Christ makes us righteous. So instead of trying to perfect ourselves, we change our mindset to accept that we are already righteous and that the good works we now do are done in thankfulness to God for making us righteous.

Changing Your Thoughts Changes Your Ways

Changing your mindset about righteousness, perfectionism, Phariseeism, means recognizing that track, that groove, in your mind

CHAPTER 51 – STOP TRYING TO BE PERFECT

that runs on a seemingly endless loop. Are you replaying events in your mind? Sometimes, I'll 'replay' events that haven't even happened. Ask God to point out these thoughts to you as soon as you start down that road, so you can change those thoughts immediately. It will take repetition, but if you ask God to help you, He will.

> *2 Corinthians 10:3-5 NIV*
> *For though we live in the world, we do not wage war as the world does.*
>
> *The weapons we fight with are not the weapons of the world. On the contrary, they* [the weapons we fight with] *have divine power to demolish strongholds.*
>
> *We demolish arguments and every pretension that sets itself up against the knowledge of God, and we take captive every thought to make it obedient to Christ.*

Strongholds are thoughts that are entrenched, those grooves or tracks I mentioned. Some strongholds are beneficial. Some are rebellion against God. You are in control of your thoughts. Just because a thought comes to your mind doesn't mean you have to keep thinking about it. We are to bring those thoughts to Christ.

Treat yourself with kindness as you're learning to change.

> *Hebrews 5:1-2 KJV*
> *For every high priest taken from among men is ordained for men in things pertaining to God, that he may offer both gifts and sacrifices for sins:*
>
> *Who* [the priests] *can have compassion on the ignorant, and on them that are out of the way; for that he himself* [the priest] *also is compassed with infirmity.*

The NLT of verse 2 says,

> *Hebrews 5:2 NLT*
> *And he is able to deal gently with ignorant and wayward people because he himself is subject to the same weaknesses.*

CHAPTER 51 – STOP TRYING TO BE PERFECT

Priests were to treat the ignorant and the wayward with kindness. Today, we are a priesthood of God.

> *1 Peter 2:5 KJV*
> *Ye also, as lively stones, are built up a spiritual house, an holy priesthood, to offer up spiritual sacrifices, acceptable to God by Jesus Christ.*

The self-righteous are ignorant and wayward. So, be kind to yourself. Be compassionate with yourself. Don't beat yourself up.

Changing your thoughts will lead to your ways changing. (Notice I didn't say that you change your ways; see Romans 12:2.) Behavior follows identity. Start to believe your righteousness in Christ and you will stop behaving as a perfectionist.

You are Righteous Now

> *Psalm 18:32 KJV*
> *It is God that girdeth me with strength, and maketh my way perfect.*

Only God can make your way perfect.

> *Ephesians 1:3-6 KJV*
> *Blessed be the God and Father of our Lord Jesus Christ, who hath blessed us with all spiritual blessings in heavenly places in Christ:*
>
> *According as he hath chosen us in him before the foundation of the world, that we should be holy and without blame before him in love:*
>
> *Having predestinated us unto the adoption of children by Jesus Christ to himself, according to the good pleasure of his will,*
>
> *To the praise of the glory of his grace, wherein he hath made us accepted in the beloved.*

Your righteousness, your acceptance, by God has everything to do with what Jesus Christ did. All you do is accept what he did. That's it. That's

CHAPTER 51 – STOP TRYING TO BE PERFECT

righteousness. No more working to prove yourself good enough for God. Jesus was the one who did that. He proved that he was good enough for God. You simply believe that he did it and God transfers (imputes, applies) Christ's righteousness to you.

> *1 Corinthians 1:30-31 KJV*
> *But of him are ye in Christ Jesus, who of God is made unto us wisdom, and righteousness, and sanctification, and redemption:*
>
> *That, according as it is written, He that glorieth, let him glory in the Lord.*

Your righteousness is of God in Christ. All glory goes to Him!

> *Psalm 118:19 KJV*
> *Open to me the gates of righteousness: I will go into them, and I will praise the LORD:*

The gate is open! Go in! Enjoy your righteousness!

> *Matthew 6:33 KJV*
> *But seek ye first the kingdom of God, and his righteousness; and all these things shall be added unto you.*

Seek God's righteousness, not your own.

You have access to God Almighty (Romans 5:2, Ephesians 2:18, Ephesians 3:12).

There are pleasures forevermore at His right hand (Psalm 16:11), where you are seated (Ephesians 2:6).

You are blameless and perfect in His sight (Ephesians 1:4, Philippians 2:15).

Stop trying to be perfect and start enjoying being a perfectly righteous child of God.

CHAPTER 52

EATING IN FAITH

It's hard to be in faith for health when you know you're doing things that contribute to sickness, for example, eating fake, chemical-laden foods and unnecessarily exposing your body to dangerous toxins. Conversely, when you eat food you know is healthy, that is, real, whole food that God made, you can have faith that you're living in harmony with God's ways for health.

God Gave Us Good Food to Eat

Adam's rebellion against God resulted in man living by his human, or sin, nature, rather than by the spirit of God. Romans 5:14 explains that death, which is the result of this sin nature, started with Adam. Sickness, which is death in part, became a part of every person's life thereafter.

God originally provided Adam and Eve with everything they needed for a healthy life in companionship with Him. He provided the best food for them.

> *Genesis 1:29 NIV*
> *Then God said, "I give you **every seed-bearing plant** on the face of the whole earth and **every tree that has fruit with seed** in it. **They will be yours for food.***

This description includes nuts, grains, legumes, and seeds. As you will recall from chapter 3, the human digestive system was designed for the way of eating God set out in Genesis 1:29.

Once man fell (Genesis 3:6), his perfect world fell apart, too. No longer was the earth properly supplying everything he needed.

> *Genesis 3:17-19 NIV*
> *To Adam he [God] said, "Because you listened to your wife and ate fruit from the tree about which I commanded you, 'You must not eat from it,' "Cursed is the ground because of you; through*

CHAPTER 52 – EATING IN FAITH

> *painful toil you will eat food from it all the days of your life.*
>
> *It will produce thorns and thistles for you, and **you will eat the plants of the field**.*
>
> *By the sweat of your brow you will eat your food until you return to the ground, since from it you were taken; for dust you are and to dust you will return."*

After the fall, God told Adam that he would eat plants. Then, after the flood of Noah, all human, animal, and plant life on land had been wiped out (except for Noah, his family, and the animals on the ark). Noah and his sons could plant crops, which would require time before they could be harvested. So, what did they eat? The only things possible to eat were the animals that had been on the ark.

> Genesis 9:1-4 NIV
> *Then God blessed Noah and his sons, saying to them, "Be fruitful and increase in number and fill the earth.*
>
> *The fear [awe] and dread of you will fall on all the beasts of the earth, and on all the birds in the sky, on every creature that moves along the ground, and on all the fish in the sea; they are given into your hands.*
>
> ***Everything that lives and moves about will be food for you. Just as I gave you the green plants, I now give you everything.***
>
> *But you must not eat meat that has its lifeblood still in it."*

Now, man was an omnivore with a body designed as an herbivore/frugivore. Therefore, God set principles regarding the eating of meat (see chapter 4).

God's Health Solution #1

After the fall of Adam, God put into motion a plan to reconcile mankind back to Himself (Genesis 3:15), but until the time that Christ came in the flesh, God in His love provided ways for man to stay healthy. One of the ways He did this was by instituting various dietary laws. God promised that if the children of Israel obeyed His laws, they would stay healthy.

> *Exodus 15:26 NIV*
> *He said, "If you listen carefully to the Lord your God and do what is right in his eyes, if you pay attention to his commands and keep all his decrees, I will not bring on you any of the diseases I brought on the Egyptians, for I am the Lord, who heals you."*

God's Health Solution #2

God's permanent solution for the health of our bodies was for His son, Jesus, to endure pain and torture so that we might be free from sin and sickness.

> *Isaiah 53:5 KJV*
> *But he was wounded for our transgressions, he was bruised for our iniquities: the chastisement of our peace was upon him; and with his stripes we are healed.*

Many people think that solution #2 eliminates the need for solution #1. However, God's solutions work best for us when we combine them. When we eat according to God's ways, with our eyes firmly fixed on the finished work of Jesus Christ, we are eating in faith.

Rebellion Revisited

Most sicknesses today are self-inflicted, meaning we bring them on ourselves by violating one or both of God's solutions. Many of God's saints feel that because they have been healed by the stripes of Jesus Christ (1 Peter 2:24), they don't need to follow God's dietary principles.

In fact, some believe that doing anything other than 'having faith' is contrary to God's will. This leads to thinking they can do/eat whatever they want and expect God will heal them. Yes, we are healed by Christ's wounds, but we also reap what we sow (Galatians 6:7).

God designed food to be fuel for the body, but today many people's lives revolve around food. We make decisions about what we eat based not

CHAPTER 52 – EATING IN FAITH

on if it will help our bodies, but if it tastes good. This is reminiscent of Eve's deception.

> Genesis 3:6 KJV
> And when the woman saw that the tree was good for food, and that it was pleasant to the eyes, and a tree to be desired to make one wise, she took of the fruit thereof, and did eat, and gave also unto her husband with her; and he did eat.

When our decisions on what foods to eat are ruled by our senses (pleasant to the eyes, pleasurable on the lips), we aren't eating in faith. We aren't taking care of, respecting, stewarding the body God has given us, the body He purchased with the blood of His Son.

Because of God's goodness and love for us, He laid out dietary principles, things that we should and should not consider to be food. Unfortunately, many of today's foods aren't really food, as God would define it. Food today has been adulterated and changed so that it no longer resembles what God made (see chapter 7).

The church today is sick and tired because we aren't eating in faith, living in harmony with God's ways regarding health. Diabetes, obesity, and cancer, among other diseases, are rampant. This ought not to be. If any group of people today should be healthy, it should be God's people.

Common Sense Eating

> 1 Timothy 5:23 KJV
> Drink no longer water, but use a little wine for thy stomach's sake and thine often infirmities.

This instruction from Paul to Timothy regarding his health was a matter of what he was consuming, of diet, of common sense. Timothy had been suffering frequent health problems, probably due to drinking contaminated water, and Paul's suggestion was to change his diet by adding some wine.

Today, our faith is being hindered because, deep down, we know we've been eating the wrong stuff. We know that the junk we eat, the potato chips and ice cream and chocolate cake, isn't good for us. If we were eating in faith, then we wouldn't be sick.

If there's that little voice in the back of your head saying, "I know I really shouldn't be eating this…" that's the spirit of God in you, prodding you to eat in faith.

Making the Change

The idea of changing one's diet can be a scary proposition. However, the anticipation of how hard it will be is almost always worse than the reality of it. In other words, the more you think about it, the harder it will seem. Once you make the change, you'll find it's much easier to live within God's guidelines for health. You can eat in faith.

CHAPTER 52 – EATING IN FAITH

CHAPTER 53

HOW THE SOUL PROSPERS

**Beloved, I wish above all things that thou mayest prosper and be in health, even as thy soul prospereth.
3 John 2 KJV**

3 John 2 is such a fundamental verse. We know that God's great desire for us is that we prosper and be in health. So, why is it that sometimes we receive and manifest what God has for us and sometimes we don't? Have you ever noticed that there's a condition to manifesting this prosperity and health? "Even as thy soul prospereth." Exactly how does the soul prosper?

Here are two different translations of 3 John 2:

> *Beloved, I wish above all things that thou mayest prosper and be in health, even as thy soul prospereth.* (KJV)

> *Beloved, I pray that all may go well with you and that you may be in good health, as it goes well with your soul.* (ESV)

I've been told that if I'm not manifesting prosperity and health, it's because of lack of faith or believing on my part, that I must have some doubt or fear. But is that what this verse says?

Let's look at the condition in this verse. "Even as your soul prospers." You can affect your entire life by taking care of one aspect, your soul. Let's see how your soul and the situations in your life are connected.

CHAPTER 53 – HOW THE SOUL PROSPERS

Defining Terms

<u>Prosper</u>

The word 'prosper' is the Greek word *euodoō*, which means "to have a prosperous, successful journey." Where does the prosperity and success in this journey come from?

> *Malachi 3:10 KJV*
> *Bring ye all the tithes into the storehouse, that there may be meat* [food] *in mine house, and prove me now herewith, saith the LORD of hosts, if I will not open you the windows of heaven, and pour you out a blessing, that there shall not be room enough to receive it.*

That's pretty clear; the blessing comes from the LORD of hosts (the LORD of the armies of heaven).

> *James 1:17 KJV*
> *Every good gift and every perfect gift is from above, and cometh down from the Father of lights, with whom is no variableness, neither shadow of turning.*

Again, very clear. Every good and perfect gift is from the Father of lights.

> *Ephesians 1:3 KJV*
> *Blessed be the God and Father of our Lord Jesus Christ, who hath blessed us with all spiritual blessings in heavenly places in Christ:*

It's very clear that ALL the blessings in life come from God. So, we're going to define prosperity as "the manifestation of God's heavenly blessings and provision here on earth."

<u>Be in Health</u>

The second thing that God desires for us in 3 John 2 is that we "be in health."

The first use of 'be in health' is in Genesis 43:28 where it's translated "in good health." The Hebrew word is *shalom*. You may be familiar with this word. It means not only peace (quiet, tranquility, contentment), but also

CHAPTER 53 – HOW THE SOUL PROSPERS

completeness, soundness (in body), welfare (health and prosperity), and friendship. It means to be whole (also called saved). I have heard it described as 'nothing missing, nothing broken.'

Psalm 42:11 shows us where health comes from.

> *Psalm 42:11 KJV*
> *Why art thou cast down, O my soul? and why art thou disquieted within me? hope thou in God: for I shall yet praise him, who is the health of my countenance, and my God.*

Bullinger's Companion Bible translates the last part as, "I shall yet praise him, who is the salvation of me, and my God."

It's also interesting to note that the Hebrew word for 'health' in this verse is *yĕshuw'ah*, which is also Hebrew for 'Jesus.' It Is Jesus who is our health.

The New International Version (NIV) of this verse is,

> *Psalm 42:11 NIV*
> *Why am I discouraged? Why is my heart so sad? I will put my hope in God! I will praise him again—my Savior and my God!*

The psalmist is talking to himself when he addresses his soul. He asks and answers his own question (haven't we all done that?). If you read the previous verses in Psalm 42, you'll see that he became discouraged by looking at his own (negative) circumstances. He was trying to figure out what to do, so he was asking himself questions to try to resolve his problem. Then, he had a light-bulb moment. He realized that his life is saved, made whole, complete, not by himself but by God.

<u>Soul</u>

First, let's note the distinction between spirit and soul.

> *1 Thessalonians 5:23 KJV*
> *And the very God of peace sanctify you wholly [all parts of you]; and I pray God your whole spirit and soul and body be preserved blameless unto the coming of our Lord Jesus Christ.*

This names three distinct parts of man: spirit, soul, and body.

CHAPTER 53 – HOW THE SOUL PROSPERS

> *Hebrews 4:12 KJV*
> *For the word of God is quick, and powerful, and sharper than any twoedged sword, piercing even to the dividing asunder of soul and spirit, and of the joints and marrow, and is a discerner of the thoughts and intents of the heart.*

The Word of God can separate the thoughts of your soul from the thoughts of your spirit.

Your soul is the part of you that gives life and movement to your body and thoughts to your mind. The heart is the innermost part of the soul.

The spirit is the gift from God when one becomes born again (see Acts 2:38). All humans and animals have soul life. Only those born again (Romans 10:9) have spirit life.

Later in this chapter, we will look more closely at HOW the soul prospers.

Even As

The words 'even as' are one Greek word *kathōs*, which means "according as, just as, in proportion as, in the degree that, since, seeing that, agreeably to the fact that." It's very important that we understand this word.

Have you ever played with a thermometer? Can you separate the thermometer from the temperature? What happens if you take the thermometer out into the sun? The temperature goes up. Can you stop it? Did you do anything to the thermometer itself other than exposing it to the sun? No.

What happens if you take it into the cold? The temperature goes down. Did you take the thermometer apart and manually change it? No.

So, we can say the thermometer's mercury will move 'even as' or according to the temperature. The temperature affects the thermometer; the thermometer can't affect or change the temperature.

Everything you're experiencing here on earth is in direct proportion to what you're experiencing in your soul. As your soul prospers, so does

CHAPTER 53 – HOW THE SOUL PROSPERS

your life. If your soul isn't prospering, then the issues of your life won't, either.

Now let's compare our souls and our prosperity in life, our blessings, the manifestation of heaven on this earth, to a thermometer. We, our lives, our souls, are the thermometer and God is the temperature. We can only be changed when we are exposed to God. We are changed by the impact God is having on our souls.

Thanks to Brent Phillips for the thermometer analogy.[1]

How the Soul Prospers

Here are some different translations of Proverbs 4:23.

> *Keep thy heart with all diligence; for out of it are the issues of life.* (KJV)

> *Guard your heart above all else, for it determines the course of your life.* (NLT)

> *Above all else, guard your heart, for everything you do flows from it.* (NIV)

Your life is built on what is flowing from you, from your heart. What goes into our hearts? Things we see, hear, and think.

Whatever is in your heart is going to build your life. The mind is the filter to your heart. If the mind is filtered in a way contrary to God's thoughts and ways, you won't be able to receive God's word and your life won't change. Jesus told us to be careful HOW we hear.

> *Luke 8:16-18 KJV*
> *No man, when he hath lighted a candle, covereth it with a vessel, or putteth it under a bed; but setteth it on a candlestick, that they which enter in may see the light.*
>
> *For nothing is secret, that shall not be made manifest; neither any thing hid, that shall not be known and come abroad.*
>
> *Take heed therefore how ye hear: for whosoever hath, to him*

CHAPTER 53 – HOW THE SOUL PROSPERS

> shall be given; and whosoever hath not, from him shall be taken even that which he seemeth to have.

This refers to the filters through which we take in information. What filter are you using? Are you filtering things through the world's standards or God's standards? God's Word should be our filter. There are filters that are at war against us, against our souls.

> *1 Peter 2:11 KJV*
> *Dearly beloved, I beseech you as strangers and pilgrims, abstain from fleshly lusts, which war against the soul;*

> *1 John 2:16 KJV*
> *For all that is in the world, the lust of the flesh, and the lust of the eyes, and the pride of life, is not of the Father, but is of the world.*

This is the source of the world's filter:

> *1 John 5:19 NIV*
> *We know... that the whole world is under the control of the evil one.*

The Evil One, aka the Devil or Satan, controls everything about this world: religion, politics, government, educational systems, the media, etc.

This is part of God's filter:

> *Psalm 101:3a KJV*
> *I will set no wicked thing before mine eyes:*

Looking at, watching, reading, or viewing wicked or evil things affects the soul and whether it prospers. What are you reading in books, newspapers, magazines, online? What are you watching on TV or movies or YouTube? What about video games? You may not think it's affecting you, but the Word of God assures you that it does.

Doing a word study of what God considers to be an abomination is very interesting. Here's an example.

CHAPTER 53 – HOW THE SOUL PROSPERS

> *Proverbs 6:16-19 KJV*
> *These six things doth the LORD hate: yea, seven are an abomination unto him:*
>
> *A proud look, a lying tongue, and hands that shed innocent blood,*
>
> *An heart that deviseth wicked imaginations, feet that be swift in running to mischief,*
>
> *A false witness that speaketh lies, and he that soweth discord among brethren.*

How many of these things are considered acceptable by today's standards, even for God's holy ones, His saints? Lying? Oh, it's just a little white lie, just in this situation. Gossip? Pride? It's okay. Is it?

Let's look at more of God's filter:

> *Philippians 4:6-9 KJV*
> *Be careful* [anxious, worried] *for nothing; but in every thing by prayer and supplication with thanksgiving let your requests be made known unto God.*
>
> *And the peace of God, which passeth all understanding, shall keep* [guard] *your hearts and minds through Christ Jesus.*
>
> *Finally, brethren, whatsoever things are true, whatsoever things are honest, whatsoever things are just, whatsoever things are pure, whatsoever things are lovely, whatsoever things are of good report; if there be any virtue, and if there be any praise, think on these things.*
>
> *Those things, which ye have both learned, and received, and heard, and seen in me, do: and the God of peace shall be with you.*

These are the things God tells us to think about. This is the filter that will lead to our souls prospering. We must feed the soul with nourishment from God.

CHAPTER 53 – HOW THE SOUL PROSPERS

Philippians 4:6 and Matthew 6:34, among others, tell us not to worry because God has promised to take care of us. But worry is very common in the world. In fact, mothers are told they're not good mothers if they don't worry about their children.

> 2 Corinthians 10:5 KJV
> Casting down imaginations, and every high thing that exalteth itself against the knowledge of God, and bringing into captivity every thought to the obedience of Christ;
>
> 2 Corinthians 10:4-5 APNT
> For the equipment of our service is not of the flesh, but of the power of God and by it, we overcome rebellious strongholds.
>
> And we pull down reasonings and all pride that elevates [itself] against the knowledge of God and we lead captive all thoughts to the obedience of Christ.

This requires diligence and action. You can't be passive about the thoughts you allow to stay in your mind if you want your soul to prosper.

If what you're seeing, hearing, and thinking is causing you to be angry, fearful, or confused, none of which are from God, you must see, hear, and think something else instead. (See chapter 1 for more information on what to think.)

The Prosperity of the Soul

> Isaiah 55:6-13 KJV
> Seek ye the LORD while he may be found, call ye upon him while he is near:
>
> Let the wicked forsake his way, and the unrighteous man his thoughts: and let him return unto the LORD, and he will have mercy upon him; and to our God, for he will abundantly pardon.
>
> For my thoughts are not your thoughts, neither are your ways my ways, saith the LORD.
>
> For as the heavens are higher than the earth, so are my ways

CHAPTER 53 – HOW THE SOUL PROSPERS

higher than your ways, and my thoughts than your thoughts.

For as the rain cometh down, and the snow from heaven, and returneth not thither, but watereth the earth, and maketh it bring forth and bud, that it may give seed to the sower, and bread to the eater:

So shall my word be that goeth forth out of my mouth: it shall not return unto me void, but it shall accomplish that which I please, and it shall prosper in the thing whereto I sent it.

For ye shall go out with joy, and be led forth with peace: the mountains and the hills shall break forth before you into singing, and all the trees of the field shall clap their hands.

Instead of the thorn shall come up the fir tree, and instead of the brier shall come up the myrtle tree: and it shall be to the LORD for a name, for an everlasting sign that shall not be cut off.

What a wonderful description of the prosperity of the soul. God's thoughts are much higher than ours. He challenges us to change our thoughts.

> *Romans 12:2 NLT*
> *Don't copy the behavior and customs of this world, but let God transform you into a new person by changing the way you think. Then you will learn to know God's will for you, which is good and pleasing and perfect.*

If you want to be transformed, change the way you think, and your life will change. We need to renew our minds; we exchange our beliefs (which are really the world's beliefs) for God's beliefs.

You're not the one who transforms you, God is. Allow Him to transform you by allowing everything that enters your heart to go through the filter of His Word.

You will know you have changed when you speak and react to things differently. When your mind has changed, your heart will change.

CHAPTER 53 – HOW THE SOUL PROSPERS

Renewing your mind lets God's Word work in your life. You have the holy spirit living in you. Change is inevitable. Through the power of God's Word, you can renew your mind and become a new person.

The question is, are you renewing your mind to the Word or the world? Garbage in, garbage out. If you don't like the harvest, change the seed.

Rejoice

Another great way to put the soul in prosperity mode is to rejoice in God. There are many verses on this subject. Let's look at a few.

> Psalm 68:3 KJV
> But let the righteous be glad; let them rejoice before God: yea, let them exceedingly rejoice.
>
> Psalm 71:23 KJV
> My lips shall greatly rejoice when I sing unto thee; and my soul, which thou hast redeemed.
>
> Philippians 4:4 KJV
> Rejoice in the Lord alway: and again I say, Rejoice.

These descriptions of rejoicing in God aren't meek and quiet. No, these people weren't afraid to raise holy hands and praise God.

Your Identity is In Christ

> 2 Corinthian 3:18 KJV
> But we all, with open face beholding as in a glass the glory of the Lord, are changed into the same image from glory to glory, even as by the Spirit of the Lord.
>
> 2 Corinthian 3:18 NLT
> So all of us who have had that veil removed can see and reflect the glory of the Lord. And the Lord—who is the Spirit—makes us more and more like him as we are changed into his glorious image.

CHAPTER 53 – HOW THE SOUL PROSPERS

> *James 1:23-25 KJV*
> *For if any be a hearer of the word, and not a doer, he is like unto a man beholding his natural face in a glass:*
>
> *For he beholdeth himself, and goeth his way, and straightway forgetteth what manner of man he was.*
>
> *But whoso looketh into the perfect law of liberty, and continueth therein, he being not a forgetful hearer, but a doer of the work, this man shall be blessed in his deed.*

Our lives reflect what we look at. If the reflection we see of ourselves is from the world, then we will manifest what the world has to offer. Anger, confusion, fear, pain, sickness, lack...

When we look into God's Word, we see back a reflection of Christ. That is who you really are. After you put the Word down, do you continue to see yourself in your mind as Christ, or do you revert back to the world's image of yourself?

The thoughts we continue to think about ourselves will manifest in our lives. Do you love yourself, do you expect blessings to hunt you down? God does. He sees you as Christ.

> *Galatians 2:20 NLT*
> *My old self has been crucified with Christ. It is no longer I who live, but Christ lives in me. So I live in this earthly body by trusting in the Son of God, who loved me and gave himself for me.*

When we think less of ourselves than what God says about us, we are passing judgment on ourselves and usually, we punish ourselves for not being perfect. We then start to expect other people to treat us in a certain way, and it becomes a self-fulfilling prophecy. It provides a negative filter through which we see everything. We have to let it go and choose to see ourselves as God sees us. When we give it to Him, He will lift it off our hearts. If you feel a burden or weight on your heart, that's a good indication that there's judgment there.

CHAPTER 53 – HOW THE SOUL PROSPERS

> *Matthew 11:28 KJV*
> *Come unto me, all ye that labour and are heavy laden, and I will give you rest.*

Change happens at the foot of the cross. As long as we make excuses for our sins (remember, whatever isn't of faith is sin – Romans 14:23), we aren't going to change. When we throw out our excuses and see ourselves as God sees us, He will change us and that sets us free from judgment and condemnation.

We empower negatives because when we believe the worst of our ourselves and our situations (poor health, anger, lack of finances, poor relationships, etc.), it becomes our reality. What you believe will happen.

> *Job 3:25 KJV*
> *For the thing which I greatly feared is come upon me, and that which I was afraid of is come unto me.*

Stop making excuses for sin. "I'm just human." "God isn't finished with me yet." (Not true; you're completely complete in Christ.) There's no godly reason for why you aren't set free, healed, prospered, etc. It all depends on what you're feeding your soul.

Putting It All Together

> *3 John 2 KJV*
> *Beloved, I wish above all things that thou mayest prosper and be in health, even as thy soul prospereth.*

Finances come from God, not from the physical realm. Good health comes from God. We may (we should) operate God's principles regarding finances and health, but they originate from a prospering soul. Then the blessings from heaven manifest.

There's no room for fear or doubt. Fear and doubt block your ability to hear God's voice. Nothing can stop the blessings when the soul is prospering. You'll manifest in the physical realm what you're experiencing in your soul.

CHAPTER 53 – HOW THE SOUL PROSPERS

Everything we want in life will come to us as a result of a prospering soul. One January, I set a theme for myself for the year: I want to live as Christ. So, I wrote down steps on how I was going to do this. I realize now that living as Christ is a manifestation of my soul prospering. That's the only thing I need to attend to. If my soul is prospering, everything else will fall in line.

Verses About the Soul

Psalm 23:3 KJV
He restoreth my soul: he leadeth me in the paths of righteousness for his name's sake.

Psalm 25:1 KJV
Unto thee, O LORD, do I lift up my soul.

Psalm 25:12-14 KJV
What man is he that feareth [is in awe of] *the LORD? him* [the man] *shall he* [God} *teach in the way that he* [God] *shall choose.*

His soul shall dwell at ease; and his seed shall inherit the earth.

The secret of the LORD is with them that fear [are in awe of] *him; and he will shew them his covenant.*

Psalm 25:20 KJV
O keep my soul, and deliver me: let me not be ashamed; for I put my trust in thee.

Psalm 33:20-21 KJV
Our soul waiteth for the LORD: he is our help and our shield.

For our heart [the innermost part of the soul] *shall rejoice in him, because we have trusted in his holy name.*

Psalm 34:2 KJV
My soul shall make her boast in the LORD: the humble shall hear thereof, and be glad.

CHAPTER 53 – HOW THE SOUL PROSPERS

> *Psalm 35:9 KJV*
> *My soul shall be joyful in the LORD: it [my soul] shall rejoice in his salvation.*

> *Psalm 41:4 KJV*
> *I said, LORD, be merciful unto me: heal my soul; for I have sinned against thee.*

If my soul is healed, physical, emotional, and mental healing will follow.

> *Psalm 42:2 KJV*
> *My soul thirsteth for God, for the living God: when shall I come and appear before God?*

I can't wait to spend time with my God.

> *Psalm 57:1 KJV*
> *[[To the chief Musician, Altaschith, Michtam of David, when he fled from Saul in the cave.]] Be merciful unto me, O God, be merciful unto me: for my soul trusteth in thee: yea, in the shadow of thy wings will I make my refuge, until these calamities be overpast.*

David's soul hid under God's wing. He didn't fear even though he was in a very scary situation. God protected his soul and thus, his physical body was safe, as well.

> *Psalm 62:1 KJV*
> *[[To the chief Musician, to Jeduthun, A Psalm of David.]] Truly my soul waiteth upon God: from him cometh my salvation [deliverance, welfare, prosperity, victory].*

> *Psalm 62:5 KJV*
> *My soul, wait thou only upon God; for my expectation [literally a cord (as an attachment); figuratively, expectancy, hope, the thing that I long for] is from him.*

Instruct your soul to wait only for God. Attach yourself to Him like He's your lifeline, your umbilical cord from which you get everything you need.

CHAPTER 53 – HOW THE SOUL PROSPERS

Psalm 63:1-8 KJV
[[A Psalm of David, when he was in the wilderness of Judah.]] O God, thou art my God; early will I seek thee: my soul thirsteth for thee, my flesh longeth for thee in a dry and thirsty land, where no water is;

To see thy power and thy glory, so as I have seen thee in the sanctuary.

Because thy lovingkindness is better than life, my lips shall praise thee.

Thus will I bless thee while I live: I will lift up my hands in thy name.

My soul shall be satisfied as with marrow [choicest, best part, abundance (of products of the land)] *and fatness* [abundance]*; and my mouth shall praise thee with joyful lips:*

When I remember thee upon my bed, and meditate on thee in the night watches.

Because thou hast been my help, therefore in the shadow of thy wings will I rejoice.

My soul followeth hard after thee: thy right hand upholdeth me.

Let your soul praise God; cling to Him as if your very life depends on it.

Psalm 66:8-9 KJV
O bless our God, ye people, and make the voice of his praise to be heard:

Which holdeth our soul in life, and suffereth not our feet to be moved.

Psalm 66:16 KJV
Come and hear, all ye that fear [are in awe of] *God, and I will declare what he hath done for my soul.*

CHAPTER 53 – HOW THE SOUL PROSPERS

Psalm 71:23 KJV
My lips shall greatly rejoice when I sing unto thee; and my soul, which thou hast redeemed.

Psalm 84:2 KJV
My soul longeth, yea, even fainteth for the courts of the LORD: my heart and my flesh crieth out for the living God.

Psalm 94:19 KJV
In the multitude of my thoughts within me thy comforts delight my soul.

Psalm 103:1-6 KJV
[[A Psalm of David.]] Bless the LORD, O my soul: and all that is within me, bless his holy name.

Bless the LORD, O my soul, and forget not all his benefits:

Who forgiveth all thine iniquities; who healeth all thy diseases;

Who redeemeth thy life from destruction; who crowneth thee with lovingkindness and tender mercies;

Who satisfieth thy mouth with good things; so that thy youth is renewed like the eagle's.

The LORD executeth righteousness and judgment for all that are oppressed.

Psalm 107:8-9 KJV
Oh that men would praise the LORD for his goodness, and for his wonderful works to the children of men!

For he satisfieth the longing soul, and filleth the hungry soul with goodness.

Psalm 116:7-8 KJV
Return unto thy rest, O my soul; for the LORD hath dealt bountifully with thee.

For thou hast delivered my soul from death, mine eyes from tears,

CHAPTER 53 – HOW THE SOUL PROSPERS

and my feet from falling.

Psalm 121:7 KJV
The LORD shall preserve thee from all evil: he shall preserve thy soul.

Psalm 130:5-6 KJV
I wait for the LORD, my soul doth wait, and in his word do I hope.

My soul waiteth for the Lord more than they that watch for the morning: I say, more than they that watch for the morning.

Psalm 138:3 KJV
In the day when I cried thou answeredst me, and strengthenedst me with strength in my soul.

Psalm 139:14 KJV
I will praise thee; for I am fearfully [awesomely] and wonderfully made: marvellous are thy works; and that my soul knoweth right well.

That's an awful lot of praising God in one's soul going on. Hmm, could this be a clue as to how the soul prospers?

Psalm 143:5-6 KJV
I remember the days of old; I meditate on all thy works; I muse on the work of thy hands.

I stretch forth my hands unto thee: my soul thirsteth after thee, as a thirsty land. Selah.

Psalm 143:8 KJV
Cause me to hear thy lovingkindness in the morning; for in thee do I trust: cause me to know the way wherein I should walk; for I lift up my soul unto thee.

Wisdom

Proverbs 2:10-11 KJV
When wisdom entereth into thine heart, and knowledge is

CHAPTER 53 – HOW THE SOUL PROSPERS

pleasant unto thy soul;

Discretion shall preserve thee, understanding shall keep thee:

Proverbs 18:7 KJV
A fool's mouth is his destruction, and his lips are the snare of his soul.

Proverbs 19:2 KJV
Also, that the soul be without knowledge, it is not good; and he that hasteth with his feet sinneth.

Proverbs 19:8 KJV
He that getteth wisdom loveth his own soul: he that keepeth understanding shall find good.

Proverbs 21:23 KJV
Whoso keepeth his mouth and his tongue keepeth his soul from troubles.

Proverbs 22:24-25 KJV
Make no friendship with an angry man; and with a furious man thou shalt not go.

Lest thou learn his ways, and get a snare to thy soul.

Proverbs 24:13-14 KJV
My son, eat thou honey, because it is good; and the honeycomb, which is sweet to thy taste:

So shall the knowledge of wisdom be unto thy soul: when thou hast found it, then there shall be a reward, and thy expectation shall not be cut off.

Proverbs 24:14 NLT
In the same way [that honey is sweet to the tongue], wisdom is sweet to your soul. If you find it, you will have a bright future, and your hopes will not be cut short.

Finding God's wisdom is sweet to the soul and brings great reward. It brings about a prospering soul whose hopes are not cut short. It will

CHAPTER 53 – HOW THE SOUL PROSPERS

manifest in prosperity and health in all areas of your life. This is God's great desire for His beloved children, which we are.

Beloved, I desire that in all respects you may experience the manifestation of God's heavenly blessing and provision and be in good health (nothing missing, nothing broken), in direct proportion and to the degree in which your mind, your will, and your emotions experience God's heavenly blessing and provision.

3 John 2

CHAPTER 53 – HOW THE SOUL PROSPERS

CHAPTER 54

HOW TO OVERCOME SELF-SABOTAGE

Have you ever started something new, whether a new job, a new lifestyle, a change in habit, a new relationship (romantic or platonic), and then suddenly, you find yourself doing stuff to undermine your new thing? Uh huh, you've fallen victim to self-sabotage. Why would we do something that may ruin everything? Here are three ways we sabotage ourselves and how to stop it.

What is Self-Sabotage?

I see self-sabotage quite often with my clients. My job is to help my clients learn which foods and products will help them restore their health and which will hurt their health. I guide them to make decisions based on the results they've told me they want to see, such as losing weight and regaining lost health. I work with them to identify the foods and products that hinder their progress and help them find new ways of being in harmony with God's ways for health.

According to *Psychology Today*,[1] behavior is said to be self-sabotaging when it "creates problems and interferes with long-standing goals." Many times, people are aware that they're putting limitations on themselves but don't know how to stop. However, many others don't realize the detrimental consequences of their behavior, and often they can't see the connection between their actions and the results (or non-results) they're getting.

Types of Self-Sabotage

Psychology Today also says that the most common self-sabotaging behaviors are "procrastination, self-medication with drugs or alcohol, comfort eating, and forms of self-injury such as cutting." Many times, we get in our own way with behaviors that contradict our stated desire or outcome.

CHAPTER 54 – HOW TO OVERCOME SELF-SABOTAGE

Procrastination

Making too many changes at once can lead to decision fatigue. If you're finding that life is too overwhelming, you'll tend to put things off, whether a current decision or new ones you know you need to make. Procrastination can become a lifestyle if you let it. It becomes easier to avoid the pain of change, so you tell yourself you'll do it later. And later. And later. Until you never do anything to accomplish your goals. Many people use procrastination to self-sabotage.

Have you ever heard the expression, 'The best way to eat an elephant is one bite at a time?' It means that you can't stuff the whole elephant in your mouth at once. The same thing is true for change. Decide to make one change at a time. Reward yourself for sticking to it. Then make another change while keeping the previous one. Pretty soon, you've eaten the whole elephant.

Comfort Eating

Comfort food is any food that provides a sense of comfort, familiarity, and well-being. Many times, we associate these foods with childhood or other carefree times. When we're experiencing emotional pain, we instinctively reach for these foods.

The biggest problem with comfort eating is that most of these foods aren't healthy and will not move you toward your health goals. If you find yourself sabotaging your goals with comfort eating, it's best to keep these foods out of your house. Instead, decide ahead of time what you can do to comfort yourself without food. If necessary, engage a friend to lean on during these times.

Ignoring the Truth

When I published an article about why bacon isn't healthy, one of the responses I got was, "I don't want to know." When you know you need to make changes, but you don't want to, you may choose to ignore the facts and pretend you don't know the truth.

Ignoring the truth doesn't work. Your subconscious knows that you're sabotaging yourself and will gnaw at you until you feel guilty and

CHAPTER 54 – HOW TO OVERCOME SELF-SABOTAGE

uncomfortable. Eventually, you will come to a place where you need to choose. You can either remain ignorant or you can confront the truth and come to accept it. The choice is yours.

How to Stop Self-Sabotage

How do you stop the train of your life from going off the rails? The first thing you must do is recognize your self-sabotaging behavior. Just acknowledging it can bring great relief. Further introspection will help you identify the things that trigger your self-sabotaging behavior. Do you always do X when Y happens? What would happen if you did Z instead? These are the questions to start asking yourself. You may also find it helpful to ask a nonjudgmental friend to help you identify your triggers.

Is it possible to avoid your triggers? If not, what can you do instead? If you always eat macaroni and cheese whenever someone belittles you (because as a child, your mama always gave you mac and cheese when you were feeling bad), what else can you do when that happens? Can you read a list you have written out ahead of time about all your great qualities? Can you call someone who will build you up? What can you do that will work for you? Is there a better way to respond?

To help let go of old patterns and establish positive new ones, I use the essential oil rosemary. See chapter 29 for information on using essential oils.

Stopping self-sabotage can free you to live the life you want to live, the life you were meant to live. Does it take guts to face yourself and your self-defeating behavior? Of course, it does. But you're worth it.

CHAPTER 54 – HOW TO OVERCOME SELF-SABOTAGE

CHAPTER 55

WORDS OF LIFE

Finding your way back to normality after dealing with leaky gut syndrome, autoimmune disorders, and other health problems can be a long but ultimately rewarding journey. And truly we are on this journey called life together with our heavenly Father God and our beloved Lord Jesus Christ. They will never leave us alone. Here are some of my favorite verses of scripture about the life God has given us to live.

> *Deuteronomy 30:19 KJV*
> *I call heaven and earth to record this day against you, that I have set before you life and death, blessing and cursing: therefore choose life, that both thou and thy seed may live:*
>
> *Deuteronomy 32:46-47 NLT*
> *He added: "Take to heart all the words of warning I have given you today. Pass them on as a command to your children so they will obey every word of these instructions.*
>
> *These instructions are not empty words—they are your life! By obeying them you will enjoy a long life in the land you will occupy when you cross the Jordan River."*
>
> *Mark 8:35 KJV*
> *For whosoever will save his life shall lose it; but whosoever shall lose his life for my sake and the gospel's, the same shall save it.*
>
> *John 1:4 KJV*
> *In him was life; and the life was the light of men.*
>
> *John 3:16 KJV*
> *For God so loved the world, that he gave his only begotten Son, that whosoever believeth in him should not perish, but have everlasting life.*
>
> *John 10:10 KJV*
> *The thief cometh not, but for to steal, and to kill, and to destroy:*

CHAPTER 55 – WORDS OF LIFE

I am come that they might have life, and that they might have it more abundantly.

John 15:13 KJV
Greater love hath no man than this, that a man lay down his life for his friends.

Romans 5:17 KJV
For if by one man's offence death reigned by one; much more they which receive abundance of grace and of the gift of righteousness shall reign in life by one, Jesus Christ.

Galatians 2:20 KJV
I am crucified with Christ: nevertheless I live; yet not I, but Christ liveth in me: and the life which I now live in the flesh I live by the faith of the Son of God, who loved me, and gave himself for me.

Philippians 2:16 KJV
Holding forth the word of life; that I may rejoice in the day of Christ, that I have not run in vain, neither laboured in vain.

Colossians 3:3 NLT
For you died to this life, and your real life is hidden with Christ in God.

Colossians 3:4 KJV
When Christ, who is our life, shall appear, then shall ye also appear with him in glory.

James 1:12 KJV
Blessed is the man that endureth temptation: for when he is tried, he shall receive the crown of life, which the Lord hath promised to them that love him.

1 John 5:12 KJV
He that hath the Son hath life; and he that hath not the Son of God hath not life.

1 John 5:20 KJV
And we know that the Son of God is come, and hath given us an

CHAPTER 55 – WORDS OF LIFE

understanding, that we may know him that is true, and we are in him that is true, even in his Son Jesus Christ. This is the true God, and eternal life.

I'm praying for and with you, my friend, as you travel this road. Please don't isolate yourself or think you're all alone. You have many fellow-travelers, myself included. You now have many tools to use to reach your goals.

CHAPTER 55 – WORDS OF LIFE

CONCLUSION

There's a lot of information packed into this book and it may take several readings to absorb it all. I encourage you to read and reread it as you continue your journey. Please realize that this is a lifetime journey. It isn't a traditional 'diet' that you start and then stop. This is a way of being in health that will serve you well throughout your life.

There may be times you experience new unpleasant symptoms and you need to revisit the Food Reintroduction Challenge. There may come a time when you can 'splurge' on occasion. After about 2 years of living the Be in Health lifestyle, I experimented with some foods I had left behind. Some didn't bother me, some did.

When you become attuned to your body, you will know exactly what causes any upset. I still don't bring sugar, dairy, grains, pork, shellfish, nightshades, or legumes into my house. If I splurge, it's a one-time thing, not a new habit.

My main purpose in living this lifestyle was not to lose weight but to restore my gut and thereby, my overall health. However, I've lost 46 pounds as of this writing and now weigh what I did when I was in my 20s. I feel better. I look better. I am better.

The most important part of being in health is your relationship with your heavenly Father God. There's a spiritual reason behind everything we see with the five senses. We can't afford to ignore either one.

Oh, dear reader, my fellow saint, my brother, my sister, I pray that you find the health and wellness in body, soul, and spirit that you are seeking.

O taste and see that the LORD is good: blessed is the man that trusteth in him. Psalm 34:8 KJV

CONCLUSION

APPENDICES

> "The problem is that we are not eating food anymore, we are eating food-like products."
> Dr. Alejandro Junger, M.D.

APPENDIX 1

COMMON GMO INGREDIENTS

Unless the item you're purchasing has both the USDA organic seal and the Non-GMO Project Verified seal, or you have written confirmation from the company that their product is both organic and GMO-free, it's best to assume that the ingredients below are GMO. This is why I prefer to consume real, whole food.

- Aspartame (also called Amino Sweet®, Equal Spoonful®, BeneVia®, E951)
- Baking Powder
- Canola Oil Oil)
- Caramel Color
- Cellulose
- Citric Acid
- Cobalamin (Vitamin B12)
- Colorose
- Condensed Milk
- Confectioner's Sugar
- Corn Flour
- Corn Masa
- Corn Meal
- Corn Oil
- Corn Syrup
- Cornstarch
- Cottonseed Oil
- Cyclodextrin
- Eystein
- Dextrin
- Dextrose
- Diacetyl
- Diglyceride
- Erythritol
- Glycerin
- Glycerol
- Glycerol Monooleate
- Glycine
- Hemicellulose
- High Fructose Corn (HFCS)
- Hydrogenated Starch
- Hydrolyzed Vegetable Protein (HVP)
- Inositol
- Inverse Syrup
- Inversol
- Invert Sugar
- Isoflavones
- Lactic Acid
- Lecithin
- Leucine
- Lysine
- Maltitol
- Malt
- Malt Syrup
- Malt Extract
- Maltodextrin
- Maltose
- Mannitol
- Methylcellulose
- Milk Powder
- Phenylalanine
- Phytic Acid
- Protein Isolate
- Shoyu
- Sorbitol
- Soy Flour
- Soy Isolates
- Soy Lecithin
- Soy Milk
- Soy Oil
- Soy Protein
- Soy Protein Isolate
- Soy Sauce
- Starch
- Stearic Acid
- Sugar (unless specified as cane sugar)
- Tamari
- Tempeh
- Teriyaki Marinades
- Textured Vegetable Protein (TVP)
- Threonine
- Trehalose

APPENDIX 1 – COMMON GMO INGREDIENTS

Equal®	Modified Starch	Triglycerides
Food Starch	Mono and Diglycerides	Vegetable Fat
Fructose (any form)	Monosodium Glutamate (MSG)	Vegetable Oil
Glucose		Vitamin B12
Glutamate	NutraSweet®	Vitamin E
Glutamic Acid	Oleic Acid	Whey
Glycerides	Tocopherols	Whey Powder
Milk Starch	Tofu	Xanthan Gum
Modified Food Starch	Eversweet™ Stevia	

Source: Herbs-Info.com[1]

APPENDIX 2

COMMON NAMES FOR SUGAR

Agave Nectar
Agave Syrup
Barley Malt
Beet Sugar
Brown Rice Syrup
Brown Sugar
Buttered Syrup
Cane Sugar
Cane Juice
Cane Juice Crystals
Carob Syrup
Confectioner's Sugar
Corn Syrup
Corn Sugar
Corn Sweetener
Corn Syrup
Corn Syrup Solids
Crystallized Fructose
Date Sugar
Dextran
Dextrose
Diastase
Diastatic Malt
Evaporated Cane Juice
Fructose
Fruit Juice
Fruit Juice Concentrate
Glucose
Glucose Solids
Golden Sugar
Golden Syrup
Grape Sugar
High Fructose Corn Syrup
Invert Sugar
Lactose
Malt
Maltodextrin
Maltose
Maple Syrup
Molasses
Raw Sugar
Refiner's Syrup
Sorghum Syrup
Sucanat®
Sucrose
Sugar
Turbinado Sugar
Yellow Sugar

Source: Herbs-Info.com [1]

APPENDIX 2 – COMMON NAMES FOR SUGAR

APPENDIX 3

COMMON CHEMICALS TO AVOID

In addition to the ingredients listed in chapter 41, I also try to avoid the following:[1]

- Agave Nectar[2]
- Aluminum zirconium and other aluminum compounds (antiperspirant and deodorant)
- Artificial nails and toxic nail polishes and removers (I use Aquarella, which is water-based.)
- Artificial sweeteners: Splenda® (sucralose), Sweet'N Low® (saccharin), Equal® and NutraSweet® (aspartame, now being called Amino Sweet®), Sunett® and Sweet One® (acesulfame potassium/acesulfame K), and neotame (known in the European Union as E961) (they alter the microbial composition of the gut)
- Benzalkonium Chloride and Benzethonium Chloride (bath, skin, personal cleanliness, and suntan products; shaving cream, eye makeup, fragrance, acne treatments, pain relief)
- Benzyl Acetate (conditioner and other cosmetic/personal care products that have a scent)
- BHA and BHT (eyeliner, eye shadow, lip gloss, lipstick, perfumes, foundation, moisturizer, skin cleanser, diaper cream)
- BPA (as well as all plastics that come in contact with food) (see replacement info in Chapter 46, Kitchen Makeover)
- Coal tar (shampoo, scalp hair treatment, soap, hair dye, lotion)
- Cocamide DEA/Lauramide DEA (shampoo, bath soap, other personal care products)
- Diethanolamine (moisturizer, sunscreen, soap, cleaner, shampoo, foundation, hair color)

APPENDIX 3 – COMMON CHEMICALS TO AVOID

- Dioxins (farm-raised fish)
- Dry cleaning chemicals (perchloroethylene or tetrachloroethylene, also known as PERC; also used as a solvent and a metal degreaser; a "likely human carcinogen" per the National Academy of Science[3])
- Ethoxylated Ceteareth/PEG Compounds (skin conditioner, emulsifiers, and other cosmetics/personal care products)
- Ethyl Acetate (nail polish, nail polish remover, basecoats, other manicuring products, mascara, perfume, teeth whitening products)
- Fabrics (top six toxic fabrics)[4]
    - "Polyester is the worst fabric you can buy. It is made from synthetic polymers that are made from esters of dihydric alcohol and terephthalic acid."
    - "Acrylic fabrics are polyacrylonitriles and may cause cancer, according to the EPA."
    - "Rayon is recycled wood pulp that must be treated with chemicals like caustic soda, ammonia, acetone, and sulphuric acid to survive regular washing and wearing."
    - "Acetate and Triacetate are made from wood fibers called cellulose and undergo extensive chemical processing to produce the finished product."
    - "Nylon is made from petroleum and is often given a permanent chemical finish that can be harmful."
    - "Anything static resistant, stain resistant, permanent press, wrinkle-free, stain proof or moth repellant. Many of the stain resistant and wrinkle-free fabrics are treated with perfluorinated chemicals (PFCs), like Teflon™."
- Food colorings
- Food preservatives

APPENDIX 3 – COMMON CHEMICALS TO AVOID

- Formaldehyde (nail polish, nail glue, eyelash glue, hair gel, baby shampoo, hair smoothing products, body soap, body wash, color cosmetics, deodorant, shaving cream)
- Formaldehyde-Releasing Preservatives (Quarternium-15, DMDM Hydantoin, Diazolidinyl Urea, Imidazolidinyl Urea, DEA, MEA, TEA) (nail polish, nail glue, eyelash glue, hair smoothing products, hair gel, baby shampoo, body wash, body soap, color cosmetics)
- Fluoride (see chapter 41)
- Fragrance (Parfum) (perfumes, colognes, deodorants, nearly every type of personal care product)
- GMO foods
- High Fructose Corn Syrup[5]
- Hormones and antibiotics (including in commercially processed meats and dairy products)
- Hydroquinone (sunscreen, hair color, anti-aging products, facial moisturizer, skin fading/lightening products, facial cleanser, moisturizers)
- Iodopropynyl Butylcarbamate (foundation, concealer, self-tanners, bronzer, mascara, eyeshadow, makeup remover, shampoo, conditioner, shaving cream, diaper cream, anti-itch and anti-rash creams, body wash, bath soak, hair dye, lip balm, moisturizer)
- Lead and Lead Compounds (lipstick, lip gloss, other lip products, eyeliner, nail color, hair dye, hair products, eye shadow, whitening toothpaste, foundation, sunscreen, blush, moisturizer, eye drops, concealer)
- Methylisothiazolinone (MI/MCI) and Methylchloroisothiazolinone (shampoo, conditioner, body wash, hair color, lotion, sunscreen, shaving cream, mascara, hairspray, makeup remover, liquid soap, baby lotion, baby shampoo, detergent)

APPENDIX 3 – COMMON CHEMICALS TO AVOID

- MSG (monosodium glutamate) and other food additives
- Oxybenzone (Benzophenone-3) (sunscreen, lotion, makeup foundation with SPF)
- Petrolatum (Petroleum) (lipstick, lip balm, hair care products, skin care products, soap)
- Pesticides
- Potassium bromates
- P-Phenylenediamine (PPD) (hair dyes – even 'natural' ones, shampoo, hairspray, other hair care products)
- Propylene Glycol (carrier for fragrance oils, cosmetic moisturizers, shampoo, engine coolants, antifreeze, paints, airplane deicer, tire sealant, rubber cleaners, polyurethane cushions, adhesives, solvents/surfactants, enamels/varnishes)
- Recombinant Bovine Growth Hormone (rBGH)
- Refined vegetable oil
- Sodium Lauryl Sulfate (SLS), Sodium Laureth Sulfate (SLES), Ammonium Lauryl Sulfate (ALS) (Scalp treatments, hair color/bleaching agents, makeup foundations, shampoo, toothpaste, body washes and cleansers, liquid hand soaps, laundry detergents, bath oils/bath salts)
- Sodium nitrate and sodium nitrite
- Talc (blush, baby powder, body/shower products, eye shadow, powder, deodorant, lotion, feminine hygiene products, foundation, face masks, lipstick)
- Teflon™ (see info in Chapter 46, Kitchen Makeover)
- Triethanolamine (perfumes and other scented body products, hair products, hair dye, shaving creams and gels, shower gel, eye serums, skin creams/lotions, makeup foundation, blush, mascara, skin cleansers, eyeshadow, eyeliner)

APPENDIX 3 – COMMON CHEMICALS TO AVOID

More information on toxins to avoid:

http://www.Immune-Health-Solutions-For-You.com/list-of-toxins.html

http://www.MindBodyGreen.com/0-8686/are-you-putting-these-18-toxic-chemicals-on-your-body-every-day.html

http://BodyEcology.com/articles/top-5-sources-of-toxins.php

APPENDIX 3 – COMMON CHEMICALS TO AVOID

INDEX

3 John 2, 1, 9, 65, 340, 341, 351, 357.
Acid Reflux/GERD, 225.
Acne/Pimples, 121, 160, 167, 172, 274.
Adaptogen, 287, 288.
Addiction, 60, 107, 176, 221, 224, 225, 226.
Adrenal Fatigue, 121, 288.
Adrenaline, 228.
Aeroponics, 163.
ALCAT Test, 167.
Allergies, 58, 84, 94, 101, 102, 105, 107, 121, 132, 162, 167, 168, 169, 177, 185, 193, 241, 263, 279, 291, 311.
  Food, 84, 94, 101, 102, 105, 107, 121, 132, 162, 167, 168, 169, 241, 279.
Aloe Vera, 179, 311.
Alzheimer's Disease, 71, 239, 241, 286, 289.
Amino Acids, 100, 151, 179, 218.
Anemia, 135, 168.
Anointing Oil, Holy, 196, 197, 199.
Anointing/Anoint, 45, 187, 188, 189, 195, 196, 197, 198, 199, 202.
Antibacterial, 102, 259, 262, 287, 288.
Antibiotics, 70, 71, 110, 120, 161, 279, 292, 377.
Anticancer, 286, 314.
Antihistamines, 185, 193.
Anti-Inflammatory, 106, 233, 234, 241, 242, 286, 287, 288, 289.
Antinutrients, 100.
Antioxidants, 219, 233, 234, 241, 242, 286, 287, 288, 289, 313, 314.
Antiviral, 102, 286, 287.
Anxiety, 16, 120, 121, 123, 130, 140, 143, 146, 167, 175, 239, 249, 266, 288, 345.
Aroma/Smell/Fragrance/Odor, 58, 111, 186, 187, 191, 192, 193, 201, 204, 259, 262, 375, 377, 378.
Aroma Freedom Technique /AFT, 201.
Aromatherapy, 193, 246.
Arsenic, 71.
Arthritis, 108, 140, 168, 219, 241, 288.
  Rheumatoid Arthritis, 120, 121, 129, 130, 135, 218.
  Osteoarthritis, 107, 218.
Artificial Sweeteners, 223, 260, 375.
Ashwagandha, 288.
Asthma, 129, 130, 135, 139, 167, 258, 288.
Astragalus, 287.
Autoimmune Disorders, 3, 84, 87, 88, 95, 105, 121, 125, 127, 129, 130, 131, 133, 135, 136, 138, 139, 141, 143, 144, 145, 149, 151, 168, 217, 218, 225,

INDEX

226, 231, 241, 249, 264, 286, 363.
Avocado, 208, 209, 210, 212, 223, 224, 232, 241, 268, 279, 297, 298, 299, 304, 305.
Axe, Dr. Josh, 106, 261, 298, 303, 307, 308, 310, 311.
Bacon, 34, 79, 109, 110, 111, 201, 268, 360.
Bacteria, 35, 65, 100, 119, 120, 125, 129, 149, 177, 179, 183, 191, 241, 274, 311.
Barber Surgeons, 47, 48, 190.
Basal Body Temperature/BBT, 145.
Baths, 46, 257, 261, 274, 375, 377, 378.
Bayer AG/Monsanto, 57, 58, 66, 71, 98, 255, 256.
Be in Health Lifestyle, 3, 4, 5, 45, 76, 146, 153, 155, 156, 159, 160, 168, 171, 205, 209, 215, 243, 273, 275, 276, 367.
Believers, see **Saints/Believers.**
Believing, see **Faith/Believing.**
Beloved, 1, 9, 19, 45, 65, 90, 250, 331, 339, 344, 350, 357, 363.
Berries, 105, 108, 208, 213, 232, 242, 269, 300, 314, 317, 319.
Bio-Engineered Food/BE, 292.
Blessing, 19, 21, 27, 30, 74, 327, 331, 334, 340, 343, 349, 350, 353, 354, 357, 363, 364, 367.
Bloating, 84, 103, 121, 150, 167, 173, 180, 209.
Blood Pressure, 80, 228, 239, 247, 286, 288.
Blood Sugar Levels, 222, 223, 225.
Blue Light, 249, 250.
Body, 3, 4, 9, 10, 11, 27, 29, 31, 33, 40, 44, 45, 59, 75, 93, 96, 99, 100, 102, 111, 121, 124, 125, 129, 130, 131, 132, 135, 136, 138, 140, 141, 143, 145, 147, 150, 151, 155, 156, 157, 159, 160, 171, 172, 173, 174, 175, 176, 177, 179, 183, 184, 185, 189, 191, 192, 193, 194, 195, 198, 199, 200, 201, 203, 205, 208, 209, 217, 219, 222, 223, 228, 229, 232, 233, 237, 238, 239, 251, 254, 263, 264, 265, 271, 273, 274, 275, 276, 286, 287, 288, 311, 313, 328, 333, 334, 335, 336, 341, 342, 349, 352, 367.
Body of Christ, 189.
Body Odor, 160, 172.
Bone Broth, 131, 156, 159, 161, 208, 210, 217, 218, 219, 223, 227, 242, 282, 299, 301, 302, 306, 307, 309, 310, 316, 317.
Bones, 11, 27, 168, 217, 218, 230, 276, 311, 313.
Bowel Movements, 150, 156, 178, 179, 181, 182, 274, 275.
Brain, 123, 124, 125, 184, 200, 201, 221, 228, 230, 232, 233, 239, 254, 276, 286, 287.
Brain Fog, 139, 140, 141, 146.
Breakfast, 101, 131, 173, 207, 208, 210, 237, 238, 243, 279.
Breastfeeding / Nursing, 58, 204, 205, 238.

INDEX

Breath/Breathe, 110, 139, 167, 190, 191, 192, 222, 251, 256, 275.
Bronchitis, 55, 167.
Butter, 89, 90, 95, 162, 214, 230, 233, 234, 241, 281.
Caffeine, 150, 225, 226, 227, 228.
Cancer, 4, 52, 53, 56, 65, 66, 69, 70, 80, 82, 87, 98, 114, 115, 161, 195, 221, 238, 241, 249, 254, 255, 256, 286, 287, 288, 291, 311, 336, 376.
   Breast, 71, 98, 99, 147.
   Colorectal/Colon, 110, 229, 230, 312.
   Ovarian, 95.
   Prostate, 94.
Candida, 120, 121.
Canola (Crop), 67, 68, 292.
   Oil, *see* **Oil: Canola.**
Capsaicin, 106, 107, 108.
Carbohydrates, 113, 156, 209, 229, 230, 231.
Carcinogen, 69, 87, 114, 162, 255, 257, 258, 289, 291, 312, 376.
Cardiovascular, *see* **Heart Health.**
Cardiovascular Disease, *see* **Heart Disease.**
Casein, 88, 95, 102, 129, 217.
   A1, 95, 96, 120, 233, 279.
   A2, 95.
Cellular Memory, 184.
Central Nervous System, 123.
Cheese, 79, 89, 90, 95, 96, 100, 213, 268, 277, 361.

Chemicals, 4, 48, 51, 55, 57, 58, 59, 60, 68, 70, 71, 79, 80, 84, 86, 96, 106, 124, 164, 185, 192, 193, 194, 234, 245, 246, 254, 257, 255, 256, 257, 258, 259, 260, 261, 262, 263, 264, 273, 277, 281, 286, 287, 312, 333, 369, 375, 376.
Chicken, 34, 71, 98, 113, 156, 207, 208, 210, 211, 213, 217, 218, 232, 268, 301, 302, 306, 307, 308, 309, 310, 315, 316, 317.
Chicken Soup, 210, 218, 307.
Cholesterol, 61, 102, 231, 232, 233, 235, 278, 286, 288, 313.
Chondroitin, 218, 219.
Chromium, 223.
Chronic Fatigue Syndrome, 140.
Church, 3, 41, 45, 46, 48, 49, 63, 64, 65, 72, 189, 190, 336.
Cilantro, 163, 210, 214, 224, 299, 302, 313, 316.
Cinnamon, 80, 131, 184, 197, 199, 208, 209, 214, 246, 279, 288, 289, 297, 298, 313.
Citrus, 168, 174, 192, 194, 269.
Clary Sage, 205, 247, 249.
Cleaners, 44, 254, 256, 257, 258, 259, 262, 264, 375, 378.
Coconut, 101, 102.
   Aminos, 214, 281, 305.
   Fat, 102.
   Flour, 85, 161, 281, 302, 303.
   Kefir/Yogurt, 177, 207, 214, 222, 281, 304, 310, 311.

383

INDEX

Milk, 96, 101, 102, 103, 176, 177, 209, 214, 283, 298, 299, 300, 303, 305, 306.
Oil, *see* **Oil: Coconut.**
Sugar, 223.
Water, 101.
Coeliac/Celiac Disease, 71, 84, 85, 87, 107, 121, 135, 292, 314
Coffee, 162, 201, 225, 226, 227, 228, 281.
Cold Turkey, 225, 226, 227.
Colitis, 167, 177, 311.
Collagen, 156, 159, 217, 218, 298, 303.
Colon Cleanse, 156, 177, 180, 181, 182, 276.
Colon/Intestines/Gut, 29, 84, 87, 88, 100, 102, 119, 120, 123, 124, 125, 129, 130, 131, 141, 145, 149, 159, 161, 168, 169, 171, 177, 179, 180, 181, 182, 186, 207, 209, 217, 225, 241, 297, 312, 367, 375.
Condemnation, 74, 136, 350.
Constipation, 121, 144, 149, 150, 182, 226, 275, 312.
Corn, 4, 67, 68, 85, 86, 89, 97, 132, 164, 168, 174, 292, 371, 373.
Oil, *see* **Oil: Corn.**
Cortisol, 225, 287, 288.
Cramps, 84, 106, 124, 150.
Crohn's Disease, 121, 177, 311.
Crucifixion/Cross, 33, 44, 186, 187, 188, 349, 350, 364.
Curcumin, 285, 286.
Cure, 48, 54, 59, 64, 75, 149, 193, 194, 205, 222.

Dairy Products, 70, 88, 89, 92, 93, 94, 95, 96, 102, 107, 120, 121, 129, 132, 150, 161, 162, 168, 174, 211, 213, 217, 233, 234, 268, 269, 278, 279, 281, 312, 367, 377.
Depression, 61, 120, 121, 123, 130, 140, 144, 146, 147, 167, 239, 260, 266.
Detoxification, 155, 160, 171, 172, 179, 219, 223, 224, 226, 227, 239, 273, 274, 275, 276, 311, 313.
Devil, *see* **Evil One.**
Devil/Evil Spirits, 136, 187.
Diabetes, 65, 82, 87, 95, 114, 115, 129, 135, 161, 221, 229, 238, 239, 269, 288, 336.
Diarrhea, 84, 103, 106, 121, 124, 149, 150, 151, 167, 177, 179, 182, 226, 311.
Digestion, 29, 35, 88, 92, 94, 95, 102, 105, 110, 119, 121, 123, 129, 150, 156, 159, 178, 179, 180, 227, 228, 230, 232, 233, 237, 238, 276, 296, 311, 313, 334.
Digestive Enzymes, 156, 177, 178, 182, 214.
Digestive System, *see* **Gastrointestinal System.**
Digestive Upset / Indigestion, 103, 121, 149, 150, 167, 180, 209, 223, 225.
Dinner, 81, 101, 113, 131, 173, 208, 210, 237, 279, 280, 295, 323.

INDEX

Dirty Dozen/Clean Fifteen, 161, 211, 242, 278.
DNA, 65, 69, 80, 184, 258.
Doctors/Physicians, 45, 46, 47, 48, 49, 50, 51, 52, 53, 54, 55, 56, 58, 59, 60, 66, 84, 85, 115, 123, 135, 139, 140, 145, 146, 147, 150, 160, 167, 168, 172, 190, 191, 192, 217, 223, 225, 235, 238, 242, 269, 278, 280.
Dopamine, 222.
Dose/Dosage, 48, 49, 51, 55, 58, 59, 146, 193.
Dreams, 160, 172, 253.
Drugs, *see* **Pharmaceutical Drugs.**
Eating Disorders, 238.
Eating Plan, 29, 155, 159, 168, 176, 207, 209, 239, 268, 269.
Eczema/Psoriasis, 106, 120, 121, 129, 130, 135, 167, 177, 311.
Edamame, 100, 269.
Eggplant, 105, 106.
Eggs, 70, 96, 131, 168, 172, 174, 176, 208, 209, 210, 213, 223, 231, 232, 268, 269, 279, 282, 297, 302, 303, 304, 309, 310.
Electrolytes, 101, 102, 224, 226.
ELISA Test, 85, 167.
Emotions, 3, 7, 9, 12, 15, 44, 123, 124, 136, 137, 155, 156, 174, 183, 194, 195, 200, 201, 202, 203, 222, 352, 357, 360.
Endocrine Disruptor, 100, 269.
Endocrine System, 99, 143, 313.
Endotoxins, 88, 119, 129, 145, 149, 274.

Energy, 53, 102, 143, 156, 195, 200, 223, 228, 230, 232, 237, 240, 265, 295.
Energy Drinks, 227.
Enteric Brain/Nervous System, 123, 125.
Environmental Working Group /EWG, 71, 261, 278, 291, 292.
Epidemic, 58, 120, 191, 221, 229.
Epigenetics, 136, 200.
Epilepsy, 247.
Esophagus, 108, 124.
Essential Oils, 2, 44, 45, 54, 135, 150, 156, 178, 179, 180, 182, 183, 184, 185, 186, 187, 189, 190, 191, 193, 194, 195, 196, 199, 201, 203, 204, 205, 206, 207, 245, 246, 247, 249, 251, 257, 258, 259, 266, 274, 286, 299, 301, 302, 303, 306, 313, 361.
   Fake/Adulterated, 194, 204, 245.
Eugenics, 55, 57.
Evil, 11, 12, 13, 15, 16, 23, 26, 27, 64, 138, 187, 344, 355.
Evil One, 2, 3, 12, 13, 14, 27, 28, 38, 63, 64, 65, 72, 73, 344.
Exercise, 46, 141, 157, 224, 265, 266, 311.
Faith/Believing, 21, 26, 33, 37, 38, 43, 63, 76, 187, 198, 252, 322, 323, 326, 327, 328, 329, 331, 332, 333, 335, 336, 337, 339, 350, 363, 364.
Fascia, 130, 139.
Fast Food, 80, 81, 82, 113, 114, 115, 268.

INDEX

Fasting, 156, 159, 175, 208, 225, 237, 238, 239, 240, 269.
   Intermittent, 208, 237, 238, 239, 240, 269.
Fat / Overweight / Obese / Fatty Tissue, 65, 72, 82, 102, 110, 114, 115, 159, 161, 171, 177, 211, 221, 225, 227, 229, 234, 238, 239, 240, 241, 276, 278, 311, 321, 322, 336, 314.
Fat Bombs, 222, 305, 306.
Father, *see* **God.**
Fatigue, 1, 121, 139, 140, 141, 144, 146, 147, 160, 172, 178, 223, 226, 288.
Fats, 88, 90, 95, 96, 101, 102, 113, 114, 150, 156, 209, 214, 223, 229, 230, 231, 232, 233, 234, 241, 242, 277, 278, 279, 300, 372.
   Healthy, 88, 101, 102, 113, 209, 223, 229, 232, 233, 234, 241, 242, 279, 300.
   Low-Fat, 101, 230.
   Monounsaturated, 232, 234, 242.
   Saturated, 95, 209, 229, 230, 231, 232, 234, 242.
   Trans, 229, 233, 234, 277, 278.
   Unhealthy, 114, 229, 233, 234, 242, 277, 278, 372.
   Unsaturated, 231, 241.
Fatty Acids, 85, 100, 101, 102, 179, 230, 231, 232, 233, 241, 278.
   Essential, 85, 179.
   Long Chain, 102, 231.
   Medium Chain, 102, 230, 232, 235.
   Medium Chain Triglyceride/ MCT, 102.
   Saturated, 101, 102.
   Short Chain, 100.
   Trans, 278.
   Unsaturated, 241.
FDA, 47, 59, 60, 67, 68, 97, 99, 102, 193, 245.
Fear/Afraid, 15, 17, 124, 136, 175, 200, 322, 339, 246, 349, 350, 352.
Fear/Awe, 11, 17, 25, 27, 31, 334, 351, 353, 355.
Fennel, 205, 214, 247, 305, 310, 313.
Fiber, 29, 102, 114, 120, 124, 181, 312, 313, 314.
Fibromyalgia, 120, 121, 129, 130, 135, 139, 140, 141, 149.
Fish, 29, 31, 34, 71, 80, 156, 161, 212, 241, 281, 334, 376.
Fish Oil Supplement, 179, 214.
Flour, 84, 85, 86, 89, 161, 180, 278, 281, 371.
   Almond, 85, 161, 281.
   Cassava, 85.
   Coconut, *see* **Coconut: Flour.**
   Einkorn, 85.
Fluoride, 162, 164, 260, 261, 377.
Folate, 61, 232.
Food Allergies, *see* **Allergies: Food.**
Food Intolerance, *see* **Allergies: Food.**
Food Reintroduction Challenge, 107, 108, 155, 159,

INDEX

161, 168, 171, 172, 175, 176, 367.
Food Sensitivity, *see* **Allergies: Food.**
Food, 1, 2, 3, 4, 27, 29, 30, 31, 35, 37, 40, 41, 58, 60, 62, 63, 64, 65, 66, 67, 68, 69, 70, 71, 72, 79, 80, 81, 82, 83, 86, 87, 88, 89, 90, 92, 93, 94, 96, 97, 98, 99, 100, 101, 105, 106, 107, 108, 111, 113, 114, 115, 120, 121, 123, 125, 127, 131, 132, 133, 136, 141, 150, 156, 159, 160, 161, 162, 163, 164, 165, 167, 168, 169, 171, 172, 173, 174, 175, 176, 177, 178, 180, 185, 195, 204, 207, 208, 209, 211, 218, 221, 222, 223, 224, 227, 228, 229, 230, 232, 233, 234, 235, 327, 238, 240, 241, 243, 246, 247, 251, 255, 262, 266, 267, 269, 273, 274, 276, 277, 278, 279, 280, 281, 282, 283, 285, 291, 292, 296, 312, 314, 333, 334, 335, 336, 340, 359, 360, 367, 369, 371, 375, 377.
Additives, 70, 131, 132, 141, 208, 234, 245, 261, 262, 281, 292, 378.
Allergies, *see* **Allergies: Food.**
Fast, *see* **Fast Food.**
Fermented, 83, 99, 100, 303.
Glyphosate, 69, 87, 114, 255.
GMO, 4, 65, 66, 67, 68, 69, 70, 71, 86, 98, 99, 114, 120, 132, 133, 162, 211, 260, 278, 279, 282, 292, 371, 377.
Healthy, 29, 30, 31, 40, 60, 71, 72, 79, 80, 81, 82, 83, 92, 97, 101, 111, 115, 125, 131, 141, 156, 175, 177, 218, 222, 224, 228, 232, 234, 235, 235, 238, 241, 243, 267, 268, 269, 273, 274, 277, 278, 279, 280, 282, 283, 291, 314, 333, 334, 371.
Industry/Supply, 3, 41, 60, 61, 63, 64, 65, 66, 67, 68, 69, 70, 71, 93, 98, 221, 292.
Non-GMO, 66, 68, 69, 81, 100, 114, 227, 278, 292.
Non-Organic, 70, 114, 161, 211, 278.
Organic, 68, 69, 70, 71, 80, 81, 100, 114, 161, 211, 213, 214, 223, 226, 241, 242, 268, 278, 279, 283, 297, 300, 302, 303, 305, 313, 314, 316, 317, 371.
Pasteurized/Unpasteurized, 79, 91, 93, 96, 132, 156, 159, 161, 180, 213, 223, 232, 281, 283, 298, 314.
Processed, *see* **Processed Food.**
Raw, 79, 91, 96, 131, 156, 159, 161, 162, 208, 209, 211, 213, 214, 223, 277, 281, 283, 287, 288, 298, 301, 314.
Sour, 91, 95, 192, 222, 223, 269.
Starchy, 86, 100, 178, 209, 212, 222, 371, 372.
Toxic, 70, 71, 100, 110, 162, 226, 227, 264, 289.
Unfermented, 100.

INDEX

Unhealthy, 1, 3, 4, 35, 60, 67, 69, 70, 71, 72, 79, 80, 81, 82, 87, 88, 98, 99, 100, 105, 106, 111, 113, 114, 115, 120, 125, 131, 132, 133, 136, 141, 177, 180, 207, 211, 221, 222, 227, 233, 234, 235, 255, 261, 262, 267, 268, 269, 273, 274, 276, 277, 278, 280, 281, 282, 292, 336, 360, 369, 377.

Food-Mood-Poop (FMP) Journal, 156, 173, 176, 295, 296.

Fool/Foolish, 19, 20, 26, 323, 356.

Forgiveness, 44, 74, 76, 136, 190, 197, 199, 201, 202, 203, 215, 250, 327, 354.

Fragrance, *see* Aroma/Smell/Fragrance/Odor.

Frankincense, 184, 187, 188, 199, 249, 274.

Free Radicals, 96, 232, 234, 239, 287.

Frequency, 53, 195, 200.

Fructose, 156, 168, 174, 213, 223, 372, 373.

Fruit, Physical, 29, 30, 45, 79, 86, 91, 96, 102, 106, 156, 163, 168, 174, 185, 208, 211, 213, 221, 223, 231, 232, 242, 247, 259, 269, 283, 285, 300, 321, 333, 373.

Fruit, Spiritual, 14, 18, 21.

Galen of Pergamon, 191.

Gallbladder, 178, 180.

Garlic, 208, 210, 212, 214, 242, 286, 287, 288, 297, 299, 300, 301, 302, 306, 307, 309, 310.

Gas, *see* Digestive Upset / Indigestion.

Gas Chambers, 55.

Gastrointestinal / Digestive System, 29, 106, 110, 121, 123, 159, 162, 177, 179, 208, 217, 219, 228, 311, 314, 333.

Gelatin, 109, 217.

Genes, 4, 62, 65, 66, 119, 129, 136, 200, 292.

Genetically Engineered / GE, 98, 133, 292.

Genetically Modified Organism / GMO, 4, 65, 66, 67, 68, 69, 70, 71, 86, 98, 99, 100, 114, 120, 132, 133, 162, 211, 260, 268, 278, 279, 282, 292, 371, 377.

GERD, see Acid Reflux/GERD.

Germ Theory of Disease, 50, 51, 191.

Germany, 48, 49, 54, 55, 56, 57, 85, 245, 255.

Ghee, 131, 162, 208, 214, 230, 233, 241, 279, 281, 304, 305.

Ginger, 179, 184, 210, 214, 242, 246, 285, 287, 288, 298, 301, 310, 313.

Glucosamine, 218, 219.

Glucose, 222, 288, 372, 373.

Glutathione, 219.

Gluten, 71, 83, 84, 85, 86, 87, 88, 107, 120, 121, 129, 161, 168, 174, 211, 214, 217, 281, 314.

INDEX

Gluten-Free, 81, 84, 85, 87, 211, 268, 277.
Gluten Sensitivity/Intolerance, *see* **Coeliac/Celiac Disease.**
Glycine, 218, 219, 371.
Glyphosate / Roundup®, 66, 68, 69, 71, 86, 87, 98, 114, 255, 256.
God/Father/LORD, 1, 2, 3, 4, 5, 7, 9, 10, 11, 12, 13, 15, 16, 17, 18, 19, 20, 21, 22, 23, 25, 26, 27, 28, 29, 30, 31, 33, 34, 35, 37, 38, 39, 40, 43, 44, 45, 50, 54, 56, 59, 62, 63, 64, 65, 66, 73, 74, 75, 76, 89, 90, 91, 109, 110, 121, 135, 136, 137, 138, 147, 153, 155, 159, 175, 185, 186, 189, 190, 191, 192, 195, 196, 197, 198, 199, 202, 204, 205, 211, 235, 237, 239, 243, 250, 253, 265, 266, 267, 285, 321, 322, 323, 324, 325, 326, 327, 328, 329, 330, 331, 332, 333, 334, 335, 336, 337, 339, 340, 341, 342, 343, 344, 345, 346, 347, 348, 349, 350, 351, 352, 353, 354, 355, 356, 357, 359, 363, 364, 365, 367.
God's Word, 14, 15, 17, 18, 21, 22, 25, 27, 37, 38, 63, 66, 73, 138, 342, 343, 344, 347, 348, 349, 355, 363, 364.
Gout, 168.
Grains, 29, 83, 84, 85, 86, 87, 88, 89, 120, 129, 132, 161, 162, 209, 211, 217, 230, 268, 279, 312, 333, 367.
  Cereal, 83, 86, 87, 88.
  Hybrid, 87.
  Refined, 86.
  Sprouted, 162.
  Unsprouted, 120.
  Whole, 86, 230.
Grass-Fed, 88, 91, 156, 161, 211, 230, 279, 281, 297, 315.
Graves' Disease, 99, 121, 129, 130, 143, 144.
Greens, Leafy, 210, 212, 222, 224, 242, 285.
Gut, *see* **Colon/Intestines/Gut.**
Gut Lining, *see* **Colon/Intestines/Gut.**
Harmony, 1, 3, 23, 26, 28, 38, 39, 195, 199, 276, 333, 336, 359.
Hashimoto's Disease, 99, 120, 121, 129, 130, 135, 144, 145, 146.
Headaches, 106, 160, 167, 172, 173, 223, 224, 226, 273.
Healing Arts, 45, 54, 56.
Health Care, 1, 3, 41, 43, 45, 46, 49, 50, 51, 53, 54, 58, 64, 204, 247.
Health Problems, 81, 105, 107, 114, 121, 135, 140, 146, 155, 159, 167, 168, 169, 171, 178, 209, 223, 254, 256, 312, 336, 363, 393.
Health/Healthy, 1, 2, 3, 4, 5, 7, 9, 10, 11, 12, 23, 26, 27, 28, 29, 33, 35, 43, 44, 46, 53, 55, 56, 59, 51, 62, 63, 65, 66, 70, 71, 72, 75, 79, 80, 82, 88, 91, 92, 97, 99, 100, 101, 102, 106, 109, 110, 113, 114, 115, 117, 121, 129, 131, 132, 133, 135, 136, 141, 145, 150, 151, 153, 155, 156, 157, 159,

INDEX

160, 161, 162, 163, 164, 165, 168, 169, 171, 174, 175, 176, 177, 179, 185, 186, 192, 193, 195, 202, 203, 204, 205, 207, 209, 217, 218, 221, 222, 223, 224, 225, 228, 229, 230, 231, 232, 233, 234, 235, 237, 238, 241, 242, 254, 263, 264, 267, 268, 269, 270, 273, 276, 277, 278, 279, 280, 285, 287, 288, 291, 292, 305, 311, 313, 314, 321, 333, 334, 335, 336, 337, 339, 340, 341, 350, 357, 359, 360, 367, 393.

Heart Attack, 80, 82, 97, 114, 147, 234, 286.

Heart Health, 99, 102, 143, 144, 177, 222, 226, 233, 234, 239, 289, 311, 314.

Heart, Emotional, 9, 10, 12, 13, 14, 16, 17, 22, 26, 27, 138, 197, 198, 199, 200, 201, 202, 252, 322, 325, 326, 341, 342, 343, 345, 347, 349, 351, 354, 355, 363.

Heart Disease, 4, 82, 95, 114, 115, 161, 229, 230, 231, 232, 233, 234, 238, 241, 265, 278, 286, 288.

Heartburn, 107, 108, 121, 124, 225.

Heavy Metals, 180, 219, 313.
Hemp, 209, 213, 241, 312.
Herbicides, 66, 98, 256.
Herbivores, 29, 30, 31, 334.
Herbs/Herbal, 44, 46, 50, 54, 56, 66, 107, 150, 162, 163, 179, 181, 183, 185, 190, 191, 192, 204, 208, 214, 246, 275, 281, 285, 313, 314, 323.

Herxheimer Reaction, 273, 274, 276.

High Fructose Corn Syrup /HFCS, 80, 223, 371, 377.

Hippocrates, 45, 119, 127, 129, 157, 276.

Histamines, 124, 185, 193.
Holocaust, 55, 57.
Honey, 79, 89, 90, 91, 92, 156, 159, 161, 213, 223, 281, 283, 298, 306, 314, 356.

Hormones, 66, 70, 71, 94, 99, ,100, 124, 143, 144, 145, 146, 147, 225, 239, 240, 247, 249, 279, 292, 377, 378.
  Bioidentical, 146, 147.
  Growth, 70, 71, 94, 239, 240, 378.
  HRT, 146, 147.
  Non-Bioidentical, 147.

Hydrogenation (process), 234.
Hypertension, 82, 114, 115, 287, 288.
Hypoglycemia, 269.
Hyssop, 184, 186, 187, 199, 205, 247.

Idaho Tansy, 247.
IG Farben, 57, 255.
IgE Test, 167.
IgG Test, 167.
Immune System, 66, 88, 114, 119, 129, 130, 131, 135, 145, 149, 159, 167, 168, 169, 171, 177, 179, 217, 218, 230, 241, 259, 286, 287, 288, 311, 313.

Immunity, 53, 232, 311.

INDEX

Immunosuppressants, 131, 141.
Indigestion, *see* Digestive Upset / Indigestion.
Industrial Waste, 54, 57, 58, 59, 192.
Inflammation, 87, 88, 95, 105, 106, 108, 119, 120, 121, 124, 139, 149, 159, 161, 167, 171, 179, 217, 218, 219, 225, 233, 234, 239, 241, 242, 263, 264, 286, 287, 288, 289.
Insomnia, 146.
Insulin, 94, 222, 225, 238, 239.
Intestinal Permeability, *see* Leaky Gut.
Intestines, *see* Colon/Intestines/Gut.
Irritable Bowel Disease/IBD, 108.
Irritable Bowel Syndrome /IBS, 103, 105, 108, 121, 129, 135, 140, 149, 150, 151, 177, 311.
Jesus Christ, 3, 7, 10, 12, 15, 16, 18, 19, 20, 21, 23, 27, 28, 33, 34, 37, 38, 39, 43, 44, 56, 64, 65, 73, 74, 75, 136, 137, 138, 155, 186, 187, 188, 189, 190, 191, 197, 198, 199, 202, 253, 323, 324, 328, 329, 330, 331, 332, 334, 335, 340, 341, 343, 345, 346, 348, 349, 350, 351, 363, 364, 365, 396.
Joints, 106, 107, 108, 168, 217, 218, 219, 276, 342.
Judgment, 19, 20, 26, 74, 136, 323, 324, 349, 350, 354.
Juniper, 184, 247.

Just/Justification, 16, 18, 76, 198, 326, 327, 328, 345.
Kale, 163, 210, 212, 242, 269, 305, 306, 307, 308, 312, 313, 314.
Kefir, 95, 103, 156, 177, 207, 214, 222, 281, 303, 304, 310, 311.
 Coconut Milk, 103, 177, 207, 214, 222, 281, 303, 304, 310, 311.
Labels, 67, 68, 70, 81, 87, 96, 99, 133, 179, 194, 204, 211, 227, 232, 235, 245, 246, 247, 256, 257, 260, 277, 291, 292.
Lactose, 94, 95, 102, 373.
Lactose Intolerance, 94, 103, 233, 311.
Law, Old Testament, 28, 33, 37, 38, 40, 76, 109, 110, 189, 197, 198, 323, 327, 328, 329, 335.
Leaky Gut Syndrome, 3, 87, 88, 95, 105, 117, 119, 120, 121, 123, 130, 133, 135, 136, 141, 149, 155, 156, 159, 162, 178, 209, 217, 225, 249, 312, 363.
Legumes, 29, 85, 88, 132, 161, 209, 231, 312, 333, 367.
L-Glutamine, 151, 179, 214, 218.
Libido, 99, 146, 147.
Lifestyle, 3, 5, 26, 45, 60, 76, 146, 155, 156, 159, 160, 168, 171, 205, 209, 215, 241, 243, 264, 273, 275, 276, 321, 359, 360, 367.
Liver, 219, 226, 230, 289.
LORD, *see* God.
Love, 1, 11, 13, 16, 18, 19, 20, 23, 33, 40, 64, 73, 89, 109, 111, 137,

391

INDEX

199, 200, 222, 243, 274, 322, 323, 324, 325, 326, 331, 334, 336, 345, 349, 356, 363, 364, 396.
Lunch, 101, 131, 173, 208, 210, 237, 279.
Lungs, 130, 164, 167, 191, 230, 256, 275.
Lupus, 120, 121, 129, 130, 135, 140.
Lyme Disease, 265.
Lymphatic System, 265.
Magnesium, 61, 102, 121, 182, 219, 222, 224, 250, 275, 314.
Malabsorption, 121, 168.
Malnutrition, 72, 115.
Maple Syrup, 213, 223, 373.
Margarine, 234.
Meal Plan, 207, 293.
Meals, 51, 82, 114, 115, 178, 179, 182, 207, 208, 237, 238, 240, 243, 268, 269, 279, 292, 293.
Meat, 30, 31, 35, 69, 71, 79, 80, 88, 97, 98, 101, 192, 209, 210, 211, 213, 262, 278, 279, 281, 297, 298, 302, 334, 377.
   Processed, see Processed Meat.
Mediator Release Testing /MRT, 167.
Medication, see Pharmaceutical Drugs.
Medicine/Medical Care, 3, 4, 41, 43, 44, 45, 46, 47, 48, 49, 50, 51, 52, 53, 54, 55, 56, 58, 59, 60, 61, 77, 119, 127, 130, 131, 140, 141, 149, 191, 193, 260, 262, 269, 271, 275, 285, 287, 288, 296.
Memory/Memories, 137, 144, 167, 184, 200, 201, 202, 203, 219, 232, 234, 239, 265, 314.
Mercola, Dr. Joseph, 100, 200, 221, 230.
Metabolism, 121, 167, 226, 228.
Miasma Theory, 191, 192, 193.
Milk Thistle, 179, 224, 275.
Milk, 71, 79, 89, 90, 91, 92, 93, 94, 95, 96, 101, 180, 192, 213, 234, 262, 277, 371, 372.
   Coconut, see Coconut: Milk.
   Cow's, 71, 90, 91, 92, 93, 94, 95, 96, 101, 103, 176, 213.
   Goat/Sheep's, 90, 91, 96, 213, 303.
   Breast/Mother's, 69, 87, 92, 255.
   Soy, 97, 100, 371.
Mind, 3, 4, 9, 10, 12, 16, 17, 25, 56, 73, 137, 138, 159, 171, 201, 202, 243, 252, 253, 325, 329, 330, 342, 343, 345, 346, 347, 349, 357.
Mind of Christ, 73, 155.
Mindset, 4, 131, 141, 267, 274, 319, 329.
Minerals, 48, 70, 83, 100, 102, 163, 217, 218, 219, 222, 233.
Monsanto, see Bayer AG/Monsanto.
Mood, 121, 123, 160, 167, 172, 173, 223, 226, 239.
Motion Sickness, 287.
MSG, 132, 372, 378.
Mucoid Plaque, 181, 182.

INDEX

Mucus, 180, 185, 193.
Multiple Sclerosis/MS, 120, 121, 129, 130, 135.
Mycotoxins, 70, 71.
Myrrh, 90, 184, 187, 188, 197, 199.
NAC (N-Acetyl Cysteine), 223, 275.
National Institutes of Health /NIH, 218, 230, 242.
Nausea, 106, 149, 160, 172, 226, 287.
Nazis, 49, 55, 56, 57.
Nervous System, 70, 123, 124, 125, 167, 228, 254, 313.
Nicotine, 106, 107.
Nightshades, 46, 105, 106, 107, 108, 132, 161, 168, 174, 316, 367.
Non-GMO Food, *see* **Food: Non-GMO.**
Non-GMO Project, 65, 68, 223, 292, 371.
Non-Organic, *see* **Food: Non-Organic.**
Non-Toxic Products/Ingredients, 258, 259, 261.
Nutrients, 61, 88, 91, 92, 96, 100, 102, 114, 123, 125, 131, 163, 165, 168, 178, 180, 218, 229, 230, 232, 275, 314.
Nutrition, 52, 60, 70, 71, 72, 83, 85, 86, 92, 95, 100, 102, 113, 114, 115, 205, 232, 268, 278, 292, 311.
Nutritional Supplements, 177, 179.

Nuts, 29, 79, 96, 107, 131, 162, 168, 172, 174, 208, 209, 213, 223, 241, 242, 269, 283, 300, 317, 333.
Obesity, *see* **Fat / Overweight / Obese.**
Odor, *see* **Aroma / Smell / Fragrance / Odor.**
Oil Pulling, 266.
Oil, 68, 86, 97, 98, 100, 101, 120, 132, 150, 156, 162, 164, 180, 194, 196, 197, 204, 208, 209, 214, 229, 230, 231, 232, 233, 234, 235, 241, 266, 275, 278, 281, 287, 297, 298, 299, 300, 301, 302, 303, 304, 305, 306, 307, 308, 309, 310, 315, 317, 371, 372, 378.
  Avocado, 156, 162, 214, 233, 281, 309, 310.
  Cannabis/Hemp, 197.
  Canola, 132, 162, 214, 230, 231, 281, 371.
  Carrier, 180, 197, 204, 287.
  Coconut, 101, 156, 162, 180, 204, 209, 214, 230, 231, 232, 233, 241, 266, 281, 297, 298, 299, 300, 301, 302, 303, 304, 305, 306, 307, 308, 309, 310, 315.
  Cod Liver, 150.
  Corn, 132, 214, 371.
  Cottonseed, 68, 132, 371.
  Extra Virgin Olive/EVOO, 156, 162, 197, 204, 208, 214, 230, 233, 234, 235, 241, 275, 281, 287, 305, 309, 310.
  Flax Seed, 150.

INDEX

Hydrogenated/Partially Hydrogenated, 120, 162, 229, 281.
Palm, 132.
Peanut, 132, 230.
Soybean, 97, 98, 100, 230, 371.
Sunflower, 132.
Vegetable, 132, 204, 214, 230, 233, 234, 278, 372, 378.
Ointments/Salves, 188, 190, 202.
Omega-3, 233, 241.
Omega-6, 233.
Operation Paperclip, 56.
Opioids, 226.
Organic, *see* Food: Organic.
Osler, Dr. William, 50, 52.
Osteoarthritis, *see* Arthritis.
Outgassing, 251.
Paracelsus, 48, 49, 51, 59, 191.
Parasite Cleanse, 178.
Parasites, 110, 178, 259.
Parkinson's Disease, 289.
Parsley, 163, 214, 297, 301, 302, 306, 307, 313, 316.
Passover, 186, 187.
Pasteurization, 93, 96.
Pasture Raised, 91, 110, 156, 161, 211, 213, 214, 223, 232, 241, 279, 281, 301, 302, 315.
Peanuts, 85, 97, 132, 162.
Perkus, Dr. Benjamin, 201.
Personal Care Products, 58, 59, 192, 254, 261, 262, 375, 376.
Pesticides, 68, 69, 83, 161, 255, 259, 278, 292, 378.
Pharmaceutical Drugs, 48, 51, 52, 53, 54, 59, 60, 61, 62, 110, 120, 150, 177, 180, 183, 185, 193, 194, 221, 222, 225, 226, 231, 235, 260, 261, 262, 266, 274, 280, 287, 288, 359.
Pharmaceutical/Drug Industry, 51, 52, 53, 57, 59, 61, 194.
Phosphorus, 102, 219, 232.
Physicians, *see* Doctors/Physicians.
Pigs/Pork, 34, 35, 109, 110, 132, 161, 213, 367.
Pilates, 266.
Plague, 47, 186, 191.
Plague Doctor, 190, 191, 192.
Plants, 29, 30, 31, 44, 45, 59, 60, 65, 66, 69, 70, 85, 86, 97, 98, 99, 105, 106, 107, 108, 163, 183, 185, 186, 217, 232, 285, 292, 333, 334.
Pneuma, 191.
Pneumonia, 54, 55, 191, 286.
Poison, 48, 49, 51, 54, 55, 58, 59, 60, 63, 69, 71, 106, 114, 192, 193, 251, 254, 257, 260, 261, 264.
Poisonous Gas, 54, 55, 192, 257.
Potassium, 61, 85, 102, 114, 219, 232, 375, 378.
Potatoes, 67, 105, 106, 108, 162, 281, 336.
Poultry, 70, 71, 161, 281.
Pregnancy, 58, 204, 205, 232, 238, 247, 287, 288.
Probiotics, 120, 156, 177, 178, 182, 214, 222, 251, 279, 311.
Processed Food, 70, 79, 80, 81, 82, 83, 86, 99, 100, 113, 115, 120, 131, 132, 160, 161, 162,

INDEX

171, 180, 211, 213, 221, 223, 226, 233, 234, 273, 277, 278, 281, 282, 292, 312, 377.
Processed Meat, 79, 80, 110, 161, 268, 281, 377.
Prosper, 1, 9, 10, 11, 22, 23, 44, 65, 74, 98, 339, 340, 341, 342, 343, 344, 345, 346, 347, 348, 350, 351, 352, 355, 356, 357.
Protein, 83, 85, 86, 87, 88, 93, 95, 97, 98, 100, 102, 113, 119, 129, 131, 145, 149, 156, 179, 208, 209, 217, 218, 230, 232, 233, 239, 241, 269, 279, 281, 298, 303, 311, 312, 371.
Psoriasis, *see* **Eczema/Psoriasis.**
Quacks, 47, 56, 59, 190.
Rash, 130, 167, 273, 274, 377.
Raw Food, *see* **Food: Raw.**
Recipes, 1, 80, 103, 131, 141, 156, 175, 176, 177, 183, 186, 207, 208, 210, 219, 222, 246, 247, 261, 282, 291, 293, 297, 298, 302, 303, 305, 306, 307, 308, 310, 315, 316, 317.
Rejection, 37, 48, 66, 136, 322.
Rejoice, 348, 351, 352, 353, 354, 364.
Renewed Mind, 138, 347, 348.
Reproductive System, 168, 291.
Respiratory System, 167.
Rest, 46, 139, 143, 147, 159, 226, 238, 239, 274.
   Mental/Spiritual, 198, 350, 354.
Restaurants, 82, 113, 115, 267, 268, 280, 292.

Restoration, 1, 3, 75, 121, 131, 133, 135, 141, 151, 153, 155, 156, 157, 159, 161, 162, 168, 177, 179, 207, 209, 210, 217, 237, 238, 242, 276, 285, 297, 304, 311, 314, 351, 359, 367.
Rheumatoid Arthritis, *see* **Arthritis.**
Rice, 71, 85, 86, 209, 312, 373.
Righteousness, 18, 21, 33, 37, 38, 39, 44, 73, 74, 75, 138, 198, 322, 323, 325, 326, 327, 328, 329, 331, 332, 335, 348, 351, 353, 354, 364.
Rosicrucianism, 48, 49.
Roundup®, *see* **Glyphosate / Roundup®.**
Sage, 205, 214, 247, 249,
Saints/Belivers, 1, 27, 28, 35, 189, 190, 335, 345, 367.
Salad Dressing, 208, 221, 235, 315, 316.
Salt, Himalayan Pink, 131, 162, 208, 214, 281, 297, 299, 301, 302, 303, 304, 305, 306, 307, 308, 309, 310, 315, 316.
Salt, Iodized/Table, 79, 80, 114, 152, 281.
Satan, *see* **Evil One.**
Sauerkraut, 96, 156, 208, 210, 222, 279, 304, 305.
Sauna, 275.
Science, 50, 53, 55, 65, 92, 109, 136, 200, 265.
Seeds, 29, 45, 66, 68, 69, 79, 83, 85, 86, 97, 162, 168, 174, 176, 183, 185, 209, 213, 223, 241, 255, 269, 275, 282, 283, 285,

297, 300, 302, 312, 313, 314, 333.
Chia, 209, 213, 241, 275, 282, 300, 312.
Flax, 176, 213, 241, 275, 282, 297, 302, 312.
Pumpkin, 213, 223, 241, 312.
Sesame, 213, 312.
Sunflower, 213, 241, 312.
Selenium, 102, 232, 233.
Self-Hate, 9, 135, 136, 200.
Self-Love, 222, 243, 274, 349.
Self-Righteousness, 39, 136, 252, 321, 322, 323, 324, 325, 326, 331, 335, 346.
Self-Sabotage, 267, 276, 359, 360, 361.
Senate, U.S., 70, 163, 229.
Serotonin, 124, 226, 287.
Shalom, 10, 44, 340.
Shellfish, 34, 35, 132, 161, 212, 367.
Shopping List, 3, 211, 212, 243, 293.
SIBO, 179.
Side Effects, 58, 59, 66, 193, 260.
Sin/Sinner, 18, 26, 33, 37, 39, 44, 75, 76, 187, 188, 321, 327, 330, 333, 335, 350, 352, 356.
Sing, 22, 199, 347, 348, 354.
Sjogren's Syndrome, 129.
Skin, 58, 121, 130, 143, 144, 146, 159, 167, 171, 204, 218, 226, 227, 232, 233, 254, 256, 257, 260, 263, 273, 274, 287, 311, 375, 376, 377, 378.

Sleep, 46, 139, 140, 141, 143, 160, 172, 218, 219, 226, 227, 228, 238, 243, 249, 250, 251, 265, 274.
Smell, *see* **Aroma/Smell/Fragrance/Odor.**
Snacks, 101, 131, 173, 175, 208, 209, 237, 238, 268, 269, 300.
Soaking/Sprouting, 162, 213, 241, 283, 300, 312.
Soda, 82, 95, 115, 162, 227, 228, 281.
Soil, 69, 70, 163, 321.
Solanine, 106.
Soul, 1, 3, 9, 10, 11, 12, 23, 26, 43, 60, 65, 74, 155, 183, 191, 192, 198, 202, 339, 341, 342, 343, 344, 345, 346, 347, 348, 350, 351, 352, 353, 354, 355, 356, 357.
Soy/Soybeans, 67, 68, 85, 86, 97, 98, 99, 100, 132, 168, 174, 209, 230, 269, 281, 292, 312, 371.
Milk, *see* **Milk: Soy.**
Oil, *see* **Oil: Soybean.**
Spices, 44, 46, 90, 190, 191, 197, 214, 242, 246, 285, 286, 287, 288, 300, 313, 315.
Spirit/Spiritual, 3, 4, 7, 9, 12, 19, 21, 23, 28, 29, 34, 38, 40, 41, 44, 49, 62, 63, 64, 74, 75, 76, 135, 136, 138, 139, 151, 155, 159, 171, 183, 187, 191, 192, 196, 197, 198, 199, 202, 203, 239, 331, 333, 337, 340, 341, 342, 348, 367.

INDEX

Standard American Diet / (SAD), 3, 88, 93, 277.
Steel Roller Mill, 83, 278.
Steroids, 61, 106, 120, 131, 141.
Stevia, 80, 161, 213, 223, 281, 297, 298, 300, 306, 314, 317, 372.
Stomach, 72, 106, 108, 115, 123, 124, 139, 150, 167, 179, 275, 287, 336.
Stomach Upset, *see* **Digestive Upset.**
Stress, 120, 124, 140, 174, 201, 203, 218, 225, 238, 241, 242, 275, 287, 288.
Stroke, 80, 82, 114, 147, 286.
Strongholds, 74, 137, 252, 253, 330, 346.
Sugar, 4, 68, 80, 100, 101, 114, 120, 131, 132, 161, 162, 178, 208, 221, 222, 223, 224, 225, 227, 239, 260, 268, 269, 281, 292, 314, 317, 367, 371, 373.
Sulfur, 30, 179, 219.
Sweet Potatoes, 86, 105, 131, 162, 208, 210, 212, 222, 223, 268, 279, 281, 315.
Symptoms, 46, 50, 53, 54, 59, 84, 88, 105, 106, 107, 108, 119, 120, 130, 131, 136, 140, 141, 143, 144, 145, 146, 147, 149, 150, 159, 160, 164, 167, 168, 171, 172, 173, 177, 185, 193, 194, 203, 218, 221, 223, 224, 226, 227, 239, 263, 264, 267, 273, 274, 275, 276, 280, 296, 311, 367.

Autoimmune Disorder, 88, 131, 149, 218, 264.
Detox/Withdrawal, 160, 168, 171, 172, 221, 223, 224, 226, 227, 273, 274, 275, 276.
Fibromyalgia, 130, 140, 141.
Food Intolerance, 167, 173, 280, 296, 311.
IBS, 149, 150, 311.
Leaky Gut Disorder, 119, 120.
Nightshade Sensitivity, 105, 106, 107, 108.
Psoriasis/Eczema, 130, 177, 311.
Thyroid Disease, 130, 143, 144, 145, 146.
Taste Buds, 131, 224.
Tea, 71, 162, 183, 210, 214, 227, 228, 242, 246, 281, 307, 308.
Teeth, 47, 160, 161, 172, 251, 254, 260, 261, 262, 266, 376, 377, 378.
Teflon™, 164, 376, 378.
Thoughts, 9, 15, 27, 22, 25, 26, 28, 73, 74, 123, 136, 137, 138, 155, 187, 201, 250, 251, 252, 253, 329, 330, 331, 342, 343, 346, 347, 349, 354.
  Toxic, *see* **Toxic: Thoughts.**
Thyroid, 99, 100, 106, 120, 121, 129, 130, 135, 140, 143, 144, 145, 146, 260, 261, 288.
  Hyper, 99, 121, 130, 143.
  Hypo, 99, 121, 130, 140, 143, 144, 145, 146, 260.
Tomatine, 106.
Tomatoes, 105, 106.
Tongue, Physical, 160, 172, 356.

INDEX

Tongue, Speech, 74, 345, 356.
Tower Garden®, 163, 164.
Toxic,
  Ingredients / Products / Food, 44, 48, 68, 171, 251, 254, 255, 256, 257, 258, 259, 260, 261, 264, 274, 375, 376, 379.
  People, 253.
  Thoughts, 187, 201, 250, 251, 252, 253, 330, 346.
Toxicity, 53, 256, 291.
  Environmental, 241,
Toxicology, 48, 256.
Toxins, 2, 4, 5, 11, 35, 62, 100, 110, 135, 150, 155, 156, 159, 160, 162, 168, 171, 172, 178, 209, 219, 226, 227, 238, 247, 251, 261, 262, 263, 264, 265, 273, 274, 275, 276, 289, 333, 379.
  Environmental, 251.
  Exposure, 2, 4, 5, 62, 155, 156, 238, 251.
  Food, 100, 110, 162, 209, 226, 251, 289, 333.
  Reducing, 4, 11, 135, 155, 156, 159, 168, 171, 251.
  Releasing, 150, 160, 172, 227, 265, 273, 274, 276.
Triggers, 87, 88, 123, 140, 158, 171, 200, 201, 228, 296, 361.
  Emotional, 201, 361.
  Environmental, 200, 201.
  Fibromyalgia, 140.
  Food, 87, 88, 168, 171, 228, 296.
Triglycerides, 102, 232, 235, 288.

Turmeric, 71, 179, 214, 224, 242, 285, 286, 299, 301, 313, 317.
Undigested Proteins, 88, 119, 129, 149.
USDA, 68, 69, 70, 93, 133, 223, 226, 229, 371,
Vaginal Dryness, 146.
Vegan Protein, 209, 312.
Vegan/Vegetarian, 102, 209, 217, 268, 312.
Vegetables, 30, 79, 94, 105, 106, 107, 108, 113, 131, 156, 159, 163, 165, 208, 209, 210, 211, 212, 214, 222, 231, 233, 242, 259, 268, 279, 282, 283, 315, 371.
Vitamins, 58, 61, 80, 83, 102, 114, 121, 179, 132, 233, 275, 313, 314, 371, 372.
  Vitamin A, 132, 233, 275, 313.
  Vitamin B, 61, 102, 121, 179, 132, 233, 313, 371, 372.
  Vitamin C, 61, 80, 102, 275, 313, 314.
  Vitamin D, 61, 233.
  Vitamin E, 61, 102, 132, 233, 275, 372.
  Vitamin K, 233, 313.
Vitiligo, 135.
Water, 62, 69, 87, 90, 91, 93, 114, 132, 150, 162, 163, 176, 179, 180, 181, 182, 204, 207, 210, 211, 214, 222, 227, 246, 247, 251, 255, 257, 258, 259, 260, 261, 262, 274, 275, 281, 282, 297, 300, 302, 304, 309, 311, 312, 314, 316, 336, 353, 375.

Pollution, 62, 69, 87, 91, 93, 114, 251, 255, 260, 261, 262, 336.
Weaning, 92, 225, 227.
Weight Gain/Loss, 72, 87, 115, 135, 144, 145, 167, 177, 229, 237, 238, 239, 260, 311, 349, 359, 367.
Wellness, 1, 2, 3, 4, 7, 9, 44, 155, 185, 203, 262, 276, 313, 367.
Wheat, 83, 84, 85, 86, 87, 89, 90, 209, 278.
  Einkorn, 84, 85, 87.
  Hybridized, 83, 84, 86.
Whey, 102, 312, 372.
Wise/Wisdom, 11, 17, 18, 20, 26, 27, 35, 205, 222, 325, 332, 336, 355, 356.
Word of God,
  see **God's Word**
Worry, 16, 22, 200, 252, 261, 345, 346.
Yeast, 70, 120, 161, 168, 174.
Yoga, 266.
Yogurt, 95, 100, 207, 222.
Zinc, 61, 120,

INDEX

ABOUT THE AUTHOR

Carol Adamy Rundle grew up in New York with her parents and two younger brothers, dreaming of being a teacher. After graduating from the State University of New York at Oswego with a Bachelor of Science degree in Elementary Education, she embarked on a teaching career.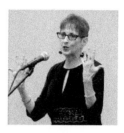

Carol has spent most of her life learning and teaching about God's love for people. As a follower of Jesus Christ, she was ordained to the non-denominational Christian ministry in 2002.

While recovering from multiple health problems (see Author's Note and Introduction), she attended the Institute of Nutritional Leadership for health coaching, so she could teach others what she had learned about being in health.

Carol lives in beautiful Tucson, Arizona with her husband, Bob. She enjoys doing counted cross stitch, researching family genealogy, and exploring the wonders of God's creation. This book is a culmination of her life-long love for God and for teaching.

Be in Health

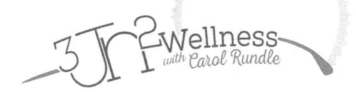

Join me on my Facebook page at Facebook.com/3Jn2Wellness.

Follow my blog at http://3Jn2Wellness.com.

Reach out to me at Carol@3Jn2Wellness.com.

ENDNOTES

Introduction
1. https://www.ncbi.nlm.nih.gov/pubmed/12610534

Chapter 3 – God's Original Eating Plan for Mankind
1. https://www.vivahealth.org.uk/wheat-eaters-or-meat-eaters/length-digestive-tract
2. https://www.livestrong.com/article/317807-sulphur-/ detox

Chapter 4 – The Dietary Laws of the Old Testament
1. Meinz, David, *Eating by the Book*, P. 225.
2. https://www.mcgill.ca/oss/article/did-you-know/rabbits-eat-their-own-poop
3. https://draxe.com/why-you-should-avoid-pork/
4. https://drericz.com/eating-shellfish/

Chapter 6 – Health Care or Sick Care?
1. https://en.wikipedia.org/wiki/Doctor_(title)
2. https://www.britannica.com/science/history-of-medicine/Hellenistic-and-Roman-medicine
3. https://www.history.com/topics/medici-family
4. https://en.wikipedia.org/wiki/History_of_medicine
5. http://mediciproject.org/medici-influence/
6. https://en.wikipedia.org/wiki/Barber_surgeon
7. https://en.wikipedia.org/wiki/Black_Death
8. https://en.wikipedia.org/wiki/Barber%27s_pole#Origin_in_barbering_and_surgery
9. https://en.wikipedia.org/wiki/Barber%27s_pole#Use_in_barbering
10. http://www.nbcnews.com/id/5319129/ns/health-health_care/t/fda-approves-leeches-medical-devices/#.WvKXU4iUs2w
11. https://en.wikipedia.org/wiki/History_of_medicine#Paracelsus
12. Webster, Charles (1995). "Paracelsus. Confronts the Saints: Miracles, Healing and the Secularization of Magic". Social History of Medicine. 8 (3): 403–21. doi:10.1093/shm/8.3.403. PMID 11609052.
13. https://en.wikipedia.org/wiki/Paracelsus
14. https://www.bl.uk/the-middle-ages/articles/medicine-diagnosis-and-treatment-in-the-middle-ages
15. Paracelsus, dritte defensio, 1538
16. Roy Porter, The Greatest Benefit to Mankind (1997), 201–11
17. https://en.wikipedia.org/wiki/Rosicrucianism
18. https://www.britannica.com/topic/Rosicrucians

ENDNOTES

19 https://en.wikipedia.org/wiki/The_Occult_Roots_of_Nazism
20 https://www.amazon.com/Occult-Roots-Nazism-Ariosophists-1890-1935/dp/0850304024
21 https://www.coursehero.com/file/p50olg/Few-effective-drugs-existed-beyond-opium-and-quinine-Folklore-cures-and/
22 https://en.wikipedia.org/wiki/The_Agnew_Clinic
23 http://journalofethics.ama-assn.org/2007/04/mhst1-0704.html
24 https://en.wikipedia.org/wiki/Joseph_Lister
25 https://en.wikipedia.org/wiki/Flexner_Report
26 https://en.wikipedia.org/wiki/The_Carnegie_Foundation_for_the_Advancement_of_Teaching
27 http://in-training.org/drugged-greed-pharmaceutical-industrys-role-us-medical-education-10639
28 https://www.ncbi.nlm.nih.gov/pubmed/21629685
29 https://www.tandfonline.com/toc/zme020/current
30 https://www.ncbi.nlm.nih.gov/pubmed/21629685
31 https://journals.lww.com/academicmedicine/Fulltext/2004/11000/Medical_Students__Exposure_to_Pharmaceutical.5.aspx
32 https://www.tandfonline.com/toc/zme020/current
33 https://journals.lww.com/academicmedicine/Fulltext/2004/11000/Medical_Students__Exposure_to_Pharmaceutical.5.aspx
34 https://www.onegreenplanet.org/natural-health/how-medical-school-funding-from-big-pharma-impacts-your-health/
35 https://www.bostonglobe.com/news/nation/2015/08/05/doctors-lobby-keep-lid-secrecy-industry-payments-for-medical-education/pP9NiZVTATh2sCygbG7V8O/story.html
36 https://clintransmed.springeropen.com/articles/10.1186/s40169-018-0193-6
37 http://www.wollheim-memorial.de/en/entstehung_der_deutschen_farbenindustrie_en
38 https://www.sciencehistory.org/distillations/magazine/a-brief-history-of-chemical-war
39 https://www.sciencehistory.org/distillations/magazine/a-brief-history-of-chemical-war
40 https://answersingenesis.org/charles-darwin/racism/darwinism-and-the-nazi-race-holocaust/
41 https://www.ushmm.org/wlc/en/article.php?ModuleId=10005143
42 https://www.ushmm.org/wlc/en/article.php?ModuleId=10005276
43 https://www.ushmm.org/wlc/en/article.php?ModuleId=10005200
44 https://www.ushmm.org/outreach/en/article.php?ModuleId=10007683
45 http://www.dailymail.co.uk/news/article-3266090/Revealed-dark-history-Hitler-s-death-camp-Nazis-murdered-psychiatric-patients-nurses-test-gas-chambers-used-mass-extermination-Jews.html
46 https://en.wikipedia.org/wiki/Religion_in_Nazi_Germany

ENDNOTES

47 https://archive.nytimes.com/www.nytimes.com/books/first/p/proctor-cancer.html?_r=2
48 https://en.wikipedia.org/wiki/Operation_Paperclip
49 https://en.wikipedia.org/wiki/Operation_Paperclip
50 https://en.wikipedia.org/wiki/IG_Farben
51 https://en.wikipedia.org/wiki/IG_Farben
52 https://en.wikipedia.org/wiki/IG_Farben
53 https://en.wikipedia.org/wiki/Petroleum_product
54 https://articles.mercola.com/sites/articles/archive/2011/02/24/are-you-or-your-family-eating-toxic-food-dyes.aspx
55 https://www.truthinaging.com/review/cosmetic-colors-and-dyes-which-ones-are-safe
56 https://wonderopolis.org/wonder/what-is-medicine-made-from
57 https://www.alternet.org/story/147318/100,000_americans_die_each_year_from_prescription_drugs_while_pharma_companies_get_rich
58 https://www.poison.org/poison-statistics-national
59 http://www.mdpi.com/1999-4923/10/1/36
60 https://chriskresser.com/why-your-genes-arent-your-destiny/

Chapter 7 – The Church. Under Assault
1 http://www.nongmoproject.org/learn-more/what-is-gmo/
2 http://responsibletechnology.org/10-reasons-to-avoid-gmos/
3 http://responsibletechnology.org/10-reasons-to-avoid-gmos/
4 http://naturalsociety.com/gmo-crop-contamination-cannot-be-stopped/
5 https://chipsahospital.org/glyphosate-a-potential-deadly-cause-of-everything-from-cancer-to-infertility-pt-1/
6 https://grist.org/article/2009-07-08-monsanto-fda-taylor/
7 https://www.coursehero.com/file/p11vn3g/Contention-6-The-biotech-industry-uses-tobacco-science-to-claim-product-safety/
8 https://www.coursehero.com/file/p7c95872/Contention-8-Independent-research-and-reporting-is-attacked-and-suppressed/
9 https://www.onegreenplanet.org/environment/how-do-gmos-impact-people-and-the-environment/
10 https://www.scientificamerican.com/article/widely-used-herbicide-linked-to-cancer/
11 https://www.ers.usda.gov/data-products/adoption-of-genetically-engineered-crops-in-the-us/recent-trends-in-ge-adoption.aspx
12 https://gmoanswers.com/current-gmo-crops
13 https://www.ecowatch.com/gmo-apples-arctic-2507751729.html
14 http://time.com/3840073/gmo-food-charts/
15 https://www.facebook.com/GMOFreeUSA/
16 https://gmoanswers.com/glyphosate-carcinogen-explained

ENDNOTES

[17] https://www.scientificamerican.com/article/newborn-babies-chemicals-exposure-bpa/
[18] https://articles.mercola.com/sites/articles/archive/2014/04/22/glyphosate-herbicide.aspx
[19] https://www.ams.usda.gov/services/organic-certification/becoming-certified
[20] https://organic.org/faqs/
[21] https://organic.org/faqs/
[22] https://thetruthaboutcancer.com/america-worst-food-quality-safety/
[23] http://betterhealththruresearch.com/USSenateDocument.htm
[24] http://www.fao.org/wairdocs/x5008e/x5008e01.htm
[25] https://thetruthaboutcancer.com/america-worst-food-quality-safety/
[26] http://www.elephantjournal.com/2015/03/are-you-celiac-gluten-intolerant-or-actually-being-poisoned/
[27] http://www.thedailybeast.com/articles/2013/03/01/our-unsafe-food-supply-is-killing-us.html
[28] http://ecowatch.com/2015/01/12/rid-planet-gmos-Roundup/
[29] https://foodrevolution.org/blog/how-to-fight-prevent-cancer-with-mushrooms/
[30] http://www.anticancerbook.com/post/Green-tea-and-mushrooms_-89-less-breast-cancer.html
[31] https://www.ncbi.nlm.nih.gov/pmc/articles/PMC2781139/
[32] http://theantimedia.org/congress-sneaks-new-monsanto-protection-act-into-sweeping-environmetal-bill/
[33] http://www.bbc.com/news/health-36518770

Chapter 9 – Why I Avoid Processed Food

[1] https://authoritynutrition.com/why-processed-meat-is-bad/
[2] https://www.livescience.com/36057-truth-nitrites-lunch-meat-preservatives.html
[3] https://www.epa.gov/sites/production/files/2014-03/documents/pahs_factsheet_cdc_2013.pdf
[4] https://www.sciencedirect.com/topics/pharmacology-toxicology-and-pharmaceutical-science/heterocyclic-amine
[5] https://www.cancer.gov/about-cancer/causes-prevention/risk/diet/cooked-meats-fact-sheet
[6] https://www.myfooddata.com/articles/what-foods-high-sodium.php
[7] https://www.myfooddata.com/articles/what-foods-high-sodium.php
[8] http://www.realfarmacy.com/annies-sells-gmo-giant-general-mills/
[9] https://www.four-h.purdue.edu/foods/Diet-Related%20Diseases.htm
[10] https://www.healthypeople.gov/2020/leading-health-indicators/2020-lhi-topics/Nutrition-Physical-Activity-and-Obesity
[11] https://www.cdc.gov/heartdisease/facts.htm

[12] https://www.helpguide.org/articles/diet-weight-loss/heart-healthy-diet-tips.htm

Chapter 10 – Wheat: The Staff of Life
[1] http://www.namamillers.org/education/wheat-milling-process/
[2] https://en.wikipedia.org/wiki/Norman_Borlaug
[3] https://celiac.org/celiac-disease/understanding-celiac-disease-2/what-is-celiac-disease/
[4] http://whfoods.org/genpage.php?tname=dailytip&dbid=388&utm_source=rss_reader&utm_medium=rss&utm_campaign=rss_feed
[5] https://www.einkorn.com/is-einkorn-flour-gluten-free/
[6] https://www.ncbi.nlm.nih.gov/pubmed/23535596
[7] https://en.wikipedia.org/wiki/List_of_edible_seeds
[8] https://dese.mo.gov/sites/default/files/whataregrains.pdf
[9] http://whfoods.org/genpage.php?tname=dailytip&dbid=388&utm_source=rss_reader&utm_medium=rss&utm_campaign=rss_feed
[10] https://lifespa.com/ancient-vs-modern-wheat-frankenwheat-myth/
[11] http://sitn.hms.harvard.edu/flash/2018/asked-whats-deal-gluten/
[12] https://www.ecowatch.com/why-is-glyphosate-sprayed-on-crops-right-before-harvest-1882187755.html
[13] https://gmoanswers.com/glyphosate-carcinogen-explained
[14] https://www.scientificamerican.com/article/newborn-babies-chemicals-exposure-bpa/
[15] https://articles.mercola.com/sites/articles/archive/2014/04/22/glyphosate-herbicide.aspx
[16] https://www.theatlantic.com/health/archive/2017/05/gluten-research/526335/
[17] https://www.webmd.com/digestive-disorders/features/leaky-gut-syndrome#1
[18] http://www.functionalps.com/blog/2011/11/20/endotoxin-and-liver-health/

Chapter 11 – Dairy Products: Yea or Nay?
[1] https://archive.org/details/everydaylifeinolooinheat
[2] http://www.fonddulacfarms.com/2-uncategorised/35-livestock-nutritionist-defends-raw-milk-safety
[3] https://archive.org/details/figuresofspeechuoobull
[4] http://www.ucl.ac.uk/news/news-articles/0908/09082801
[5] http://www.truth-out.org/news/item/31835-the-surprising-history-of-milk
[6] https://io.wp.com/www.3jn2wellness.com/wp-content/uploads/2017/05/Milk-Infographic.gif?ssl=1
[7] https://www.motherjones.com/environment/2014/03/a1-milk-a2-milk-america/
[8] https://bodyecology.com/articles/healing-leaky-gut

ENDNOTES

9. https://www.mygenefood.com/dairy-dangers-sheep-goat-dairy-healthier-cow-dairy/
10. https://draxe.com/raw-milk-benefits/
11. https://bodyecology.com/articles/avoid_pasteurized_foods.php

Chapter 12 – Soy.: Friend or Foe?
1. http://ncsoy.org/media-resources/history-of-soybeans/
2. https://en.wikipedia.org/wiki/Genetically_modified_soybean
3. https://www.ers.usda.gov/data-products/adoption-of-genetically-engineered-crops-in-the-us/recent-trends-in-ge-adoption.aspx
4. https://modernfarmer.com/2016/02/imported-edamame/
5. https://www.goodhousekeeping.com/health/diet-nutrition/a20707020/is-soy-good-or-bad-for-you/
6. https://www.ncbi.nlm.nih.gov/pmc/articles/PMC3930722/
7. https://onlinelibrary.wiley.com/doi/abs/10.1002/cncr.30615
8. https://academic.oup.com/jcem/article-lookup/doi/10.1210/jc.2015-3473
9. https://www.ncbi.nlm.nih.gov/pmc/articles/PMC3139237/
10. http://lpi.oregonstate.edu/mic/dietary-factors/phytochemicals/soy-isoflavones#food-sources
11. http://www.menopause.org/docs/default-source/2014/soy-vms-equol.pdf
12. http://www.heart.org/idc/groups/heart-public/@wcm/@adv/documents/downloadable/ucm_312848.pdf
13. https://www.fda.gov/NewsEvents/Newsroom/PressAnnouncements/ucm582744.htm
14. https://www.globalhealingcenter.com/natural-health/5-ways-soy-upsets-hormone-balance/#references
15. https://www.ncbi.nlm.nih.gov/pmc/articles/PMC3443957/
16. Valladares L, Garrido A, Sierralta W. Soy isoflavones and human health: breast cancer and puberty timing. Rev Med Chil. 2012 Apr;140(4):512-6. doi: 10.4067/S0034-98872012000400014.
17. https://www.niehs.nih.gov/health/topics/agents/sya-soy-formula/
18. Siepmann T, Roofeh J, Kiefer FW, Edelson DG. Hypogonadism and erectile dysfunction associated with soy product consumption. Nutrition. 2011 Jul-Aug;27(7-8):859-62. doi: 10.1016/j.nut.2010.10.018.
19. Chavarro JE, Toth TL, Sadio SM, Hauser R. Soy food and isoflavone intake in relation to semen quality parameters among men from an infertility clinic. Hum Reprod. 2008 Nov;23(11):2584-90. doi: 10.1093/humrep/den243.
20. Russo J, Russo IH. The role of estrogen in the initiation of breast cancer.. J Steroid Biochem Mol Biol. 2006 Dec;102(1-5):89-96.
21. https://www.zerobreastcancer.org/research/bcerc_factsheets_phytoestrogen_genistein.pdf
22. https://www.ncbi.nlm.nih.gov/pmc/articles/PMC5646220/
23. https://www.ncbi.nlm.nih.gov/pubmed/16571087

24 Doerge, D.; Chang, H. Inactivation of thyroid peroxidase by soy. isoflavones, in vitro and in vivo. J. Chromatogr. B Anal. Technol. Biomed. Life Sci. 2002, 777, 269–279.
25 https://articles.mercola.com/sites/articles/archive/2017/11/13/soy-health-food-or-not.aspx
26 https://articles.mercola.com/sites/articles/archive/2017/11/13/soy-health-food-or-not.aspx
27 https://articles.mercola.com/sites/articles/archive/2016/07/18/health-benefits-fermented-foods.aspx
28 https://www.niehs.nih.gov/health/topics/agents/sya-soy-formula/

Chapter 13 – The Advantages of Coconut Milk
1 https://draxe.com/coconut-milk-nutrition/
2 https://www.bbcgoodfood.com/howto/guide/ingredient-focus-coconut-milk
3 https://www.ncbi.nlm.nih.gov/pubmed/12634436
4 https://www.westonaprice.org/health-topics/soy-alert/the-brilliance-and-courage-of-dr-mary-enig/
5 https://www.ncbi.nlm.nih.gov/pubmed/24282632
6 https://www.livestrong.com/article/523545-is-coconut-milk-good-for-the-bowels/

Chapter 14 – Avoiding Nightshades
1 https://en.wikipedia.org/wiki/Solanine
2 https://en.wikipedia.org/wiki/Acetylcholinesterase_inhibitor
3 https://en.wikipedia.org/wiki/Solanine#Symptoms
4 https://draxe.com/nightshade-vegetables/
5 https://www.sciencedirect.com/science/article/pii/0738081X9190078Y
6 https://www.sciencedirect.com/science/article/pii/S0014299913008200
7 https://www.ncbi.nlm.nih.gov/pubmed/24941673
8 https://draxe.com/nightshade-vegetables/
9 https://draxe.com/nightshade-vegetables/
10 https://www.ncbi.nlm.nih.gov/pubmed/12479649
11 https://www.webmd.com/arthritis/features/arthritis-diet-claims-fact-fiction#1
12 https://www.ncbi.nlm.nih.gov/pubmed/10632656

Chapter 15 – Just Say No to Bacon
1 https://en.wikipedia.org/wiki/List_of_IARC_Group_1_carcinogens
2 https://en.wikipedia.org/wiki/List_of_IARC_Group_1_carcinogens
3 https://www.splendidtable.org/story/inside-the-factory-farm-where-97-of-us-pigs-are-raised

ENDNOTES

Chapter 16 – The Dangers of Fast Food
1. https://www.cnpp.usda.gov/healthyeatingindex
2. https://responsibletechnology.org/10-reasons-to-avoid-gmos/
3. https://www.reuters.com/investigates/special-report/who-iarc-glyphosate/
4. https://www.scientificamerican.com/article/newborn-babies-chemicals-exposure-bpa/
5. http://www.careersinpublichealth.net/comparing-fast-food-nutrition
6. https://www.four-h.purdue.edu/foods/Diet-Related%20Diseases.htm
7. https://www.healthypeople.gov/2020/leading-health-indicators/2020-lhi-topics/Nutrition-Physical-Activity-and-Obesity
8. https://www.cdc.gov/heartdisease/facts.htm
9. https://www.helpguide.org/articles/diet-weight-loss/heart-healthy-diet-tips.htm
10. https://www.thesimpledollar.com/dont-eat-out-as-often-188365/
11. https://www.csmonitor.com/Business/The-Simple-Dollar/2012/0710/Common-dollars-and-sense-Eating-less-fast-food-does-a-body-good
12. http://www.bbc.com/news/health-36518770

Chapter 17 – "All Disease Begins in the Gut"
1. https://www.ncbi.nlm.nih.gov/pmc/articles/PMC3637398/
2. https://www.ncbi.nlm.nih.gov/pubmed/25162769
3. https://www.ncbi.nlm.nih.gov/pubmed/?term=intestinal+permeability
4. https://www.ncbi.nlm.nih.gov/pubmed/25695388
5. https://www.google.com/webhp?sourceid=chrome-instant&ion=1&espv=2&ie=UTF-8#q=International+Journal+of+ gastroenterology+and+ Hepatology+2006
6. http://foodintegritynow.org/2015/05/27/leaky-gut-is-it-becoming-an-epidemic/

Chapter 18 – Your Gut: Your Second Brain
1. https://www.hopkinsmedicine.org/health/healthy_aging/healthy_body/the-brain-gut-connection
2. http://www.hopkinsmedicine.org/health/healthy_aging/healthy_body/the-brain-gut-connection
3. http://www.psyking.net/id17.htm
4. http://www.psyking.net/id36.htm
5. http://www.psyking.net/id36.htm
6. https://www.eeb.ucla.edu/evmed/indivfaculty.php?f=mayer

Chapter 19 – Why Does the Body Attack Itself?
1. https://en.wikipedia.org/wiki/Autoimmunity
2. https://www.ncbi.nlm.nih.gov/pmc/articles/PMC3637398/
3. https://www.ncbi.nlm.nih.gov/pubmed/25162769

4. https://www.ncbi.nlm.nih.gov/pubmed/?term=intestinal+permeability
5. https://www.ncbi.nlm.nih.gov/pubmed/25695388
6. https://www.google.com/webhp?sourceid=chrome-instant&ion=1&espv=2&ie=UTF-8#q=International+Journal+of+Gastroenterology+and+Hepatology+2006
7. http://www.nongmoproject.org/gmo-facts/
8. http://articles.mercola.com/sites/articles/archive/2009/04/21/msg-is-this-silent-killer-lurking-in-your-kitchen-cabinets.Aspx
9. http://bodyecology.com/articles/avoid_pasteurized_foods.php
10. http://www.ecowatch.com/house-passes-dark-act-banning-states-from-requiring-gmo-labels-on-food- 1882075093. Html

Chapter 21 – I Hurt All Over. Do I Have Fibromyalgia?
1. https://www.fasciablaster.com/blogs/blog/fascia
2. http://blog.arthritis.org/living-with-arthritis/symptoms-fibromyalgia-triggers-treatment/
1. https://www.healthline.com/health/common-thyroid-disorders
2. https://thyroidpharmacist.com/
3. https://thyroidpharmacist.com/resources/
4. https://drchristianson.com/basal-body-temperature-for-thyroid-function-a-comprehensive-guide/
5. https://thyroidpharmacist.com/articles/top-9-things-id-say-to-a-friend-newly-diagnosed-with-hashimotos/
6. https://thyroidpharmacist.com/articles/what-to-do-if-your-tsh-is-normal-and-you-are-anything-but/
7. JAMA. 2002 Jul 17;288(3):321-33
8. JAMA. 2004 Apr 14;291(14):1701-12
9. https://www.foreverhealth.com/blogs/forever-health/69756997-a-brief-history-of-hormone-replacement-therapy
10. Breast Cancer Res Treat. 2008 Jan;107(1):103-11

Chapter 23 – What Can Be Done About IBS
1. https://www.ncbi.nlm.nih.gov/pubmed/25162769
2. https://www.ncbi.nlm.nih.gov/pubmed/?term=intestinal+permeability
3. https://www.ncbi.nlm.nih.gov/pubmed/25695388
4. https://tinyurl.com/icp-myyl
5. https://tinyurl.com/ComfortTone-yl
6. https://tinyurl.com/AlkaLime-YL
7. https://tinyurl.com/AlkaLime-YL

Chapter 25 – How I Changed What I Eat
1. https://draxe.com/eating-tilapia-is-worse-than-eating-bacon/
2. http://www.ewg.org/foodnews/

ENDNOTES

3. http://www.thegraciouspantry.com/organic-vs-sustainable/
4. http://draxe.com/sprout/
5. https://www.drweil.com/diet-nutrition/food-safety/perplexed-about-peanuts/
6. https://www.mindbodygreen.com/0-13454/3-reasons-no-one-should-be-on-a-raw-foods-diet.html
7. http://www.bottledwater.org/fluoride
8. http://www.npr.org/2011/03/02/134196209/study-most-plastics-leach-hormone-like-chemicals
9. http://www.drmitraray.com/q-a/q-and-a-the-tower-garden/
10. http://betterhealththruresearch.com/USSenateDocument.htm
11. http://tibbs.unc.edu/ask-a-toxicologist-is-it-safe-to-use-teflon-pans/
12. http://tibbs.unc.edu/ask-a-toxicologist-is-it-safe-to-use-teflon-pans/
13. http://www.globalhealingcenter.com/natural-health/why-you-should-never-microwave-your-food/

Chapter 26 – Food Allergy or Food Intolerance?
1. https://www.allergyscope.com/?gclid=CjwKEAjw1Iq6BRDYtK-9OjdmBESJABlz0Y7onBiYMaqx7wXm9aaZ_tYq5-imOJyiJ6iQDb35JY8rhoCaXXw_wcB

Chapter 28 – Cleansing and Maintaining the Colon
1. https://www.healthline.com/nutrition/8-health-benefits-of-probiotics#section7
2. https://www.cbsnews.com/news/parasites-causing-infections-in-the-us-cdc-says/
3. https://tinyurl.com/ParaFree-YL
4. https://tinyurl.com/spearmintEO-YL
5. https://tinyurl.com/PeppermintEO-YL
6. https://tinyurl.com/super-B-yl
7. http://tinyurl.com/sulfurzyme
8. https://www.psychologytoday.com/us/blog/in-the-zone/201204/what-are-the-real-differences-between-epa-and-dha
9. http://www.listentoyourgut.com/symptoms/16/diarrhea.html
10. https://tinyurl.com/GingerVitality
11. https://tinyurl.com/PeppermintEO-YL
12. https://tinyurl.com/DigizeVitality
13. https://tinyurl.com/LemonEO-Vitality
14. https://tinyurl.com/spearmintEO-YL
15. Deardeuff, LeAnne, *Inner Transformations Using Essential Oils.*
16. Deardeuff, LeAnne, *Inner Transformations Using Essential Oils.*
17. https://tinyurl.com/CleansingKitTrio
18. https://amzn.to/2rCRWK4

ENDNOTES

Chapter 29 – Benefits of Essential Oils for Body, Soul, and Spirit
1. https://www.rebootedmom.com/how-do-essential-oils-affect-emotions/
2. https://en.wikipedia.org/wiki/Ebers_Papyrus
3. https://www.curezone.org/forums/fm.asp?i=839144
4. Stewart, David, *Healing Oils of the Bible*, p. 30.
5. https://www.curezone.org/forums/fm.asp?i=839144
6. Stewart, David, *Healing Oils of the Bible*, p. 268.
7. http://www.faithfuldroppers.com/2016/05/hyssop/
8. Stewart, David, *Healing Oils of the Bible*, p. 141ff.
9. https://en.wikipedia.org/wiki/Plague_doctor
10. https://en.wikipedia.org/wiki/Miasma_theory
11. https://en.wikipedia.org/wiki/Plague_doctor
12. https://en.wikipedia.org/wiki/Galen
13. https://en.wikipedia.org/wiki/Galen
14. http://essentialoilsacademy.com/history/
15. https://www.omicsonline.org/open-access/detecting-essential-oil-adulteration-jreac.1000132.php?aid=40867
16. https://en.wikipedia.org/wiki/Resonance
17. https://mychronicrelief.com/holy-anointing-oil-cannabis/
18. https://www.telegraph.co.uk/news/science/science-news/10486479/Phobias-may-be-memories-passed-down-in-genes-from-ancestors.html
19. https://articles.mercola.com/sites/articles/archive/2015/03/14/trapped-emotional-energy.aspx
20. https://aroma-freedom.myshopify.com/pages/about-us
21. Magiera, Janet M., *The Armor of Victory*, p. 134-135.

Chapter 31 – My Shopping List
1. https://www.produceretailer.com/article/news-article/2018-dirty-dozen-and-clean-15-lists-released

Chapter 32 – The Amazing Health Benefits of Bone Broth
1. https://www.yogajournal.com/practice/ask-expert-vegetarian-bone-broth
2. https://www.foodrenegade.com/gelatin-inflammation/
3. https://www.ncbi.nlm.nih.gov/pubmed/8378772
4. https://well.blogs.nytimes.com/2007/10/12/the-science-of-chicken-soup/
5. https://www.nih.gov/
6. https://blog.kettleandfire.com/bone-broth-balances-glycine-and-methionine/
7. http://medmetricsrx.com/bone-broth-optimal-health-5-benefits-need-know/
8. https://www.cdc.gov/prc/index.htm
9. https://draxe.com/the-healing-power-of-bone-broth-for-digestion-arthritis-and-cellulite/

ENDNOTES

Chapter 33 – How to Overcome a Sugar Addiction
10. https://draxe.com/anti-inflammatory-foods/
11. https://www.westonaprice.org/health-topics/why-broth-is-beautiful-essential-roles-for-proline-glycine-and-gelatin/
1. https://articles.mercola.com/sites/articles/archive/2016/04/23/cut-down-sugar-consumption.aspx
2. https://www.youtube.com/watch?v=p2yCGuaI6c8
3. https://www.medicalnewstoday.com/articles/320156.php
4. https://www.mindbodygreen.com/articles/how-to-stop-sugar-cravings
5. https://www.ncbi.nlm.nih.gov/pmc/articles/PMC5569266/
6. https://www.webmd.com/healthy-aging/features/exercise-lower-blood-sugar#1
7. https://www.mindbodygreen.com/0-14004/12-ways-to-beat-sugar-cravings-for-good.html
8. https://www.mindbodygreen.com/0-29973/this-snack-reverses-aging-and-takes-less-than-5-minutes-to-make.html
9. https://www.mindbodygreen.com/articles/how-to-stop-sugar-cravings
10. https://www.mindbodygreen.com/0-14004/12-ways-to-beat-sugar-cravings-for-good.html
11. https://www.mindbodygreen.com/articles/how-to-stop-sugar-cravings

Chapter 34 – How to Quit Coffee
1. http://www.sarahwilson.com/2015/02/10-reasons-why-coffee-might-not-be-great-if-you-have-autoimmune-disease/
2. https://www.huffingtonpost.com/dr-mark-hyman/quit-coffee_b_1598108.html
3. https://yurielkaim.com/cortisol-and-belly-fat/
4. https://coffeeconfidential.org/health/decaffeination/
5. https://www.naabt.org/faq_answers.cfm?ID=25
6. https://www.caffeineinformer.com/my-caffeine-detox
7. http://the.republicoftea.com/library/caffeine-in-tea/how-many-milligrams-of-caffeine-is-in-decaffeinated-green-tea/
8. https://www.livestrong.com/article/433642-does-coffee-really-give-you-energy/
9. https://www.prevention.com/health/a20473995/quit-caffeine-0/
10. https://www.womenshealthmag.com/health/a19982674/why-coffee-makes-you-poop/
11. https://www.prevention.com/health/a20473995/quit-caffeine-0/
12. https://www.caffeineinformer.com/benefits-quitting-caffeine

Chapter 35 – Why (The Right Kind of) Fat is Healthy
1. https://www.cdc.gov/obesity/data/prevalence-maps.html
2. http://catalog.hathitrust.org/Record/007418251

ENDNOTES

3. https://www.helpguide.org/articles/healthy-eating/choosing-healthy-fats.htm
4. https://academic.oup.com/ajcn/article/91/3/535/4597110
5. https://healthyforgood.heart.org/Eat-smart/Articles/Trans-Fat#.WK3tO_krI2w
6. https://jamanetwork.com/journals/jama/fullarticle/202340
7. https://articles.mercola.com/sites/articles/archive/2009/09/22/7-reasons-to-eat-more-saturated-fat.aspx
8. http://circ.ahajournals.org/content/early/2017/06/15/CIR.0000000000000510
9. http://blogs.plos.org/absolutely-maybe/2017/06/28/saturated-biases-where-the-aha-advice-on-coconut-oil-went-wrong/
10. http://observer.com/2017/06/new-study-coconut-oil-ldl-cholesterol-levels/
11. https://www.bmj.com/content/346/bmj.e8539
12. https://academic.oup.com/ajcn/article-abstract/36/4/617/4693514
13. https://www.ncbi.nlm.nih.gov/pubmed/18400720
14. https://www.ncbi.nlm.nih.gov/pubmed/11023005
15. https://www.incredibleegg.org/eggcyclopedia/c/color/
16. https://www.healthline.com/health/high-cholesterol/foods-to-increase-hdl
17. https://draxe.com/vitamin-e-benefits/
18. https://draxe.com/mct-oil/
19. https://bodyecology.com/articles/benefits_of_real_butter.php
20. https://www.sciencedirect.com/science/article/pii/S002203027784068X
21. https://draxe.com/ghee-benefits/
22. https://en.wikipedia.org/wiki/Margarine
23. https://www.ncbi.nlm.nih.gov/pubmed/28729812
24. https://www.healthline.com/nutrition/butter-vs-margarine
25. http://www.nejm.org/doi/full/10.1056/NEJMoa1200303?query=featured_home&
26. https://draxe.com/olive-oil-benefits/
27. http://olivecenter.ucdavis.edu/research/files/report041211finalreduced.pdf
28. http://fortune.com/2015/06/24/olive-oil-brands-lawsuits/

Chapter 36 – The Surprising Benefits of Intermittent Fasting

1. https://www.facebook.com/RawFoodForDummies/
2. https://www.ncbi.nlm.nih.gov/pubmed/28115234
3. https://news.yale.edu/2015/02/16/anti-inflammatory-mechanism-dieting-and-fasting-revealed
4. https://www.rd.com/health/wellness/intermittent-fasting-benefits/
5. https://www.rd.com/health/wellness/intermittent-fasting-benefits/
6. https://www.sciencedaily.com/releases/2017/02/170223124259.htm
7. https://www.rd.com/health/wellness/intermittent-fasting-benefits/
8. https://www.linkedin.com/pulse/5-psychological-benefits-fasting-sarah-halabi

ENDNOTES

9. http://www.psy-journal.com/article/S0165-1781(12)00815-3/abstract
10. https://www.ncbi.nlm.nih.gov/pmc/articles/PMC4931830/
11. https://medium.com/@drbradysalcido/6-surprising-brain-power-benefits-of-intermittent-fasting-49ad1bc39e04
12. http://web.stanford.edu/group/hopes/cgi-bin/hopes_test/brain-derived-neurotrophic-factor-bdnf/
13. https://proteinpower.com/drmike/2006/09/13/fast-way-to-better-health/

Chapter 37 – The 10 Best Anti-Inflammation Foods
1. https://bodyecology.com/articles/inflammation_cause_of_disease_how_to_prevent.php
2. https://www.ncbi.nlm.nih.gov/pubmed/24613207?dopt=Abstract
3. https://www.medicalnewstoday.com/articles/9978.php
4. https://draxe.com/sprout/
5. Harvard Women's Health Watch, 2015
6. https://draxe.com/anti-inflammatory-foods/
7. https://www.ewg.org/foodnews/
8. https://www.ncbi.nlm.nih.gov/pmc/articles/PMC4425174/
9. https://www.ncbi.nlm.nih.gov/pmc/articles/PMC4258329/
10. https://www.drweil.com/diet-nutrition/anti-inflammatory-diet-pyramid/dr-weils-anti-inflammatory-food-pyramid/
11. https://www.biosourcenaturals.com/pure-essential-oils/essential-oils-considered-safe-by-the-fda/

Chapter 39 – How to Cook with Essential Oils.
2. http://www.raindroptraining.com/messenger/v2n2.html

Chapter 40 – Hacks That Help Me Sleep
1. https://www.medicalnewstoday.com/articles/320554.php
2. https://www.npr.org/sections/health-shots/2015/09/01/436385137/aim-for-at-least-7-hours-of-sleep-nightly-to-fend-off-a-cold
3. https://justgetflux.com/
4. http://www.sleepcycle.com/
5. https://itunes.apple.com/us/app/koala-web-browser-sleep-better/id788474204?mt=8

Chapter 42 – Reducing Toxin Exposure
1. https://www.lifehack.org/articles/communication/12-toxic-thoughts-you-need-drop-for-better-life.html
2. https://cfpub.epa.gov/roe/chapter/air/indoorair.cfm
3. http://www.stlucieco.gov/home/showdocument?id=498
4. https://www.cdc.gov/nchs/data/databriefs/db196.htm
5. https://draxe.com/indoor-air-quality-natural-solutions/

ENDNOTES

6. https://cfpub.epa.gov/roe/chapter/air/indoorair.cfm
7. http://www.enviroalternatives.com/nontoxichome.html
8. http://www.enviroalternatives.com/nontoxichome.html
9. https://www.ewg.org/news/news-releases/2010/03/05/chairman-rush-chemicals-umbilical-cord-blood---including-pbts---need
10. https://www.opb.org/news/blog/ecotrope/replacing-toxic-products-with-green-chemistry/
11. https://www.bloomberg.com/news/articles/2018-05-25/bayer-said-to-win-u-s-antitrust-nod-for-monsanto-deal-next-week
12. https://www.huffingtonpost.com/entry/monsanto-bayer-merge_us_5afeef96e4b07309e0578b5e
13. http://press.bayer.com/baynews/baynews.nsf/id/2018-0164-EN
14. https://www.ecowatch.com/monsantos-glyphosate-most-heavily-used-weed-killer-in-history-1882164311.html
15. https://gmoanswers.com/glyphosate-carcinogen-explained
16. https://www.scientificamerican.com/article/newborn-babies-chemicals-exposure-bpa/
17. https://articles.mercola.com/sites/articles/archive/2014/04/22/glyphosate-herbicide.aspx
18. https://www.theguardian.com/business/2018/aug/10/monsanto-trial-cancer-dewayne-johnson-ruling?CMP=Share_iOSApp_Other
19. https://www.theguardian.com/us-news/2018/may/08/weedkiller-tests-monsanto-health-dangers-active-ingredient
20. https://articles.mercola.com/sites/articles/archive/2011/12/21/are-you-slowly-killing-your-family-with-hidden-dioxane-in-your-laundry-detergent.aspx
21. http://www.ehaontario.ca/
22. https://www.epa.gov/hw/defining-hazardous-waste-listed-characteristic-and-mixed-radiological-wastes
23. http://www.dailymail.co.uk/femail/article-3220306/Why-air-fresheners-scented-candles-wreck-health-cause-cancerous-DNA-mutations-asthma.html
24. https://www.theguardian.com/lifeandstyle/2015/feb/10/phthalates-plastics-chemicals-research-analysis
25. https://www.consumerreports.org/cro/news/2014/10/5-reasons-to-skip-antibacterial-soap/index.htm
26. https://slsfree.net/
27. https://jech.bmj.com/
28. http://bestfolkmedicine.com/2018/07/scientists-found-fluoride-hypothyroidism-depression-weight-gain/
29. http://fluoridealert.org/issues/dental-products/toothpastes/
30. https://realnewsaustralia.com/2018/06/29/fluoridation-is-mass-medication-nz-supreme-court-rules/

ENDNOTES

31 http://ewg.org
32 https://www.huffingtonpost.com/vanessa-cunningham/dangerous-beauty-products_b_4168587.html
33 https://www.huffingtonpost.com/tim-elmore/what-3-tattoo-trends-teach-us-about-millennials_b_5440360.html
34 https://www.mayoclinic.org/healthy-lifestyle/adult-health/in-depth/tattoos-and-piercings/art-20045067
35 https://en.wikipedia.org/wiki/Granuloma

Chapter 42 – The Body Was Made to Move
1. https://hovrpro.com/blogs/news/10-side-effects-of-sitting-all-day
2. http://www.acefitness.org/acefit/healthy-living-article/60/1478/why-do-muscles-tighten-up/
3. http://www.eurekalert.org/pub_releases/2012-02/ps-pay020812.php
4. http://www.bmj.com/content/347/bmj.f5577
5. http://www.aasmnet.org/jcsm/ViewAbstract.aspx?pid=29078
6. http://well.blogs.nytimes.com/2008/02/29/the-cure-for-exhaustion-more-exercise/
7. http://journals.lww.com/nursingresearchonline/Abstract/1994/07000/The_Effect_of_Low_Intensity_Aerobic_Exercise_on.4.aspx
8. http://www.health.harvard.edu/blog/regular-exercise-changes-brain-improve-memory-thinking-skills-201404097110
9. https://books.google.com/books?hl=en&lr=&id=wCmCAgAAQBAJ&oi=fnd&pg=PA88 &dq=exercise+increases+self+confidence&ots=RKEOzku ODP&sig= mov8hGqo1 Jsl-DM maWTxyilsnSs#v=onepage&q&f=false
10. http://well.blogs.nytimes.com/2009/10/14/phys-ed-does-exercise-boost-immunity/?r=0
11. https://hbr.org/2014/10/regular-exercise-is-part-of-your-job/
12. http://well.blogs.nytimes.com/2014/04/02/how-exercise-can-help-you-live-longer/
13. http://wellnessmama.com/7866/oil-pulling/

Chapter 43 – How to Eat Healthy When Eating Out
1. http://www.globalhealingcenter.com/natural-health/5-ways-soy-upsets-hormone-balance/

Chapter 44 – What is a Herxheimer Reaction?
1. http://www.silver-colloids.com/Pubs/herxheimer.html
2. https://www.jillcarnahan.com/2012/11/17/tips-for-dealing-with-herxheimer-or-die-off-reactions/
3. Brian R. Clement, *Hippocrates Life Force: Superior Health and Longevity*.

ENDNOTES

Chapter 45 – Is Healthy Food Really Too Expensive?
1. https://en.wikipedia.org/wiki/Trans_fat
2. https://www.mayoclinic.org/diseases-conditions/high-blood-cholesterol/in-depth/trans-fat/art-20046114
3. https://www.ewg.org/foodnews/

Chapter 47 – 6 Spices to Improve and Maintain Health
1. http://lpi.oregonstate.edu/mic/dietary-factors/phytochemicals/curcumin
2. http://lpi.oregonstate.edu/mic/glossary#antioxidant
3. http://lpi.oregonstate.edu/mic/glossary#inflammation
4. http://www.hopkinsmedicine.org/news/publications/johns_hopkins_health/summer_2013/a_simple_spice_that_may_battle_cancer
5. http://content.iospress.com/articles/journal-of-alzheimers-disease/jad00606
6. http://www.ncbi.nlm.nih.gov/pubmed/12676044
7. http://www.ncbi.nlm.nih.gov/pmc/articles/PMC3918523/
8. https://tinyurl.com/BlackPepperEO
9. http://www.webmd.com/vitamins-supplements/ingredientmono-300-garlic.aspx?activeingredientid=300
10. http://www.cancer.gov/about-cancer/causes-prevention/risk/diet/garlic-fact-sheet
11. https://www.sciencedaily.com/releases/2014/02/140218124538.htm
12. http://draxe.com/natural-ear-infection-remedies/
13. http://draxe.com/5-raw-garlic-benefits-reversing-disease/
14. http://draxe.com/hair-loss-remedies/
15. http://www.drweil.com/drw/u/REM00002/Astragalus-Dr-Weils-Herbal-Remedies.html
16. http://umm.edu/health/medical/altmed/herb/astragalus
17. http://www.ncbi.nlm.nih.gov/pubmed/14724098
18. http://www.ncbi.nlm.nih.gov/pubmed/8580483
19. http://draxe.com/7-adaptogen-herbs-to-lower-cortisol/
20. http://umm.edu/health/medical/altmed/herb/ginger
21. http://www.prevention.com/health-conditions/chemotherapy
22. http://www.ncbi.nlm.nih.gov/pubmed/15630214
23. https://books.google.com/books?id=YDAAAAMBAJ&pg=PA196&lpg=PA196&dq= ginger+study+cruise+ship&source=bl&ots=R3apQIjrXc&sig= kUc6bYEI28aNMUnc5k boabjoyjU&hl=en&sa=X&ved=0ahUKEwjG4ej Yna3MAhVKzGMKHX32BhIQ6AEINzAE#v=onepage&q=ginger %20study% 20cruise% 20ship&f=false
24. http://umm.edu/health/medical/altmed/herb/ginger
25. http://www.arthritis.org/living-with-arthritis/treatments/natural/supplements-herbs/guide/ginger.php
26. http://www.webmd.com/colorectal-cancer/news/20111011/ginger-may-have-cancer-fighting-qualities

ENDNOTES

[27] http://www.webmd.com/vitamins-supplements/ingredientmono-953-ashwagandha.aspx?activeingredientid=953&
[28] https://www.psychologytoday.com/blog/inner-source/201401/ashwaganda-anxiety
[29] http://www.lifeextension.com/protocols/emotional-health/stress-management/page-02
[30] http://www.naturalnews.com/032025_Ashwagandha_thyroid.html
[31] http://www.livestrong.com/article/492102-ashwagandha-for-adrenal-fatigue/
[32] https://www.organicfacts.net/health-benefits/herbs-and-spices/health-benefits-of-ashwagandha-or-indian-ginseng.html
[33] http://www.medicinehunter.com/adaptogens
[34] http://en.mr-ginseng.com/ashwagandha/#Ashwagandha_Dosage
[35] http://care.diabetesjournals.org/content/26/12/3215.full
[36] http://www.ncbi.nlm.nih.gov/pmc/articles/PMC4003790/
[37] http://www.ncbi.nlm.nih.gov/pmc/articles/PMC4003790/
[38] http://www.ncbi.nlm.nih.gov/pubmed/19433898
[39] http://www.ncbi.nlm.nih.gov/pubmed/24946862
[40] http://www.ncbi.nlm.nih.gov/pubmed/8834832
[41] https://www.thespruceeats.com/what-is-cassia-1807003

Chapter 48 – Apps to Help Us Get and Stay Healthy
[1] https://www.consumerreports.org/cro/magazine/2015/02/gmo-foods-what-you-need-to-know/index.htm

Chapter 50 – Gut-Restoring Recipes
[1] https://bodyecology.com/digestive-health-kefir-starter.html
[2] https://tinyurl.com/PeppermintEO-YL
[3] https://www.mindbodygreen.com/0-29973/this-snack-reverses-aging-and-takes-less-than-5-minutes-to-make.html
[4] https://draxe.com/kefir-benefits/
[5] https://www.healthline.com/nutrition/8-health-benefits-of-probiotics#section7
[6] https://melmagazine.com/youre-eating-way-too-much-protein-3a3c3eb7e4c7
[7] http://www.onegreenplanet.org/vegan-food/how-to-add-clean-protein-to-your-smoothie-without-a-powder/
[8] https://www.doctoroz.com/blog/jodi-sawyer-rn/why-fiber-so-important
[9] https://www.shape.com/healthy-eating/diet-tips/10-best-leafy-greens
[10] https://wholenewmom.com/recipes/autoimmune-protocol-aip-taco-seasoning-no-nightshades-seeds/

ENDNOTES

Chapter 53 – How Does the Soul Prosper?
1. https://www.youtube.com/watch?v=4yGNjXlAVg8

Chapter 54 – How to Overcome Self-Sabotage
1. https://www.psychologytoday.com/basics/self-sabotage

Appendix 1 – Common GMO Ingredients
1. http://www.herbs-info.com/blog/common-gmo-ingredients-you-may-not-know-about-eye-opening/

Appendix 2 – Common Names for Sugar
1. http://www.herbs-info.com/blog/3-vital-steps-to-control-your-sugar-consumption-and-related-health-problems/
1. http://www.herbs-info.com/blog/the-dirty-30-a-list-of-toxic-beauty-product-ingredients-to-avoid/
2. https://draxe.com/agave-nectar/
3. https://www.webmd.com/cancer/news/20100209/dry-cleaning-chemical-likely-causes-cancer#1
4. https://bodyecology.com/articles/top_6_fabrics_you_should_avoid_wearing.php
5. http://drhyman.com/blog/2011/05/13/5-reasons-high-fructose-corn-syrup-will-kill-you/

ENDNOTES

CPSIA information can be obtained
at www.ICGtesting.com
Printed in the USA
FSHW021044151218
54501FS